Handbook of Dermatological Drug Therapy

Handbook of Dermatological Drug Therapy

Uday Khopkar
Ex-Professor and Head of Dermatology
KEM Hospital and Seth GS Medical College
and Consultant Dermatologist
Mumbai

Sushil Pande
Professor of Dermatology
NKP Salve Institute of Medical Sciences and Research Centre
Nagpur

K. C. Nischal
Director
Nirmal Skin and Hair Clinic
Bengaluru

Akansha Chadha
Assistant Professor
TN Medical College and BYL Nair Charitable Hospital
Mumbai

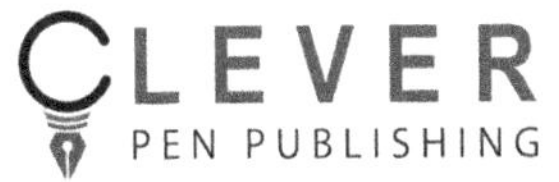

Clever Pen Publishing

Handbook of Dermatological Drug Therapy
Khopkar, Pande, Nischal and Chada

First Edition 2007
Reprinted 2008
Reprinted 2010
Reprinted 2011
Reprinted 2012
Second Edition 2022

Medical knowledge is constantly changing. As new information becomes available, changes in treatment, procedures, equipment and the use of drugs become necessary. The authors, editors, contributors and the publisher have, as far as it is possible, taken care to ensure that the information given in this text is accurate and up-to-date. However, readers are strongly advised to confirm that the information, especially with regard to drug dose/usage, complies with current legislation and standards of practice.

Published by

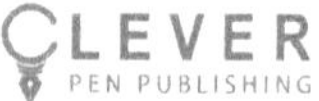

Clever Pen Publishing
D-2, Neelkanth Business Park Co-op. Premises Society Ltd.
Nathani Road, Vidyavihar (West)
Mumbai 400086
Mob. : 09867 268945 / 09867 214519
E-mail : cleverpen9@gmail.com

ISBN 978-93-92215-07-0

Printed in India

Dedicated with gratitude to the astute clinician

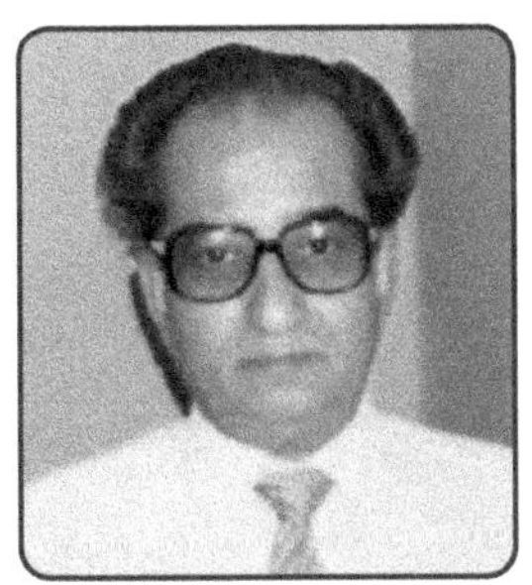

Late Dr. V. R. Mehta

(17-01-1929 – 02-02-2018)

Who initiated me to the field of Dermatopathology

– Uday Khopkar

Foreword

I am pleased to write a foreword for *'Dermatological Drug Therapy'* written by Professor Dr. Uday Khopkar and his colleagues. The book is designed to serve the purpose of providing a source of ready reference for postgraduates and practicing dermatologists in India. I hope that the book will satisfy a long-felt need of postgraduate students in dermatology and will definitely help students prepare for the practical examination in dermatology in a more systematic manner.

The book acquaints the reader with the full gamut of dermatotherapeutics including topical and systemic therapy of skin disorders and many neglected areas like wound care. It is written succinctly, yet not missing the essentials and inclusive of topics of common interest to young dermatologists such as cosmeceuticals, chemical peels, dermal fillers, botulin toxin, and lasers.

Authentic information of magnitude and relevance is presented in a readable fashion in this book by Dr. Khopkar for the benefit of postgraduate students and practitioners. I know Dr. Khopkar as an academician and a clinician and I perceive this book to be a continuation of his sincere effort to uplift the standard of postgraduate education in dermatology in India.

Obviously this is not a book discussing detailed management of cutaneous disorders in depth. This is because the focus and emphasis of this book is on the drugs. Besides, the book presupposes adequate knowledge of clinical dermatology.

Overall, it is a commendable effort! I congratulate Dr. Khopkar and his colleagues for enriching Indian dermatological literature by writing such a useful book and wish this publication all success.

Dr. R. G. Valia
Emeritus Professor of Dermatology
LTM Medical College and LTMG Hospital
Sion, Mumbai

Preface to the Second Edition

I am pleased to present this revised and fully updated second edition of the Handbook of Drugs in Dermatology. I am indebted to my co-authors for sharing my passion for accuracy and comprehensiveness in this work. I note with satisfaction that the text has been completely overhauled in line with the wishes of my mentor, Late Dr. VR Mehta, but without disturbing the basic structure of the handbook. Dr. Akansha and Dr. Sushil have worked untiringly with me to update the chapters on drugs while Dr. Nischal has looked after the chapters on cosmetic dermatology.

I am grateful to my publisher, **Mr. Rajesh Bhalani** and **Mrs. Harsha Shah** from **Clever Pen Publishing** for making persistent efforts to complete the book in time, in spite of the challenges of a pandemic and without whose prodding this second edition may not have materialized.

Finally, I am thankful to the readers whose insistent queries about availability of the book motivated me to finally come out with another edition after 15 long years. I hope that our painstaking efforts will not go un-noticed by discerning readers. Finally I wish and hope that this handbook will remain a companion for students and practitioners in their clinics at least in the near future.

In gratitude for all the affection showered on me,

Uday Khopkar

Preface to the First Edition

It gives me great pleasure to present this short text on dermatologic therapeutics. The idea of writing this simple book was given to me by Bhalani Publishers. I could only bring it to fruition through the help of my younger colleagues, Dr. Sushil Pande and Dr. K. C. Nischal, whose enthusiasm during this project knew no bounds.

The book is meant to be a companion to dermatology practitioners and residents who may have difficulty in accessing bigger books in the outpatient clinic. The emphasis has been on providing the right amount of clinically relevant information on the commonly used therapies in dermatology.

The book is divided in natural sections on systemic agents and topicals used in dermatology and sexually transmitted infections. Although most of the commonly used drugs are covered, no attempt has been made to make the book comprehensive. This is because several textbooks are available on the subject that could be referred to by the more avid readers. No references have been provided as the information is derived from well-known texts on the subject. An appendix on commonly used instruments in dermatology has been added for the benefit of the postgraduates.

I would appreciate feedback from readers regarding any errors of omission or commission in this text so that we can make it more complete and correct.

Uday Khopkar

How to Use this Book

This book may be used in two modes :

- Referring to the basics of a drug while prescribing; and
- Thorough reading for practical examinations.

While finding a particular drug before prescribing, easiest way is to check in the alphabetical index at the back. However, for systematic reading before examinations, one may read the whole chapter. Tables have been prepared for ease of reading and understanding.

Each chapter gives an initial classification of the drugs in that group followed by a detailed discussion on each. Occasionally, when too many drugs are in a group, the relevant information has been placed either in a Table, or when the information is common to all the drugs in that group, at the beginning of the discussion on that group of drugs.

Mechanism of action of drugs have been highlighted in a box as this information is frequently difficult to remember.

Contents

Foreword ... *v*
Preface ... *vii*
How to Use this Book ... *ix*
Contents ... *xi-xii*

SECTION 1 : SYSTEMIC AGENTS

1. Systemic Antibacterials ... 3-41
2. Systemic Antifungals ... 42-63
3. Systemic Antiviral Agents ... 64-72
4. Antiretroviral Drugs ... 73-101
5. Systemic Antiparasitic Agents ... 102-116
6. Antileprosy Drugs ... 117-132
7. Antituberculous Agents ... 133-147
8. Oral and Injectable Steroids ... 148-161
9. Non-steroidal Immunosuppressive Drugs ... 162-177
10. Oral Retinoids ... 178-186
11. Systemic Photoprotective Agents ... 187-193
12. Psoralens, PUVA and Phototherapy ... 194-207
13. Immunobiologicals ... 208-232
14. Vitamins and Trace Elements ... 233-254
15. Antihistamines and Mast Cell Stabilizers ... 255-265
16. Miscellaneous Agents ... 266-285

SECTION 2 : TOPICAL AGENTS

17. Principles of Topical Therapy ... 286-297
18. Topical Antibacterials ... 298-308

19. Topical Antifungals ... 309-315
20. Topical Antivirals ... 316-324
21. Topical Antiparasitic Agents ... 325-334
22. Topical and Intralesional Corticosteroids ... 335-343
23. Topical Immunomodulators ... 344-354
24. Topical Retinoids ... 355-359
25. Sunscreens ... 360-367
26. Hypopigmenting Agents ... 368-375
27. Moisturizers and Keratolytic Agents ... 376-385
28. Miscellaneous Topical Agents ... 386-398
29. Cosmeceuticals ... 399-411
30. Commonly Used Chemical Agents in Dermatological Practice ... 412-420
31. Chemical Peels ... 421-436
32. Wound Care Products ... 437-454
33. Baths ... 455-461
34. Dermal Fillers ... 462-465
35. Botulinum Toxin ... 466-471

APPENDIXES

Appendix I : Office Aids in Dermatological Practice 472-480
Appendix II : Common Instruments in Dermatological Procedures ... 481-505
Appendix III : Apparatuses in Dermatological Practice 506-559

Index ... 560-570

x=x=x=x=x

Section 1

Systemic Agents

1
Systemic Antibacterials

The various classes of commonly used antibacterials in dermatology are :

1. Sulfonamides and cotrimoxazole
2. Penicillins and cephalosporins
3. Aminoglycosides
4. Tetracyclines
5. Macrolides
6. Oxazolidinones
7. Fluoroquinolones

COTRIMOXAZOLE (TRIMETHOPRIM-SULFAMETHOXAZOLE) :

Cotrimoxazole is a fixed dose ratio of 1:5 of trimethoprim (TMP) to sulfamethoxazole (SMX).

MECHANISM OF ACTION :
Sulfamethoxazole (SMX) competes with PABA of bacteria while trimethoprim is an inhibitor of dihydrofolate reductase enzyme.

INDICATIONS :

1. Nocardial actinomycetoma.
2. STIs like chancroid, granuloma inguinale, and lymphogranuloma inguinale.
3. Treatment option for cat scratch disease, toxoplasmosis, melioidosis, pyoderma, atypical mycobacterial infections (mainly M. marinum infection).

4. Pediculosis.
5. Diarrhea caused by Isospora belli in AIDS patients.
6. Prophylaxis against P. carinii infection and toxoplasmosis in AIDS patients.

MECHANISM OF BACTERIAL RESISTANCE :

Mutational or plasmid mediated acquisition of dihydrofolate reductase with low affinity for the drug.

DOSES :

SEPTRAN or BACTRIM TMP 80 mg + SMX 400 mg single-strength (SS) tablet. Also available as double strength tablets.

PREGNANCY CATEGORY – B :

SIDE EFFECTS :

Systemic :

GI disturbances, agranulocytosis, crystalluria, interstitial nephritis, unconjugated hyperbilirubinemia, and methemoglobinemia.

Cutaneous :

Maculopapular rash (more common in HIV infections), fixed drug eruption, Stevens-Johnson's syndrome, toxic epidermal necrolysis, etc. (Table 1.1)

KEY POINTS :

- Cotrimoxazole depletes normal bacterial flora in the gut of lice on which it is dependent, thereby useful in pediculosis.
- TMP-SMX is also useful for the treatment of gram negative folliculitis in patients with acne and in mixed bacterial infection. It may also be used for uncomplicated methicillin resistant staphylococcus aureus infections

TABLE 1.1 : **Indications and doses of cotrimoxazole in dermatovenereology**

Indication	Doses
P. carinii	**Tablet :** Cotrimoxazole DS 4-6 times 2-3 weeks for treatment **Tablet :** Cotrimoxazole DS o.d. for prophylaxis
Toxoplasmosis	**Tablet :** Cotrimoxazole DS o.d. for prophylaxis
Chancroid	**Tablet :** Cotrimoxazole DS b.i.d. 2 weeks
Donovanosis	Cotrimoxazole SS 2 tablets b.i.d. 2 weeks
Lymphogranuloma venereum	Cotrimoxazole SS 2 tablets b.i.d. 2 weeks
Nocardial mycetoma	Cotrimoxazole DS 1-2 tablets b.i.d. x 3-6 months
Community acquired uncomplicated MRSA	Cotrimoxazole DS 1 tablet b.i.d. X 2 weeks
Gram negative folliculitis in patients with acne	Cotrimoxazole DS 1 tablet b.i.d. x 2 weeks

- TMP-SMX has more incidence of adverse drug reactions in HIV positive patients due to slow acetylation.
- Elderly patients, AIDS are the risk factors for bone marrow toxicity with cotrimoxazole.
- Adequate hydration is required during cotrimoxazole therapy to avoid nephrolithiasis. Dose should be reduced in moderate-to-severe renal impairment.
- Thrombocytopenia can occur when cotrimoxazole is concurrently used with diuretics.
- Cotrimoxazole desensitization or inducing tolerance is achieved by giving TMP-SMX orally, starting with 0.4 mg TMP and 2 mg of SMX, followed by incremental dose to achieve full dose of TMP/SMX at the end of 5 days. Development of clinical tolerance of TMP/SMX for more than 10 days can be labeled as "successful cotrimoxazole desensitization". It is usually required in HIV-positive individuals, sensitive to cotrimoxazole to allow its use for prophylaxis against P. carinii.

PENICILLINS :

Penicillins are the beta-lactam antibiotics. Natural penicillins include Benzyl penicillin or penicillin-G and its preparations. Attachment of other side chains to the beta-lactam ring results in semisynthetic penicillins.

Semisynthetic penicillins include the commonly used ampicillin and amoxicillin (aminopenicillins), methicillin and cloxacillin (penicillinase-resistant penicillins), ticarcillin (carboxypenicillins), piperacillin (ureidopenicillins), and clavulanic acid and sulbactam (beta-lactamase inhibitors). They are particularly used for skin and soft tissue infections.

> MECHANISM OF ACTION :
>
> **Penicillins interfere with the bacterial cell wall synthesis by inhibiting cross-linking transpeptidases.**

INDICATIONS :

Common indications of all penicillins in dermatology include :

1. Skin and soft tissue infections.
2. Sexually transmitted diseases.

SIDE EFFECTS :

Systemic :

1. Hypersensitivity is the most feared side effect, manifestations of which include rash, urticaria, fever, itching, serum sickness, angioneurotic edema, and anaphylaxis.
2. Jarisch-Herxheimer reaction observed when penicillin is used particularly during early syphilis is characterized by fever and constitutional symptoms like sweating, etc. It is most likely due to the release of bacterial endotoxins or immunologically mediated reaction that subsides within 24 h. It can be prevented by prophylactic administration

of systemic steroids, prednisolone 20 mg o.d. 2-3 days prior to administration of penicillin.

3. Diarrhea is the most common side effect of ampicillin.
4. Accidental injection of procaine penicillin into a vessel leads to mental confusion, visual and auditory hallucination, perceived changes of body shape, swelling of tongue, fear of impending death, dizziness, headache, and hypotension. (Hoigne syndrome or procaine psychosis.) This pseudoanaphylactic shock does not require discontinuation of penicillin treatment.

Cutaneous :

1. Urticaria/Angioedema.
2. Maculopapular rash (ampicillin and amoxicillin).
3. Erythema multiforme/Stevens-Johnson's syndrome/Toxic epidermal necrolysis.
4. Fixed drug eruptions.
5. Acute exanthematous pustulosis.
6. Leukocytoclastic vasculitis.
7. Photo-onycholysis.

PREGNANCY CATEGORY – B :

BACTERIAL RESISTANCE :

Mechanisms of bacterial resistance include :

1. Production of beta-lactamase, which opens the beta-lactam ring of penicillin, is the most important mechanism of penicillin resistance. Enzyme penicillinase is also produced by Gram-negative bacilli, *e.g. Neisseria gonorrheae.* This type of resistance is plasmid mediated.
2. Low affinity of target enzymes for penicillins.
3. Variable permeability of penicillins through "porin" channels of Gram-negative bacilli.

TABLE 1.2 : **Indications of penicillins in dermatovenereology**

Drug	Dose
Syphilis :	
Procaine penicillin	1.2 MU i.m. for 10 days in early and latent syphilis.
Crystalline penicillin	2-4 MU 4 hourly i.v. for 10-14 days in immunocompromised with neurosyphilis.
Crystalline penicillin	50,000 IU/kg 8 hourly i.v. for 10 days in early prenatal syphilis.
Benzathine penicillin	2.4 MU deep i.m. single dose in early syphilis and three doses 1 week apart in late syphilis.
Gonorrhea :	
Procaine penicillin	Single dose of 4.8 MU along with 1 g probenecid oral.
Crystalline penicillin (in gonococcal septicemia and disseminated gonococcal infection).	75,000-100,000 U/kg/day in six divided doses for 10 days.
Fusospirochetal infections, *e.g.* phagedena, noma.	Crystalline penicillin 50,000 IU/kg 6-8 hourly i.v. for 3-5 days followed by oral penicillins.
Actinomycosis :	
Centrofacial cases	1-6 million units/day of Penicillin G aqueous IV for 4 weeks.
Thoracic and abdominal disease	10-20 million units/day of Penicillin G aqueous IV divided q4-6 hr x 6 weeks.
Skin and soft tissue infections :	
Cloxacillin (beta-lactamase producing staphylococci).	0.25-0.5 g oral/i.m./i.v. 6 hourly, 25-50 mg/kg/day in children.
Ampicillin (staphylococci/streptococci/mixed infections).	0.5-2 g oral/i.m./i.v. 6 hourly, 25-50 mg/kg/day in children.
Amoxicillin (staphylococci/streptococci/mixed infections).	0.5-2 g oral/i.m./i.v. 6 hourly, 25-50 mg/kg/day in children.
Amoxicillin-clavulanic acid (beta-lactamase producing staphylococci/streptococci/mixed infections).	625 mg oral/i.v. 12 hourly 7 days.
Ampicillin-sulbactam (beta-lactamase producing staphylococci/streptococci/mixed infections).	Ampicillin 1 g + sulbactam 0.5 g i.m. 8 hourly days.
Piperacillin	100-150 mg/kg/day in three divided doses i.m./i.v.

Beta-lactamase-resistant penicillins are cloxacillin and methicillin. More commonly, drugs acting against beta-lactamase are combined with penicillins to make them effective against these organisms. These include clavulanic acid (combined with amoxicillin) and sulbactam (combined with ampicillin). (Table 1.2)

Drug Interactions of Penicillins :

Drug 1	Drug 2	Interactions
Penicillin	Probenacid	Renal excretion of penicillin prolonged
Amoxicillin	Ethinyl estradiol	Low risk of contraceptive failure
Amoxicillin	Warfarin	Increased levels of warfarin and increased INR
Amoxycillin	Tetracycline, doxycycline	Decreased effect of amoxicillin due to pharmacodynamic antagonism

Key Points :

- Antibacterial spectrum of the penicillins mainly includes Gram-positive cocci and bacilli although the Gram-negative Neisseria species is also sensitive to penicillin-G. Ticarcillin and piperacillin are the penicillins with potent anti-pseudomonal activity.
- Intradermal test with benzylpenicilloyl-polylysine is essentially required prior to the intramuscular or intravenous administration of penicillins due to the potential risk of fatal anaphylaxis. Cross-reactions can occur between penicillin and cephalosporins.
- **Procedure of penicillin sensitivity testing :**
    i. ***Required supplies for sensitivity testing :*** penicillin sensitivity test is associated with a risk of anaphylaxis and should always be done in an intensive care unit. Patients should not undergo penicillin sensitivity testing if they have a history of severe skin reaction like Stevens-Johnson syndrome or toxic epidermal necrolysis, as it may reactivate the disease. Reagents required are benzylpenicilloyl-polylysine injection,

dilute solution of penicillin G (10,000 U/ml), histamine for positive control and sterile normal saline for negative control.

ii. ***Performing scratch testing :*** Volar aspect of forearm is cleaned with spirit swab. Sites for all 4 reagents is marked with a pen and a drop of each benzylpenicilloyl-polylysine injection, dilute solution of penicillin G (10,000 U/ml), histamine for positive control and sterile normal saline for negative control is placed in their respective sites. The surface of the skin is then scratched over the drop using minimal pressure. Results are read after 15 min. The histamine site should always be positive in order for the test to be valid. An induration of greater than 3 mm than the negative saline site in either the benzylpenicilloyl-polylysine injection site or penicillin G site indicates a positive allergy test. If the induration is less than 3 mm in both the two sites, then it is safe to move on to intradermal test.

iii. ***Intradermal testing :*** Done when the scratch test is negative. It is usually performed on the forearm opposite to the side of the scratch test or on the back of the arm. With the help of a 26G or 28G tuberculin syringe a 2-3 mm bleb is raised at two sites for benzylpenicilloyl-polylysine injection and penicillin G each and one site for sterile normal saline. Histamine is not used in intradermal test. The perimeter of the bleb is circled with a pen and growth beyond original bleb size is watched for. Results are read after 15-20 min. A positive test is indicated by a significant increase in bleb size with a wheal diameter for 3 mm or more than the control. Itching and flare are usually present. If the wheal is only slightly larger than the original bleb size or if there is discordant result between the duplicate placements, a repeat test is advised and concordance of 3 out of 4 is taken as positive.

iv. ***Offering an optional oral challenge :*** The oral antibiotic of choice is given as an oral challenge and patient is observed for one hour.

- **Management of anaphylaxis :**
  i. Prompt stoppage of the drug.
  ii. Maintenance of airway, breathing, and circulation (ABC), Head low position to increase blood flow to brain and lateral position to prevent aspiration are the quick measures to be undertaken. Intravenous fluids (to replenish intravascular fluid loss) should be given.
  iii. Injection of epinephrine (natural antagonist of histamine) 0.3 cc (1:1000) subcutaneously. It may be required to repeat at 20-min intervals.
  iv. Injection of hydrocortisone 100 mg stat. (corrects hypotension, bronchospasm, and prevents further release of histamine).
  v. Antihistamines like diphenhydramine 50-100 mg intramuscular or intravenously is the ancillary method for treating urticaria-angioedema.
- Ampicillin and amoxicillin have high incidence of maculopapular rash in patients of infectious mononucleosis, AIDS, and lymphocytic leukemia.
- Clavulanic acid is beta-lactamase inhibitor which is combined with penicillin group of antibiotics to overcome antibiotic resistance in bacteria that secrete beta-lactamase. Usually combined with amoxicillin and ticarcillin. Although it has minimal intrinsic antibacterial activity, it acts as suicide inhibitor and binds to serine residue of beta-lactamase enzyme, permanently inactivating it. Adverse effects like cholestatic jaundice and acute hepatitis may occur during therapy or shortly after. Similarly Sulbactam is an irreversible inhibitor of beta-lactamase. It can inhibit most forms of beta-lactamase except ampC cephalosporinase. Hence it offers little

protection against Pseudomonas aeruginosa, Citrobacter, Enterobacter and Serratia. It has been combined with cefoperazone and ampicillin.

Penicillin Desensitization :

Penicillin desensitization is required in following conditions :

1. Congenital syphilis with allergy to penicillin.
2. Pregnant woman with syphilis and allergy to penicillin.
3. Disseminated gonococcal infection secondary to strains of gonococci, only sensitive to penicillin in a patient allergic to penicillin.

Penicillin desensitization is done by oral administration of increasing doses of penicillin-G, beginning with 100 U or 60 μg, at 15-min intervals over a period of 4-6 h. At the end of the procedure, the full dose of parenteral penicillin-G or ampicillin can be administered with successful desensitization. All emergency medications and resuscitation measures should be kept ready prior to the procedure for the management of anaphylaxis should the situation arise.

CEPHALOSPORINS :

Cephalosporins are beta-lactam antibiotics similar to penicillin. The attachment of other side chains to the beta-lactam ring results in semisynthetic cephalosporins.

Mechanism Of Action :

Cephalosporins interfere with the bacterial cell synthesis. Attachment of different side chains to the beta-lactam ring explains the difference in potency and resistance of cephalosporins to that of penicillins.

Indications :

Common indications of cephalosporins in dermatology include:

1. Skin and soft tissue infections.
2. Sexually transmitted diseases.

SIDE EFFECTS :

Systemic :

1. Hypersensitivity.
2. Nausea, Vomiting and Diarrhea.
3. Fever, Eosinophilia and increased transaminases.
4. Stevens-Johnson syndrome and toxic epidermal necrolysis.
5. Pseudomembranous colitis.
6. Nephrotoxicity (highest with cephaloridine).
7. Hypoprothrombinemia and increased INR.
8. Disulfiram-like reaction (cefoperazone).

Cutaneous :

1. Urticaria/Angioedema.
2. Acute exanthematous pustulosis.

PREGNANCY CATEGORY – B :

BACTERIAL RESISTANCE :

Mechanisms of bacterial resistance include :

1. Production of beta-lactamase (cephalosporinase).
2. Low affinity of target enzymes.
3. Alteration of target proteins. (Tables 1.3 & 1.4)

DRUG INTERACTIONS OF CEPHALOSPORINS :

Drug 1	Drug 2	Interactions
Cefadroxil, cephalexin, cefuroxime, ceftazidime, cefotaxime	BCG and Typhoid vaccine	Decreased efficacy of vaccine due to pharmacodynamic antagonism.
Cefadroxil , cephalexin, cefuroxime, ceftazidime, cefotaxime	Ethinyl estradiol	Low risk of contraceptive failure.

TABLE 1.3 : **Classification and spectrum of cephalosporins**

	Spectrum	Oral	Parenteral
First generation	Gram-positive cocci and nonenterococcal streptococci	Cephalexin; Cefadroxil	Cefazolin
Second generation	Decreased Gram-positive and increased Gram-negative activity as compared to 1st generation cephalosporins	Cefaclor; Cefuroxime proaxetil	Cefuroxime; Cefoxitin
Third generation	Less Gram-positive and greatly increased Gram-negative spectrum including antipseudomonal activity	Cefixime; Cefpodoxime proaxetil	Cefotaxime; Ceftriaxone; Ceftazidime; Cefoperazone
Fourth generation	Gram-negative including pseudomonas and Gram-positive action; is more resistant to hydrolysis by beta-lactamases	—	Cefepime; Cefpirome

TABLE 1.4 : **Indications of cephalosporins in dermatovenereology**

Indication	Dose
Skin and soft tissue infections	Cefadroxil 500 mg twice a day for 5 days Cephalexin 250 mg 4 times a day for 5 days Cefazolin 0.5-1 g IV q6-8 hr.
Actinomycosis and nocardial mycetoma	Ceftriaxone 6-12 months.
Syphilis	Ceftriaxone 1 g daily 10 days (unknown efficacy data).
Gonorrhea	Ceftriaxone 250 mg i.m. single dose. Cefotaxime 1 g i.m. single dose. Cefpodoxime proaxetil 100 mg oral. Cefixime 400 mg oral single dose.
Pelvic inflammatory disease :	
Outpatient regimen	Ceftriaxone 250 mg i.m. (plus doxycycline 100 mg b.i.d. 14 days).
Inpatient regimen	Cefoxitin 2 g i.v. 8 hourly (plus doxycycline 100 mg b.i.d. 14 days).
Chancroid	Ceftriaxone 250 mg i.m. single dose.
Donovanosis	Ceftriaxone 1 g i.m. in 2 ml of 1% lignocaine 10 days.

Drug 1	Drug 2	Interactions
Cefadroxil, cephalexin, cefuroxime, ceftazidime, cefotaxime	Amoxicillin, ampicillin, penicillin G	Both drugs increase levels of each other by decreasing renal clearance
Ceftriaxone	Warfarin	Increased INR
Ceftriaxone	Heparin	Increased chances of bleeding due to pharmacodynamics synergism.
Ceftriaxone	Calcium chloride, calcium gluconate, calcium citrate.	Flush IV infusion lines after calcium infusion and before ceftriaxone. Risk of ceftriaxone-calcium precipitation. Never use calcium containing solution like Ringer's lactate with ceftriaxone

KEY POINTS :

- Gram-negative antibacterial spectrum of the cephalosporins increases from first to fourth generations. Ceftazidime has the most potent antipseudomonal activity.
- Fourth generation cefalosporins are more resistant to hydrolysis by beta-lactamases.
- Cross-reactions can occur between penicillin and cephalosporins.

AMINOGLYCOSIDES :

Aminoglycosides are the bactericidal antibiotics, mainly effective against Gram-negative bacteria. Aminoglycosides include streptomycin, gentamicin, kanamycin, tobramycin, amikacin, sisomicin, and netilmicin.

MECHANISM OF ACTION :

Aminoglycosides inhibit bacterial protein synthesis by binding to 30-50S interface except for streptomycin, which only binds to the 30S ribosomal subunit.

> The cidal action of aminoglycosides is probably due to secondary changes in the integrity of bacterial cell membrane.

INDICATIONS :

1. Mainly against infections caused by Gram-negative bacteria.
2. Tuberculosis : streptomycin, amikacin, and kanamycin.
3. Actinomycetoma : streptomycin and amikacin.
4. Tularemia.
5. Sexually transmitted diseases : streptomycin.

ADVERSE EFFECTS :

1. Ototoxicity includes cochlear damage caused by all aminoglycosides except for kanamycin, which causes vestibular toxicity.
2. Nephrotoxicity
3. Neuromuscular blockade most likely due to neomycin and streptomycin and least likely with tobramycin.

KEY POINTS :

- Aminoglycosides should not be mixed with any other drug in the same syringe or bottle.
- Aminoglycosides should be avoided in pregnancy due to the risk of fetal ototoxicity.
- Concurrent use of other ototoxic drugs like minocycline, cisplatin, or furosemide should be avoided. Hearing loss caused by aminoglycosides is irreversible.
- Concurrent use of other nephrotoxic drugs like amphotericin-B, vancomycin, cisplatin, or cyclosporine should be avoided.
- Muscle relaxants should be used cautiously in patients on aminoglycoside therapy as they can produce muscle paralysis.

- Resistance to aminoglycosides is either due to mutation or plasmid mediated.
- Aminoglycosides when given parenterally may cause systemic contact dermatitis in patients sensitized to topical aminoglycosides.

STREPTOMYCIN :

The oldest aminoglycoside antibiotic.

MECHANISM OF ACTION AND INDICATIONS :
Similar to that of aminoglycosides (described earlier).

DOSES AND PREPARATIONS :

Ambistryn-S, Streptonex (streptomycin sulphate) 0.75 g, 1 g dry powder per vial for injection.

TABLE 1.5 : **Indications of streptomycin in dermatovenereology**

Indication	Doses and Duration
Acute infections	0.75 gm. o.d. for 7 days
Tuberculosis	0.75 gm. o.d. for 60 days
Actinomycetoma	0.75 gm. o.d. till it heals
Donovanosis	0.75 gm. b.i.d. for 10 days
Chancroid	0.75 gm. o.d. for 7 days

PREGNANCY CATEGORY – D :

KEY POINTS :

- Streptomycin is the least nephrotoxic aminoglycoside; it is excreted unchanged in urine.
- Certain mutants grown in the presence of streptomycin becomes dependent on it; this may be significant in tuberculosis.

GENTAMICIN :

The commonly used aminoglycoside antibiotic.

Mechanism Of Action And Indications :

Similar to that of aminoglycosides, except it is not effective against *M. tuberculosis.*

Doses And Preparations :

- Gentamicin 80 mg i.m./i.v. 8 hourly.
- GENTICYN, GENTASPORIN 20, 40, 80 mg/vial injection; 0.3% eye/ear drops, 0.1% cream.

PREGNANCY CATEGORY – C :

Key Points :

- Gentamicin has a broader spectrum of action, however is not effective against *M. tuberculosis.*
- Single-daily-dose regimen is proposed for gentamicin, efficacy of which is not established.
- Gentamicin inhibits *Staphylococcus aureus* more efficiently than *Streptococcus pyogenes.*
- Topical use of gentamicin is discouraged due to risk of sensitization and development of resistance.

AMIKACIN :

The semisynthetic derivative of kanamycin.

Mechanism Of Action And Indications :

Similar to that of aminoglycosides (*see* page 11).

Doses And Preparations :

- Amikacin 15 mg/kg/day in two divided doses; 500 mg 12 hourly IM or IV for 2 months in actinomycetoma.
- AMICIN, MIKACIN 100, 250 mg, 500 mg/2 ml injection.

PREGNANCY CATEGORY – D :

KEY POINT :

- Amikacin, being resistant to aminoglycoside inactivating enzymes of bacteria, is one of the most potent aminoglycosides.

SPECTINOMYCIN :

Bacteriostatic antibiotic chemically related to aminoglycosides.

MECHANISM OF ACTION :

Similar to that of aminoglycosides (*see* page 11).

INDICATIONS :

1. Complicated gonococcal infections.
2. Gonococcal infections during pregnancy.
3. Chancroid.

DOSES AND PREPARATIONS :

- 2 g i.m. stat single dose.
- 2 g i.m. o.d. 3 days in disseminated gonococcal infections (DGI).
- TOGAMYCIN 2 g vial.

PREGNANCY CATEGORY – B :

SIDE EFFECTS :

Fever and urticaria.

TETRACYCLINES :

Tetracyclines include chlortetracycline, oxytetracycline, minocycline, doxycycline, demeclocycline, and tetracycline.

MECHANISM OF ACTION :

Tetracyclines act by inhibiting bacterial protein synthesis by binding to 30S ribosomal subunit.

INDICATIONS :

1. Acne vulgaris.
2. Acne rosacea.
3. Sexually transmitted infections.

CONTRAINDICATIONS :

- Pregnancy and lactation.
- Children below 12 years of age as it causes growth retardation and brownish teeth discoloration.
- Hypersensitivity.

PREGNANCY CATEGORY – D :

KEY POINTS :

- Tetracycline has antiinflammatory action.
- Demeclocycline is the most phototoxic tetracycline.

TETRACYCLINE :

Tetracycline is the widely used prototype of the tetracyclines.

INDICATIONS :

Similar to that of tetracyclines; owing to its antiinflammatory effect it is used in bullous pemphigoid and in acute and chronic parapsoriasis.

DOSES AND PREPARATIONS :

- 1-2 g daily in four divided doses, 20–40 mg/kg daily in divided doses
- HOSTACYCLINE 250 mg, 500 mg tab, TERRAMYCIN injection 50 mg/ml (10 ml vial).

TABLE 1.6 : **Indications of tetracycline in dermatovenereology**

Indications	Doses
Acne vulgaris	500 mg q.i.d. 1-3 months.
Rosacea	250-500 mg q.i.d. 2-4 weeks.
Bullous Pemphigoid	500 mg q.i.d. x 2-8 weeks.
Pityriasis lichenoides	500 mg q.i.d. x 2-4 weeks.
Early syphilis	500 mg q.i.d. 2 weeks (in penicillin allergy).
Late syphilis	500 mg q.i.d. 4 weeks (in penicillin allergy).
Chancroid	500 mg q.i.d. 10 days.
Chlamydial urethritis	500 mg q.i.d. 2 weeks.
Donovanosis	500 mg q.i.d. 6-8 weeks.
LGV	500 mg q.i.d. 6-8 weeks.

SIDE EFFECTS :

Systemic :

GI disturbances, tooth discoloration, enamel hypoplasia, and superinfections.

Cutaneous :

Phototoxic drug reactions and photoonycholysis.

KEY POINT :

Tetracycline-resistant strains of Propionibacterium acnes are also resistant to doxycycline but not to minocycline.

DOXYCYCLINE :

Doxycycline, which belongs to tetracyclines group is commonly used because of its convenient dose schedule.

MECHANISM OF ACTION :

Similar to that of tetracyclines, but do not have antiinflammatory action.

INDICATIONS :

Similar to that of tetracycline.

DOSES AND PREPARATIONS :

- 100 mg b.i.d. for 1-3 days followed by 100 mg once daily for severe infections 100 mg twice daily.
- DOXY-1 100 mg tab, MARTIDOX 100 mg tab.

SIDE EFFECTS :

Systemic :

GI disturbances particularly esophagitis, tooth discoloration, and enamel hypoplasia.

Cutaneous :

Phototoxic drug reactions and photoonycholysis.

KEY POINTS :

1. It is well absorbed from the gut, even after the food. Milk, antacids, magnesium, calcium, iron reduces the absorption of doxycycline.
2. Doxycycline is the safest tetracycline in renal failure being exclusively excreted in the gastrointestinal tract.

MINOCYCLINE :

Minocycline is a tetracycline antibiotic mainly used for inflammatory acne vulgaris in dermatology.

MECHANISM OF ACTION :

Similar to that of tetracycline, and also supposed to have antiinflammatory effect.

INDICATIONS :

Similar to that of tetracycline, but additionally used in leprosy, actinomycetoma and atypical mycobacterial infections particularly *M. marinum* infection. Apart from antiinfective agent it is also used as non-specific anti-inflammatory agent for the treatment of inflammatory disorders like pyoderma gangrenosum, vasculitis, etc.

DOSES AND PREPARATIONS :

- 100 mg Once or twice daily, 45/65 ER (extended release formulation) for acne.
- MINOZ 50/100 mg , MINYM ER 45/65 mg Tablets, CYANOMYCIN 50 mg, 100 mg cap.

SIDE EFFECTS :

Systemic :

Dizziness and vertigo, GI disturbances, yellow-gray brown colored tooth discoloration, enamel hypoplasia, autoimmune hepatitis, and drug hypersensitivity syndrome, drug induced lupus, pseudotumor cerebri

Cutaneous :

Pigmentation-brown-black hyperpigmentation may occur in varying patterns affecting :

- photoexposed areas.
- lesional skin pigmentation including scars.
- pretibial.
- diffuse (muddy skin syndrome).

Biopsy demonstrates the black pigment of drug metabolite-protein complex chelated with calcium in dendritic cells and extracellularly throughout the dermis. The othere side effects are :

- Phototoxic drug reactions.
- Drug-induced SLE (2 years after minocycline).

KEY POINTS :

- It is well absorbed from the gut, even after the food. Milk, antacids, iron reduces the absorption of minocycline.
- Minocycline owing to its proposed antiinflammatory effects, has been tried with variable success in conditions like sarcoidosis, pyoderma gangrenosum, etc.
- Minocycline has a potential to cause autoimmunity and thus has chances of autoimmune hepatitis, drug hypersensitivity syndrome.

TIGECYCLINE :

Tigecycline is a newer tetracycline antibiotic.

MECHANISM OF ACTION :

Similar to that of tetracycline.

INDICATIONS :

- Complicated skin and skin structure infections (cSSI).
- Complicated intra-abdominal infections and Community-acquired bacterial pneumonia.

DOSES AND PREPARATIONS :

- Inj TYGACIL 50 mg lyophilized powder for reconstitution in a single-dose 5 mL vial.
- Initial dose of 100 mg, followed by 50 mg every 12 hours administered intravenously over approximately 30 to 60 minutes.

SIDE EFFECTS :

Systemic :

- The most common adverse reactions (incidence > 5%) are nausea, vomiting, diarrhea, abdominal pain, headache, and increased SGPT.

- If used in children during tooth development may cause permanent discoloration of the teeth.

Cutaneous :

Hypersensitivity reactions.

KEY POINTS :

Anticoagulation test should be monitored if tigecycline is administered to patients receiving warfarin.

MACROLIDES :

Macrolides are the group of antibiotics mainly effective against Gram-positive organisms. They are known as macrolides as they contain a large lactone ring in their chemical structure.

Erythromycin is a prototype of macrolides. Lincomycin and clindamycin (a deviature of lincomycin) are not macrolides structurally. The newer macrolides of great dermatological importance include azithromycin, roxithromycin, and clarithromycin.

MECHANISM OF ACTION :

Inhibits bacterial protein synthesis by binding to 50 S ribosomal subunit.

INDICATIONS :

1. Skin and soft tissue infections particularly in patients allergic to penicillins.
2. Sexually transmitted diseases like chancroid, nongonococcal urethritis due to *Ureaplasma urealyticum,* syphilis in pregnant women or those sensitive to penicillins and donovanosis.
3. For the treatment of streptococcal infections, which may coexist with guttate psoriasis in children or

leukocytoclastic vasculitis, erythema nodosum, scleroderma, or other similar dermatologic conditions thought to be precipitated by streptococcal infections.

SIDE EFFECTS :

Erythromycin **:** Nausea, vomiting, abdominal pain with high doses. Cholestatic hepatitis, is seen with erythromycin estolate only and is more common if given during pregnancy.

Clindamycin : Pseudomembranous colitis caused by *Clostridium difficile.*

ERYTHROMYCIN :

Erythromycin, a macrolide, is bacteriostatic or bactericidal drug depending upon its concentration.

MECHANISM OF ACTION AND INDICATIONS :

Similar to other macrolides, but also used for its proposed antiinflammatory effects.

DOSES AND PREPARATIONS :

- Erythromycin 500 mg q.i.d. 30-40 mg/kg in divided doses.
- ELTOCIN (erythromycin estolate) 500 mg enteric-coated tablet.

TABLE 1.7 : **Indications of erythromycin in dermatovenereology**

Indications	Doses
Skin jnfections with pyogenic bacteria	250 - 500 mg q.i.d. x 1-2 weeks
Acne vulgaris	250 – 500 mg q.i.d. x 4-8 weeks
Early syphilis (in pregnancy)	500 mg q.i.d. 2-3 weeks
Chancroid	500 mg q.i.d. 7 days
Gonorrhea (pregnancy and penicillin allergy)	500 mg q.i.d. 4-7 days
Nongonococcal urethritis	500 mg q.i.d. 7-14 days
Donovanosis	500 mg q.i.d. 14-21 days
Lymphogranuloma venereum	500 mg q.i.d. 14-21 days

- ERYTHROCIN (erythromycin stearate) 500 mg enteric-coated tablet, ERYTHROCIN sus. (60 ml) 100 mg/5 ml, inj. 100 mg/2 ml vial.

PREGNANCY CATEGORY – B :

KEY POINTS :

- Erythromycin is partly destroyed by gastric acid, hence needs to be given in the form of enteric-coated tablet. Estolate, an ester form, is more resistant for gastric inactivation with better absorption.
- Levels of erythromycin decreases by 6-8 h necessitating periodic dosing at 6 hourly intervals.
- CSF penetration of erythromycin is poor; however, adequate during meningeal inflammation.
- Erythromycin estolate is responsible for cholestatic hepatitis associated with erythromycin. It clears within 1 week of discontinuation of therapy. It is more common when the drug is given during pregnancy.
- Apart from antibacterial effects used for skin infections, acne vulgaris, acne rosacea; erythromycin is also used in bullous pemphigoid (probably antiinflammatory action similar to tetracycline) in combination with niacinamide.
- Erythromycin may increase blood levels of many other drugs as it inhibits cytochrome P450 enzyme.

ROXITHROMYCIN :

A macrolide antibiotic.

MECHANISM OF ACTION AND INDICATIONS :

Similar to other macrolides.

DOSES AND PREPARATIONS :

- Roxithromycin 150 mg twice a day.
- ROXEPTIN, ROXID 150 mg tablet.

Key Points :

- Convenient twice daily dosing allows better GIT tolerance and better compliance.
- Roxithromycin does not have antiinflammatory effect unlike erythromycin.
- Roxithromycin is not used in the treatment of STDs.

AZITHROMYCIN :

Newer macrolide antibiotic.

Mechanism Of Action And Indications :
Similar to other macrolides, however it posseses increased activity against Gram-negative organisms and atypical mycobacteria.

Doses And Preparations :

- 500 mg o.d., 10 mg/kg in divided doses.
- AZIWIN, AZIFAST 250 or 500 mg tablet.

TABLE 1.8 : **Indications of azithromycin in dermatovenereology**

Indications	Doses
Skin and soft tissue infections	500 mg o.d. 3-5 days
Acne vulgaris	500 mg b.i.d. 3-5 days in every fortnight pulse
Chancroid	1 g stat
Gonorrhea	1 g stat
Donovanosis and LGV infections	1 g o.d. 21 days

PREGNANCY CATEGORY – B :

Key Points :

- Azithromycin has an advantage of expanded spectrum, better tolerability, less drug interactions as compared to other macrolides. Other advantages include long duration of action better tissue penetration and longer post-antibiotic effect.

- Azithromycin causes time-dependent killing of microorganisms with moderate to prolonged effect. Post-antibiotic effect of azithromycin is because of reduction of cell surface hydrophobicity and increased bacterial phagocytosis independent of antimicrobial action. This permits pulse therapy of azithromycin.

CLARITHROMYCIN :

Newer macrolide antibiotic with extended activity against mycobacterial infections.

MECHANISM OF ACTION :
Similar to other macrolides.

INDICATIONS :

Apart from uses similar to that of erythromycin, the drug is used :

1. As an antileprosy drug. When other drugs are not tolerated or for dapsone or rifampicin resistant leprosy.
2. As an effective antituberculous drug against atypical mycobacterial infections and multi-drug resistant tuberculosis.
3. To eradicate *H. pylori* infection.
4. An effective alternative for treatment of skin & soft tissue infections (SSTIs).

DOSES AND PREPARATIONS :

- 250-500 mg b.i.d.
- CLARIBID 250, 500 mg tablet, CRIXAN susp. 125 mg/5 ml.

PREGNANCY CATEGORY – C :

Side Effects :

Nausea, vomiting, diarrhea, abdominal pain, and dyspepsia.

Key Points :

- Clarithromycin can increase the levels of theophylline and carbamazepine.
- Dose adjustments of clarithromycin is needed in elderly with impaired renal function.

TELITHROMYCIN :

It is a ketolide antibiotic that is related to macrolides and is mainly used against many macrolide-resistant strains that are susceptible to telithromycin. Dose of telithromycin is 800 mg once daily.

CLINDAMYCIN :

Clindamycin is a derivative of lincomycin with extended activity against anaerobic infections.

Mechanism Of Action And Indications :

Similar to other macrolides. Effective against Staphylococci, Streptococci, Gram positive anaerobes (except C. Difficile) and gram negative anaerobes, Corynebacterium sp.

Doses And Preparations :

- 150-300 mg q.i.d.
- CLINCIN 150, 300 mg tab, 300 mg/2 ml injection.

PREGNANCY CATEGORY – B :

Side Effects :

Systemic :

Pseudomembranous colitis, nausea, vomiting, diarrhea, abdominal pain, hepatitis, and eosinophilia.

Cutaneous :

Urticaria and rash.

KEY POINTS :

- Erythromycin acts as an antagonist of clindamycin while gentamicin has synergistic effect.
- Clindamycin, active against MRSA, has good tissue penetration (97%) and tolerability profile, and the ability to inhibit production of bacterial toxins common in CA-MRSA infection.
- Pseudomembranous colitis is the most noted and feared side effect of clindamycin caused by *Clostridium difficile.* It responds to vancomycin or metronidazole.

VANCOMYCIN :

Complex glycopeptide antibiotic of bactericidal nature mainly effective against Gram-positive cocci and some Gram-positive bacilli.

MECHANISM OF ACTION :

It inhibits cell wall synthesis and RNA synthesis.

INDICATIONS :

1. Resistant skin and soft tissue infections, including methicillin-resistant staphylococcal aureus (MRSA) infections. (more frequently, hospital acquired infections).
2. Pseudomembranous colitis.

DOSES AND PREPARATIONS :

- 1 g 12 hourly i.v infusion over 100 min for 7-10 days or 10 mg/kg 6 hourly by slow i.v. infusion over 60 min for 7-10 days; MRSA infections 1 gm 12 hourly for 10-14 days; Pseudomembranous colitis 125 mg 6 hourly for 7-14 days.
- VANCOLID 500 mg, 1 g vial.

PREGNANCY CATEGORY – C :

SIDE EFFECTS :

Systemic :

Nephrotoxicity, drug fever, and deafness.

Cutaneous :

Flushing, red man syndrome (with rapid intravenous infusion).

KEY POINTS :

- Vancomycin is the drug of choice for MRSA infections and pseudomembranous colitis.
- BUN and serum creatinine should be strictly monitored in patients on vancomycin therapy.
- Oritavancin, a derivative of vancomycin, has extended bactericidal activity against MRSA and daptomycin non-susceptible VRE (vancomycin resistant enterococcus) . Single intravenous dose of oritavancin was non-inferior to twice-daily vancomycin.

TEICOPLANIN (TARGOCID®) :

- A newer glycopeptide antibiotic that is similar to vancomycin. Indications are similar to that of vancomycin. However, it has a longer half life (t½) permitting once daily dosage.
- Dalbavancin, a derivative of a teicoplanin-like natural antibiotic has antimicrobial activity against almost all clinical MRSA isolates.

OXAZOLIDINONES :

LINEZOLID :

An oxazolidinone antibiotic is effective against gram positive organisms (including methicillin resistant Staphylococcus aureus, MRSA) and Enterococcus spp.

MECHANISM OF ACTION :

Inhibits protein synthesis by binding to 50S ribosomal subunit.

INDICATIONS :

1. Skin and soft issue infections (complicated and uncomplicated) including those caused by MRSA.
2. Hospital acquired skin and soft tissue infections including Vancomycin resistant and multi-drug resistant infections.
3. Atypical mycobacterial infection.

SIDE EFFECTS :

Thrombocytopenia, neutropenia.

DOSES AND PREPARATIONS :

- LINOX 600 mg Tab, LINID; 2 mg/ml, 300 ml or 600 ml vial, 600 mg BD orally or intravenously.

KEY POINTS :

- Linezolid has an advantage over vancomycin as it does not require dose adjustment in renal dysfunction.
- It is a preferred drug in necrotizing fasciitis as it inhibits bacterial toxin production similar to clindamycin.
- The oxazolidinones are particularly helpful for the treatment of necrotizing fasciitis since they inhibit the production of bacterial pyrogenic endotoxins.

TEDIZOLID :

A newer oxazolidinone antibiotic with once daily dosage.

MECHANISM OF ACTION :

Tedizolid phosphate is the prodrug of tedizolid, an antibacterial agent.

INDICATIONS :

- Acute bacterial skin and skin structure infections (ABSSSI) caused by designated susceptible bacteria.

SIDE EFFECTS :

- Nausea, headache, diarrhea, infusion- or injection-related adverse reactions, vomiting, and dizziness.

DOSES AND PREPARATIONS :

- SILVEXTRO™ 200 mg administered once daily orally or as an intravenous (IV) infusion over 1 hour for six days
- For injection : 200 mg, sterile, lyophilized powder in single-use vial for reconstitution for intravenous infusion; Tablet : 200 mg

KEY POINTS :

- Tedizoild (when administered orally) can increase the plasma concentrations of orally administered Breast Cancer Resistance Protein BCRP substrates. Monitor for adverse reactions related to the concomitant BCRP substrates if coadministration cannot be avoided.

FLUOROQUINOLONES :

Fluoroquinolones (FQs) are quinolone antimicrobials having one or more fluorine substitutes. Additional "fluoro" and other substitutes extend the microbial activity and confer metabolic stability. First generation FQs include ciprofloxacin, ofloxacin, norfloxacin, and pefloxacin, while lomefloxacin, sparfloxacin, and amifloxacin are second generation fluoroquinolones.

MECHANISM OF ACTION :

Fluoroquinolones inhibit bacterial protein synthesis by interfering with bacterial DNA gyrase, which prevents uncoiling of DNA that is necessary for multiplication.

INDICATIONS :

Common indications of all fluoroquinolones in dermatology include :

1. Skin and soft tissue infections.
2. Leprosy : ofloxacin and sparfloxacin.
3. Sexually transmitted diseases.
4. Tuberculosis (second-line antituberculous drug).
5. Rhinoscleroma.

SIDE EFFECTS :

1. Nausea, vomiting, and diarrhea.
2. Arthropathy of weight bearing joints in children (not proven adequately).
3. Photosensitivity especially sparfloxacin.
4. Hypersensitivity.

PREGNANCY CATEGORY – C :

BACTERIAL RESISTANCE :

Mechanisms of bacterial resistance include :

1. Chromosomal mutation producing a DNA gyrase with reduced affinity for fluoroquinolones.
2. Reduced permeability of the bacterial membranes to the drug.

TABLE 1.9 : **Indications of fluoroquinolones in dermatovenereology**

Examples of FQs used in dermatovenereology	Dose
Nongonococcal urethritis (NGU) : Ofloxacin TARIVID 200 mg tablet Sparfloxacin SPARLOX 200 mg tablet	 100 mg b.i.d. for 7 days 300 mg b.i.d. or 100 mg o.d. for 6 days
Chancroid : Ciprofloxacin CIPLOX 500 mg tablet	 500 mg single dose
Donovanosis : Norfloxacin NORFLOX 400 mg tablet	 400 mg b.i.d. for 7 days
Gonorrhea : Ciprofloxacin	 250 mg single dose
Skin and soft tissue infections : Ciprofloxacin	 500 mg b.i.d. for 7 days
Tuberculosis : Ciprofloxacin (second-line antituberculous agent) Ofloxacin (second-line antituberculous agent)	 750 mg b.i.d. for 2 years 400 mg od for 2 years
Leprosy (experimental, not in common use) : Ofloxacin Sparfloxacin	 400 mg o.d. as a part of newer regimen 200 mg o.d.

Doses And Preparations :

Key Points :

- Antacids, sucralfate and iron salts reduce absorption of fluoroquinolones.
- Fluoroquinolones can cause cartilage damage in weight bearing joints; hence it is contraindicated in children below 10 years of age and during pregnancy.
- Sparfloxacin can cause phototoxic reactions. Ofloxacin is the least phototoxic. Fluoroquinolones can be given at night to avoid phototoxicity.
- Ciprofloxacin and ofloxacin are most commonly used for the treatment of mycobacterial infections of the skin, while

ofloxacin, pefloxacin, sparfloxacin, and moxifloxacin are proposed for use in leprosy.

- Sparfloxacin, galifloxacin, moxifloxacin and levofloxacin may prolong QT interval on ECG which may precipitate polymorphic ventricular tachycardia *(Torsad de pointes).*

ANTIBIOTICS ON THE HORIZON :

NEWER ANTIBIOTICS :

CARBAPENEMS :

Carbapenems are beta lactam antibiotics that are effective against extended spectrum beta lactamase (ESBL) strains of gram negative organisms, especially E. coli, that are resistant to aminoglycosides or fluoroquinolones. Hence, they are extremely useful in serious infections due to these organisms. Imipenem, meropenem and doripenem are some of the molecules in current use. They act by preventing formation of peptidoglycan needed for cell wall formation of bacteria. They are used as injectables as a last hope in patients with gram negative septicemia not responding to injectable combinations of third generation cephalosporins or synthetic penicillin or aminoglycosides. New improved versions of carbapenems are under research.

FAROPENEM :

Faropenem is an orally effective penem (not a carbapenem) that is useful for gram negative as well as gram positive infections but is not effective against MRSA or vancomycin resistant gram negative infections. In contrast, meropenem is effective against these bacteria and is therefore used for serious infections caused by them. Faropenem is used in skin and soft tissue infections in a dosage of 200 mg two to three times daily. Side effects of faropenem include gastrointestinal intolerance, hypersensitivity including pseudo anaphylactic reaction, rashes including Stevens Johnson syndrome, rhabdomyolysis and rarely, agranulocytosis. Hence, caution is needed in its use in skin infections. It is mainly used in resistant upper and lower respiratory and urinary tract infections.

DAPTOMYCIN :

Daptomycin is a lipopeptide antibacterial.

MECHANISM OF ACTION :

Daptomycin binds to bacterial membranes and causes a rapid depolarization of membrane potential. This loss of membrane potential causes inhibition of DNA, RNA, and protein synthesis, which results in bacterial cell death.

INDICATIONS :

- Complicated skin and skin structure infections (cSSSI).
- Staphylococcus aureus bloodstream infections (bacteremia), including those with right-sided infective endocarditis.

DOSES AND PREPARATIONS :

- Inj CUBICIN™ 500 mg lyophilized powder for reconstitution in a single-use vial.
- Daptomycin 4 mg/kg should be administered intravenously in 0.9% sodium chloride injection once every 24 hours for 7 days.

PREGNANCY CATEGORY – B :

SIDE EFFECTS :

Systemic :

- Abnormal liver function tests, elevated creatinine phsophokinase (CPK) levels, dyspnea, and pneumonia.
- Myopathy and rhabdomyolysis : Monitor CPK levels and follow muscle pain or weakness; if elevated CPK or myopathy occurs, consider discontinuation of daptomycin.

Cutaneous :

Hypersensitivity reactions may occur.

KEY POINT :

- No preservative or bacteriostatic agent is present in this product, hence daptomycin injection has to be given immediately after reconstitution.

FOSFOMYCIN :

A synthetic, broad spectrum, bactericidal antibiotic.

MECHANISM OF ACTION :

Fosfomycin is a bactericidal antibiotic that interferes with cell wall synthesis in both **Gram-positive** and **Gram-negative bacteria** by inhibiting the initial step involving **phosphoenolpyruvate synthetase**.

INDICATIONS :

- Fosfomycin due to its excellent tissue penetration and in vitro bactericidal activity has been advocated for MRSA infection. However, more clinical data is needed to be available.
- Fosfomycin is indicated only for the treatment of uncomplicated urinary tract infections (acute cystitis) in women due to susceptible strains of Escherichia coli and Enterococcus fecalis.

DOSES AND PREPARATIONS :

MONUROL 3 gm sachet.

- Fosfomycin should be taken orally. Pour the entire contents of a single-dose sachet into 3 to 4 ounces of water (½ cup) and stir to dissolve. Do not use hot water. It should be taken immediately after dissolving in water.
- Fosphomycin is available as a single-dose sachet containing the equivalent of 3 grams of fosfomycin.

PREGNANCY CATEGORY – B :

SIDE EFFECTS :

Systemic :

Diarrhea, headache, vaginitis, nausea, rhinitis, back pain, dysmenorrhea, pharyngitis.

Cutaneous : rash.

KEY POINTS :

- When coadministered with fosfomycin, metoclopramide, a drug which increases gastrointestinal motility, lowers the serum concentration and urinary excretion of fosfomycin. Other drugs that increase gastrointestinal motility may produce similar effects.

CEFTAROLINE :

QUINUPRISTIN/DALFOPRISTIN :

1. Ceftaroline, a new generation cephalosporin with clinically meaningful activity against MRSA, is approved for the treatment of cSSTIs and community-acquired pneumonia. Over 90% of MRSA isolates were found to be susceptible to ceftaroline. Ceftaroline has also shown potent antimicrobial activity against a large number of SSTI-associated bacterial isolates including MRSA (80.6% susceptibility) from South Africa and Asia-Pacific region.

   The safety profile of ceftaroline was consistent with cephalosporin class. The most common adverse events observed were diarrhea, nausea, and rash. Administration of ceftaroline demonstrated no significant effect on the intestinal flora in healthy participants, and thus, risk of C. difficile-related diarrhea is low. Ceftaroline (every 8 or 12 hour dosing schedule) is a viable option for treating cSSTIs due to Gram-negative and Gram-positive (with MRSA) infections or following failure of vancomycin therapy.

2. Oritavancin and dalbavancin are lipoglycopeptides (approved by US FDA in 2014) with the pharmacokinetic advantage of extended plasma half-life, enabling single-dose regimens.

   Oritavancin, a derivative of vancomycin, has extended bactericidal activity against MRSA and daptomycin non-susceptible VRE. Single iv dose, oritavancin, was non-inferior to twice-daily vancomycin resistant (7-to-10 day course) in two Phase III studies of ABSSSI caused by Gram-positive pathogens.

   Dalbavancin, a derivative of a teicoplanin-like natural antibiotic has antimicrobial activity against almost all clinical MRSA isolates. Once-weekly iv dalbavancin was non-inferior to twice-daily vancomycin followed by oral linezolid with comparable success rates in ABSSSI as demonstrated in a pooled analysis. Dalbavancin and oritavancin have similar safety profiles as vancomycin. In clinical studies, the most commonly reported adverse events were headache, nausea, diarrhea, and vomiting. The elimination of multidose and multiday regimen and lower propensity for resistance development are potential benefits of dalbavancin and oritavancin treatments.

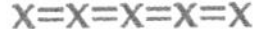

2
Systemic Antifungals

CLASSIFICATION OF ANTIFUNGALS :

1. **Antifungal antibiotics :**
   a. Polyenes : amphotericin B, nystatin, hamycin and natamycin
   b. Echinocandins : capsofungin, micafungin, anidulofungin
   c. Heterocyclic benzofuran : griseofulvin
2. Antimetabolite : flucytosine.
3. Azoles
   a. Imidazoles : ketoconazole.
   b. Triazole : fluconazole, Itraconazole, voriconazole, posaconazole.
4. Allylamine : terbinafine and naftifine.
5. Benzylamine : butenafine.

Ergosterol synthesis pathway and site of action of some antifungal drugs :

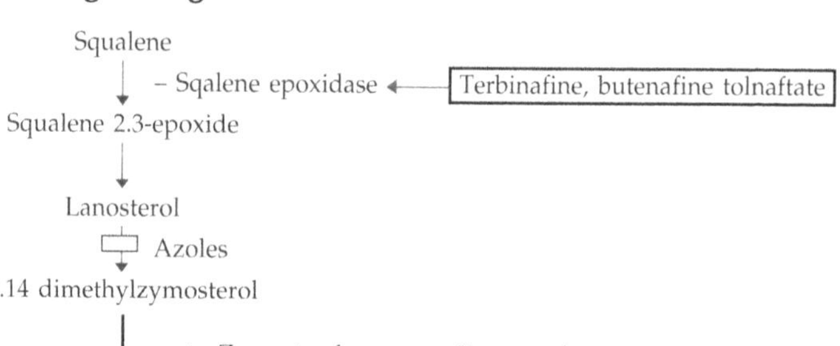

Antifungals can also be classified based on their Mechanism of Action as follows :

Mechanism of action	Antifungal drug
Fungal cell wall synthesis inhibitors	Ecchinocandins like Capsofungin, Micafungin etc.
Bind to fungal cell membrane ergosterol forming pores	Amphotericin B, Nystatin
Inhibition of ergosterol + lanosterol synthesis	Terbinafine, Naftifine, Butenafine
Inhibition of ergosterol synthesis	Azoles
Inhibition of nucleic acid synthesis	5-Flucytosine
Inhibition of fungal mitosis through disruption of microtubules	Griseofulvin

GRISEOFULVIN :

Griseofulvin, a heterocyclic benzofuran antibiotic, is most commonly used for fungal infections of the skin caused by dermatophytes.

MECHANISM OF ACTION :

Fungistatic drug interferes with mitosis to form multinucleated, stunted, and curled hyphae (hence called the "curling factor").

Indications for Griseofulvin (or Oral Antifungals) in Dermatophyte infections :

1. Tinea capitis.
2. Tinea pedis and tinea manuum (optional).
3. Tinea corporis that is either :
   a. Widespread, or relcalcitrant or recurrent,
   b. Has underlying predisposing factor like diabetes mellitus, immunosuppressive therapy, or HIV infection, or

c. Is not responding to topical antifungals,

d. Combined with oral azoles these days to exert additional antifungal effect through different MOA.

4. **Tinea unguium** : However, newer oral antifungals like terbinafine and itraconazole are preferred for tinea unguium because of their higher efficacy in nail infections.

DOSES AND PREPARATIONS :

- 250 mg twice a day (micronized) or 375 mg once a day (ultra-micronized) for an ordinary adult, 10 mg/kg/day (micronized) for children.
- GRISOVIN FP (micronized) 125 mg tablet; GRIS-OD 375 mg tablet (ultra-micronized); GRISACTIN FORTE 250 mg tablet.

PREGNANCY CATEGORY – C DURATION OF THERAPY :

TABLE 2.1 : **Duration of griseofulvin therapy in dermatophytosis**

Body skin	4 weeks
Hair	4-6 weeks
Palms and soles	6-8 weeks
Finger nails	6-12 months
Toe nails	12-18 months

ADVERSE EFFECTS :

Systemic :

- Headache, the commonest.
- GIT disturbances.
- Transient leukopenia.
- Peripheral neuritis.
- Albuminuria (without renal damage).
- Hepatotoxicity (contraindicated in severe liver disease).

Cutaneous :

- Fixed drug eruption, photoallergic dermatitis, and lichenoid drug eruption.
- Precipitation of acute intermittent porphyria or lupus erythematosus.

Key Points :

- Gastrointestinal absorption of griseofulvin depends upon the particle size and presence of fat in the food. Phenobarbitone reduces the absorption of griseofulvin.
- Duration of treatment depends on the site of infection, thickness of SC, its turnover rate, and immunological status.
- Since this is a fungistatic drug, fungus persists in already infected keratin till it is shed off. Excretion in the sweat is a major route of delivery of griseofulvin in the skin.
- Ineffective against pityrosporum, candidal, molds, and deep mycotic infections.
- Griseofulvin is an antifungal of choice in patients with renal failure.
- Griseofulvin can cause alcohol intolerance.
- Griseofulvin reduces efficacy of oral contraceptive pills.

FLUCONAZOLE :

Broad-spectrum triazole antifungal; it is also somewhat effective against some Gram-positive and anaerobic bacteria.

Mechanism Of Action :

Inhibits fungal ergosterol synthesis by blocking fungal enzyme lanosterol 14-demethylase.

Mechanism of antibacterial action remains unexplained.

Indications :

1. Cryptococcal meningitis and coccidioidal meningitis.

2. Mucocutaneous/Disseminated candidiasis.
3. Candidiasis including oropharyngeal, vaginal, and mucocutaneous candidiasis (except *C. krusei*).
4. Dermatophyte infections of the skin, hair, and nail.
5. Pityrosporum ovale infections.
6. Histoplasmosis, paracoccidioidomycosis and sporotrichosis.
7. Fungal keratitis.

Doses And Preparations :

Varies widely as per the indication and stated in Table 2. In most instances, 2-6 mg/kg/day is required.

- ZOCON, FUSYS 50, 100, 150, 200 mg tablets.
- ZOCON 200 mg/100 ml intravenous infusion for systemic infections, dose same as oral.
- SYSCAN 0.3% eye drops for fungal keratitis.

PREGNANCY CATEGORY – C :

Doses And Duration :

TABLE 2.2 : **Doses and duration of fluconazole therapy in fungal infections**

Dermatophyte and cutaneous candidiasis	150 mg/wk for 4-6 weeks used to be effective in the past. However, higher dosages are used now in view of increasing MIC levels to fluconazole. Doses may vary from 150 mg twice a week to 150 mg alternate days or even 100-150 mg daily.
Vaginal candidiasis and candidial balanoposthitis	150 mg single dose or repeat for 3 weeks in cases of recurrences or uncorrectable predisposing factor
Cryptococcosis and Cryptococcal meningitis	400 mg o.d. 8-10 weeks in non-AIDS patients. In AIDS patients, 200 mg o.d. (suppressive dose) after i.v. amphotericin B + flucytosine (5-FC).
Onychomycosis	150 mg/wk till "cure" (not more than 1 year).
Pityriasis versicolor	400 mg stat (repeat after 2 weeks).

ADVERSE EFFECTS :

Systemic :

Well tolerated; side effects may occur like nausea, vomiting, abdominal pain, headache, thrombocytopenia, and raised creatinine levels.

Cutaneous :

Fixed drug eruption, Maculopapular rash (rare).

KEY POINTS :

- Of the orally administered fluconazole, 94% is absorbed; oral bioavailability is not affected by food or gastric pH; 80% of fluconazole is excreted unchanged in urine.
- Longer half life of fluconazole (25-30 h) permits its single dose and once weekly regimen.
- Penetration in brain and CSF is good, hence used for cryptococcal meningitis.
- Unlike ketoconazole, it does not inhibit steroid synthesis and hence is not antiandrogenic (no gynecomastia).
- Can cause elevation of hepatic transaminases in HIV patients being used in higher doses for prolonged periods for cryptococcosis.
- Plasma levels of fluconazole is reduced by rifampicin and enhanced by zidovudine.
- Fluconazole potentiates hypoglycemic effects of tolbutamide and glipizide.

ITRACONAZOLE :

Broad-spectrum azole antifungal with fungistatic action that also includes moulds like *Aspergillus* and *Mucor.*

Mechanism Of Action :

Inhibits fungal ergosterol synthesis like other azoles.

Indications :

1. Subcutaneous mycoses like eumycetoma and chromoblastomycosis (drug of choice).
2. Systemic mycoses not associated with meningitis like blastomycosis and paracoccidioidomycosis (drug of choice).
3. Aspergillosis and mucormycosis (partially effective and 2nd drug of choice).
4. Pityrosporum ovale infections.
5. Dermatophyte infections of the skin, hair, and nail.
6. Candidiasis.

Doses And Preparations :

- 100-200 mg b.i.d., 3-5 mg/kg/day.
- CANDITRAL/CANDISTAT 100 mg capsule; ITRA 100 mg capsules containing granules or pellets of sizes varying from 0.5 mm to 1.5 mm. Efficacy of absorption is shown to be related to uniform pellet size, consumption one hour before food and gastric acidity.
- Inj Sporinox 25 ml Ampoule (to be diluted with 50 ml of 0.9 NS to make 75 ml-discard 15 ml of reconstituted solution to obtain 60 ml containing 3.33 mg/mL = 200 mg Itraconazole. It is slowly infused intravenously over 60 minutes).
- Syntran SB 50 mg capsules contain super bioavailable drug equivalento to 100 mg of regular itraconazole.

PREGNANCY CATEGORY – C :

Doses And Duration :

TABLE 2.3 : **Doses and duration of ordinary (O) and super-bioavailable (SB) itraconazole therapy in superficial fungal infections**

Dermatophytosis treatment naive	O : 100 mg twice daily for 4-6 weeks SB : 50 mg twice daily for 4-6 weeks
Dermatophytosis recalcitrant	O : 200 mg twice daily for 6-8 weeks SB : 100 mg two times daily for 4-6 weeks
Fingernail onychomycosis	O : 200 mg twice daily for one week per month for 2 months
Toenail onychomycosis	O : 200 mg twice daily for one week per month for 3 months
Vaginal candidiasis	O : 600 mg single dose or 100 mg BD for a week
Oral candidiasis	O : 100 mg BD for 15 days
Pirtyriasis versicolor	O : Single dose of 400 mg or 100 BD for a week
Histoplasmosis, cryptococcosis, eumycotic mycetoma, blastomycosis, phycomycosis, chromoblastomycosis, and much less effective against mucormycosis, aspergillosis	O : 200 mg BD or higher for several months

Adverse Effects :

Systemic :

More side effects as compared to fluconazole. In superficial mycoses, incidence of side effects are upto 7% while when used for systemic mycoses, it is upto 16.2%.

- Nausea, abdominal pain, constipation. At higher doses gastritis, bloating, diarrhea are common.
- Dizziness, headache,
- Hypokalemia (in higher doses),
- Negative inotropic effect on cardiac muscles leading to congestive cardiac failure,

- Hepatitis (higher doses and for longer duration of time may be associated with transient elevation of transaminases. Relatively contra-indicated in patient with hepatic impairment.

Cutaneous :

Skin rash and cutaneous vasculitis is reported.

DRUG INTERACTIONS :

Most of these are related to inhibition of cytochrome P450 3A4 CC-3.

1. Phenytoin, rifampicin, H_2 blockers decrease plasma concentration of itraconazole.
2. Increases concentration of cyclosporine and warfarin.
3. Itraconazole and hypolipidemic drugs, *i.e.* "statins" can lead to rhabdomyolysis.
4. Itraconazole and terfenadine, astemizole, cisapride can cause ventricular tachycardia.
5. Contraindicated if patient is on antiarrhythmic drugs like disopyramide, dofetilide, dronedarone, quinidine.
6. Itraconazole and nifedipine : peripheral edema and negative inotropic effect on the heart.

REMARKS :

- Itraconazole is a weak base that ionizes at low pH, hence gastric acidity is required. Oral absorption of itraconazole is enhanced by food or gastric acid. Use of proton pump inhibitors, ranitidine or antacids decrease efficacy of Itraconazole when administered together. On the other hand, use of acidic beverages will enhance absorption.
- Super-bioavailable preparation of itraconazole is now available and this has more uniform absorption that is not affected by food, gastric acidity or consumption of proton pump inhibitors.

- Unlike fluconazole, penetration of itraconazole in brain and CSF is poor.
- Itraconzale is detectable in the sebum after 4 days of administration of 200 mg/d of the dose while it is detectable in the sweat in 24 hours. However, unlike griseofulvin, excretion through sweat is minor route of delivery to the skin. In the nail, it reaches to the distal nail bed in 7 days time. In the nail, it remains for 6-9 months after cessation of Itraconazole pulse therapy.
- As Itraconazole inhibits ergosterol synthesis but still leading to formation of lanosterol which forms weak cell membrane of fungus, chances of recurrences following Itraconazole discontinuation are higher.
- Itraconazole may persist in stratum corneum for 3–4 weeks after discontinuation justifying pulse therapy of itraconazole. The extensive protein binding of itraconazole ensures that its concentration at the site of infection remains higher than the corresponding plasma concentration for several days. Based on this property of itraconazole, it is recommended to use in pulse therapy for the management of dermatophytosis including onychomycosis.
- Unlike ketoconazole, it does not inhibit steroid synthesis and hence does not have antiandrogenic effects like gynecomastia, loss of libido or oligospermia.

KETOCONAZOLE :

First oral broad-spectrum antifungal with mechanism of action similar to that of other azoles.

INDICATIONS :

1. Widespread dermatophytosis (as an effective alternative to griseofulvin).
2. Candidiasis.

3. Pityrosporum ovale infections.
4. Less serious systemic mycoses (preferred over amphotericin due to low cost and toxicity).
5. Systemic mycoses in combination with amphotericin or flucytosine particularly cryptococcosis, histoplasmosis, and blastomycosis.
6. Dermal leishmaniasis and *kala azar.*

DOSES AND PREPARATIONS :

- 200 mg o.d./b.i.d., 3-6 mg/kg o.d.
- HYPHORAL 200 mg tab, NIZRAL 2% cream, NIZRAL 2% shampoo.

PREGNANCY CATEGORY – C :

DRUG INTERACTIONS :

- H_2 blockers, proton pump inhibitors, and antacids decrease oral absorption.
- Phenytoin and rifampicin-decrease plasma concentration of ketoconazole.
- Ketoconazole concentration of cyclosporine and warfarin, sulfonylureas.

ADVERSE EFFECTS :

Systemic :

More side effects like nausea and vomiting-the most common, anorexia, headache, paresthesia. Loss of libido, gynecomastia, hair loss, oligospermia-antiandrogenic effect.

Cutaneous :

Rash and alopecia.

KEY POINTS :

- Oral absorption of ketoconazole is enhanced by gastric acid.

- Penetration in brain and CSF is poor unlike in fluconazole.
- Ketoconazole inhibits conversion of cholesterol to steroid hormones like testosterone and cortisol and thus has many anti-androgenic side effects like gynecomastia.
- Ketoconazole is not a preferred drug for fungal infections because of its antiandrogenic side effects and potential drug interactions, but still can be used for candidal, dermatophyte, and pityrosporum infections for short period of time.

TERBINAFINE :

Oral and topical broad-spectrum allylamine antifungal.

MECHANISM OF ACTION :

Fungicidal drug, Inhibits squalene epoxidase, leading to accumulation of intracellular squalene and deficient ergosterol synthesis with subsequent fungal cell death.

Drug reaches the body surface through diffusion from dermal vasculature and via sebum to the hair follicle.

INDICATIONS :

1. Widespread dermatophytosis (as an effective alternative to griseofulvin) with Dermatophytosis. However, in the last few years widespread resistance to terbinafine has emerged in many parts of India reducing its utility.
2. Candidiasis (less effective than other alternative anticandidal drugs like fluconazole).

DOSES AND PREPARATIONS :

- 250 mg o.d., children < 20 kg : 62.5 mg/day div q.o.d.; children > 20 kg : 125 mg/day div q.o.d.
- ZIMIG, SEBIFFIN 250 mg tab, TERBEST, TERBO 2% cream.

PREGNANCY CATEGORY – B :

Doses And Duration :

TABLE 2.4 : **Doses and duration of terbinafine therapy in fungal infections**

Dermatophytosis	250 mg b.i.d. for 2-4 weeks-tinea corporis/tinea cruris. 250 mg b.i.d. for 4-6 weeks-tinea pedis 250 mg daily for 4-6 weeks-tinea capitis.
Finger nail onychomycosis	200 mg o.d. for 6 weeks – 3 months 200 mg b.i.d. for 7 consecutive days/per month 2 months.
Toe nail onychomycosis	200 mg o.d. for 6 weeks – 3 months 200 mg b.i.d. for 7 consecutive days/per month 3 months.
Cutaneous candidiasis (not routinely recommended)	250 mg once daily for 2-4 weeks.

Adverse Effects :

Systemic :

Mild gastrointestinal disturbances, deranged hepatic function (idiosyncratic) and renal function.

Cutaneous :

Skin rash, autoimmune hepatitis, precipitation of lupus erythematosus. Acute generalised exanthematous pustulosis and dyschromatosis are also reported.

Key Points :

- 70-80% oral absorption, not significantly affected by presence of food.
- Being lipophilic, it accumulates in keratinous tissues and is present in the tissues long after it is withdrawn. This is the basis of terbinafine pulse therapy.
- It is less effective against candida and pityrosporum infections particularly when used topically.

- Rifampicin increases elimination of terbinafine.
- Caution should be exerted when terbinafine is used with anti-arrhythmics and antidepressants as terbinafine inhibits the CYP2D6-mediated metabolism of these drugs
- Terbinafine resistance is now well established in India with increasing MIC values for terbinafine. Resistance to effective fungicidal drug like terbinafine could be the main cause of pandemic of dermatophytosis in country like India.

AMPHOTERICIN B (AMB) :

Broad-spectrum polyene macrolide antibiotic is the most potent antifungal agent for systemic mycoses.

MECHANISM OF ACTION :

Fungicidal drug at high concentrations and static at lower concentrations.

High affinity for fungal ergosterol, forms "micropore" in fungal cell membrane through which ions, amino acids, and other water-soluble substances move out.

Markedly increases cell permeability.

Cholesterol, present in host cell membranes, closely resembles fungal ergosterol and thus explains the high toxicity of AMB in humans.

INDICATIONS :

1. Disseminated candidiasis, cryptococcosis, and coccidioidomycosis (in combination with 5-flucytosine).
2. Histoplasmosis (in combination with itraconazole or ketoconazole).
3. Aspergillosis and mucormycosis (drug of choice).
4. Disseminated sporotrichosis.

5. Chromoblastomycosis.
6. Paracoccidioidomycosis (second drug of choice).
7. Leishmaniasis (reserve drug).

DOSES AND PREPARATIONS :

- 1.5-5 mg/kg/day for 6-12 weeks (available in powdered form to be dissolved in 5% dextrose).
- FUNGISOME 10, 25, 50 mg vial.

PREGNANCY CATEGORY – B :

LIPOSOMAL AMB : NEW LIPID FORMULATIONS (Dose 3-5 mg/kg/day).

AMB is incorporated into lipid formulations to reduce toxicity and enhance efficacy. This allows higher dose to be used without increasing the toxicity. Currently, three such lipid formulations are available and are more expensive than ordinary amphotericin B, which seems to be their only disadvantage.

AmBisome – incorporates AMB with liposomes.

Abelact – ribbons of lipids interspersed with AMB.

Amphocil – AMB colloidal suspension.

AMPHOLIP 10, 50, 100 mg liquid for injection.

ADVERSE EFFECTS :

Systemic :

Nephrotoxicity-most serious (dose > 5 mg/day may produce irreversible renal damage), nausea and vomiting, fever, chills, hypokalemia, thrombophlebitis, thrombocytopenia, and anaphylaxis.

Cutaneous :

Hypersensitivity.

KEY POINTS :

- Is not absorbed enterally; hence can be given orally for intestinal candidiasis.
- Penetration in brain and CSF is poor (but extremely effective in fungal meningitis when combined with 5-FC).
- Antihistamines and intravenous hydrocortisone 100 mg is routinely given prior to the administration of AMB to avoid hypersensitivity reactions.
- Drug should be preferably given through the central intravenous line due to the risk of thrombophlebitis.
- Intravenous or oral K^+ supplementation is necessary with monitoring of serum K^+ levels during AMB administration. Daily monitoring of blood urea nitrogen and creatinine is mandatory. If they show elevation, dose should be maintained or reduced as per situation.
- Drug concentration achieved in infected skin is very low, and hence ineffective against superficial fungal infections.
- Start with a test dose of 1 mg on day 1. If there is no hypersensitivity, increase to 0.5 mg/kg/day. If no other side effects, the dose can be steadily increased (except in candidiasis) to reach a maximum of 1 mg/kg/day. For serious infections, one can dispense with the test dose and start with the higher dose.

FLUCYTOSINE (5-FC) :

Pyrimidine antimetabolite, narrow-spectrum fungistatic.

MECHANISM OF ACTION :

It is taken up by fungal cells and converted into 5-fluorouracil and then to 5-fluorodeoxyuridylic acid, which is an inhibitor of thymidylate synthesis.

SPECTRUM :

Cryptococcus neoformans, strains causing chromoblastomycosis, a few species of *Candida* and *Aspergillus.*

INDICATIONS :

- Chromoblastomycosis.
- Meningeal and nonmeningeal cryptococcosis and disseminated candidiasis (synergistic action with AMB).

ADVERSE EFFECTS :

Myelosuppression, GI disturbances, mild and reversible liver dysfunction.

DOSE AND PREPARATIONS :

100-150 mg/kg/day in four divided doses orally.

PREGNANCY CATEGORY – B (No confirmed data available) :

KEY POINTS :

- Since this is a narrow-spectrum fungistatic, it is mainly used as an adjuvant drug and not as a sole therapy.
- CSF penetration is excellent, hence it is combined with AMB in fungal meningitis.
- Mammalian bone marrow cells have the capacity to convert 5-FC to 5-FU, and this explains marrow toxicity with flucytosine. Concurrent use of other myelosuppressive drugs should be avoided.

NEWER SYSTEMIC ANTIFUNGAL AGENTS :

Newer antifungal agents that are used for systemic administration have evolved significantly in the last few years for the treatment of systemic mycoses like mucormycosis, aspergillosis, candidemia, disseminated histoplasmosis, cryptococcosis and other opportunistic fungal infection causing life threatening multisystem involvement. These are however used by critical care physicians in the intensive care set up. Such systemic mycoses are common in following conditions :

1) Neutropenic patients.
2) Patients on cancer chemotherapy or immunosuppressives following organ transplantation.
3) Late stage HIV/AIDS or even during the recent SARS-COV-2 pandemic.
4) Uncontrolled diabetes.

Dermatologists should be aware of these antifungals. Some of these new antifungals like echinocandins and newer azoles are discussed below.

ECHINOCANDINS :

Drugs belonging to echinocandins group are frequently used for systemic mycoses. These include drugs like caspofungin, micafungin and anidulafungin.

Mechanism Of Action :

It inhibits fungal cell wall synthesis.

Spectrum :

Candida species, Aspergillus species.

Indications :

- Candidemia.
- Aspergillosis.

Adverse Effects :

Hypersensitivity, infusion reactions, hepatic dysfunction.

Dose And Preparations :

INJ CANCIDASTM (Capsofungin) 70 mg, 50 mg vial) , INJ MYCAMINETM (Micafungin) 50 mg, 100 mg, INJ ERAXIS TM.

Anidulafungin 50 mg vial.

Capsofungin loading dose is 70 mg on the first day followed by daily 50 mg for at least 14 days.

PREGNANCY CATEGORY – C (No confirmed data available):

KEY POINTS :

- Echinocandins are cost effective and safer than amphotericin B and flucytosine.
- All these echinocandins have to be reconstituted with suitable diluent (like 0.9 normal saline) to form reconstituted solutions. Dosages are as per mg/ml of reconstituted solution.
- Cyclosporine increases levels of caspofungin by 35% while rifampicin reduce capsofungin levels.

VORICONAZOLE :

Oral broad-spectrum antifungal with mechanism of action similar to that of other azoles.

INDICATIONS :

1. Invasive aspergillosis.
2. Invasive Candidiasis.
3. Fusariosis, Scedosporiosis.
4. Systemic mycoses like cryptococcosis, histoplasmosis, and blastomycosis.
5. Widespread dermatophytosis (when Itraconazole is not tolerated or not effective). However, this indication is contested by experts as the drug is similar in mechanism of action, efficacy and failure rates to itraconazole but is far more expensive.

DOSES AND PREPARATIONS :

- Tablets : 50 mg, 200 mg twice daily is the common adult dose; but per kg dose is 9 mg/kg/dose.

- For Oral Suspension : after reconstitution 200 mg/5 ml.
- For Injection : lyophilized powder containing 200 mg voriconazole and 3200 mg of sulfobutyl ether beta-cyclodextrin sodium (SBECD); after reconstitution 10 mg/mL of voriconazole and 160 mg/mL of SBECD.

PREGNANCY CATEGORY – D :

DRUG INTERACTIONS :

Same as AZOLES.

ADVERSE EFFECTS :

Systemic :

Same as azoles.

Cutaneous :

Photosensitivity is common especially in children. Alopecia, urticaria, Erythema multiforme, eczema, fixed drug reaction, Stevens Johnson syndrome is reported.

KEY POINTS :

- The MIC ranges of voriconazole, fluconazole, and griseofulvin, were 0.002 to 0.06 µg/ml, 0.25 to 32 µg/ml, and 0.125 to 2.0 µg/ml, respectively in a study of dermatophyte susceptibility done in 2006 in India. The drug used by some dermatologists in India with claims of good results. However the drug is not approved by US FDA for use in dermatophytosis.
- Voriconazole can cause blurring of vision and sensitivity to light. Hence it is advisable not to drive in the night and operate machines after taking voriconazole. Also it is advisable to avoid direct sunlight due to risk of photosensitivity.

POSACONAZOLE :

Systemic broad-spectrum antifungal with mechanism of action similar to that of other azoles.

Indications :

1. Prophylaxsis of Invasive aspergillosis and Invasive Candidiasis.
2. Candidiasis refractory to Itraconazole and fluconazole.

Doses And Preparations :

- Delayed release Tablets : 100 mg (300 mg BD for a single day followed by 300 OD to be continued thereafter).
- Injection is available 300 mg. Dosages similar as for oral delayed release tablet.
- Oral suspension given as 200 mg (5 ml) three times a day.

PREGNANCY CATEGORY NO DATA AVAILABLE :

Drug Interactions :

Same as AZOLES.

Adverse Effects :

Systemic :

- Arrhythmias and QTc Prolongation.
- Diarrhea, nausea, fever, vomiting, headache, coughing, and hypokalemia.
- Hepatic toxicity.

Cutaneous :

Hypersensitivity reactions.

Key Points :

- Advise patients to take posaconazole delayed-release

tablets with food. Tablets must be swallowed whole and not divided, crushed, or chewed.

- Oral Suspension of posaconazole should be taken during or immediately (*i.e.* within 20 minutes) following a full meal. In patients who cannot eat a full meal, each dose of oral suspension should be administered with a liquid nutritional supplement or an acidic carbonated beverage (*e.g.* ginger ale) in order to enhance absorption.

x=x=x=x=x

3

Systemic Antiviral Agents

CLASSIFICATION :

1. Antihuman herpes virus (anti-HHV) drugs Acyclovir, Famcyclovir, Valacyclovir, Foscarnet.
2. Anti-CMV drugs Ganciclovir, Cidofovir.
3. Antiretroviral drugs : refer chapter "Antiretroviral Agents" for details.

ACYCLOVIR :

Acyclovir is an antiviral agent commonly used against infections caused by herpes viruses namely HSV-1, HSV-2, and Varicella-Zoster virus (VZV).

MECHANISM OF ACTION :

Acyclovir $\xrightarrow{\text{Viral thymidine kinase (TK)}}$ Acyclovir monophosphate (AMP)

Acyclovir monophosphate (AMP) $\xrightarrow{\text{Cellular kinase}}$ Acyclovir triphosphate

Acyclovir triphosphate inhibits viral DNA polymerase inhibiting DNA synthesis.

INDICATIONS :

ACYCLOVIR

1. Primary herpes simplex infections that include herpetic gingivostomatitis/herpes genitalis/eczema herpeticum/herpetic whitlow/herpes manuum and gladiatorum, neonatal herpes simplex infections/herpeticum keratitis/herpetic meningoencephalitis, and recurrent HSV

infections like herpes labialis and recurrent herpes genitalis.

2. VZV infections include chicken pox and herpes zoster. If initiated early, antiviral agents may reduce chances of developing post-herpetic neuralgia.

DOSES AND PREPARATIONS :

- ZOVIRAX, OCUVIR 200 mg tablet, 400 mg tablet, 800 mg tablet.
- ACIVIR 100 ml/vial containing 25 mg/ml injection, ACIVIR 3% ointment.

TABLE 3.1 : **Doses and duration of acyclovir for herpetic infections**

Primary HSV infections	200 mg 5 times a day for 7 days
Herpetic meningoencephalitis	5-10 mg/kg i.v. 8 hourly 10 days
Secondary HSV infection	200 mg 5 times a day for 5 days
Prophylaxis for HSV infections	400 mg b.i.d. (for 1-2 years).
Chickenpox	800 mg 5 times a day for 5-7 days
Herpes zoster	800 mg 5 times a day for 5-7 days
Herpes zoster in immunocompromised	10 mg/kg IV 8 hourly for 7-10 days

PREGNANCY CATEGORY – B :

ADVERSE EFFECTS :

Systemic :

- Hypersensitivity.
- Headache, nausea, malaise (when given orally).
- Rash, sweating, hypotension, vomiting (in few patients when given intravenously).

Cutaneous :

Not reported when given orally. Burning can occur after topical application.

KEY POINTS :

- Creatinine clearance is calculated by the formula : Creatinine clearance (CrCl) = (140-age) x Wt/Serum creat. x 72.
- In case of renal failure, acyclovir dose is calculated according to the Table :

CrCl 10-25 mL/min	800 mg PO q8hr
CrCl 0-10 mL/min	800 mg PO q12hr

- 20-30% GI absorption orally, not significantly affected by the presence of food.
- Increased sensitivity of HSV to acyclovir as compared to VZV permits lower doses of acyclovir in HSV infections.
- Acyclovir is unlikely to be effective against HHV-3 (EBV) and HHV-4 (CMV) infections.
- Use of acyclovir during chicken pox does not prevent development of immunity.
- Treatment of primary herpes infections does not prevent recurrences, as virus remains dormant in sensory ganglion and therefore is not killed by acyclovir.
- Duration of the treatment of herpes infections by acyclovir is longer in immunocompromised patients and depends on clinical response.
- Since acyclovir, valacyclovir, and famcyclovir are excreted unchanged in urine, the dose of acyclovir, valacyclovir, and famcyclovir is to be reduced to one-10th in case of renal failure.
- Topical acyclovir is neither toxic nor effective.
- Absent or decreased production of viral thymidine kinase, known as TK– strains is the most common mechanism of acyclovir resistance.

VALACYCLOVIR :

Valacyclovir is 1-valyl ester of acyclovir.

MECHANISM OF ACTION AND INDICATIONS :

Similar to that of acyclovir.

DOSES AND PREPARATIONS :

- VALCIVIR 500 mg tablet.

TABLE 3.2 : **Doses and duration of valacyclovir in herpetic infections**

Primary HSV infections	1000 mg b.i.d. for 10 days
Recurrent HSV infection	500 mg b.i.d. for 5 days
Prophylaxis for HSV infections	1000 mg o.d. (for 1-2 years)
Chickenpox	1000 mg TDS for 5 days
Herpes zoster	1000 mg TDS for 5 days

PREGNANCY CATEGORY – B :

ADVERSE EFFECTS :

Systemic :

Hypersensitivity, headache, nausea and vomiting.

KEY POINTS :

- Valacyclovir has 45-50% oral bioavailability.
- Convenient dosage schedule allows better compliance in patients treated with valacyclovir.
- Efficacy and safety profile of valacyclovir is not proven in immunocompromised patients.

FAMCYCLOVIR :

Famcyclovir is prodrug of penciclovir, an acyclic nucleoside.

MECHANISM OF ACTION AND INDICATIONS :

Similar to that of acyclovir.

Doses And Preparations :

- VIROVIR, FAMTRAX 250, 500 mg tablets.

TABLE 3.3 : **Doses and duration of famcyclovir**

Primary HSV infections	250 mg TDS for 10 days
Recurrent HSV infection	125 mg b.i.d. for 5 days
Prophylaxis for HSV infections	250 mg b.i.d. (for 1-2 years)
Chickenpox and Herpes Zoster	500 mg TDS for 5-7 days

PREGNANCY CATEGORY – B :

Adverse Effects :

Systemic :

Headache, nausea, and hypersensitivity.

Key Points :

- Famcyclovir has 80-90% oral bioavailability, resulting in quicker onset of action.
- Convenient dosage schedule allows better compliance of patients treated with famcyclovir.
- Famcyclovir is the preferred drug for infections due to VZV in immunocompromised patients.
- Famcyclovir supposedly has some role in preventing postherpetic neuralgia (PHN) following herpes zoster infection.

FOSCARNET :

Foscarnet is a synthetic nonnucleoside analog.

Mechanism Of Action :

Directly inhibits DNA polymerase without the activation by cellular or viral kinases.

INDICATIONS :

Acyclovir-resistant mucocutaneous HSV infections.

DOSES AND PREPARATIONS :

- 40 mg/kg 8 hourly for 10-42 days.
- Vial : 2.4 g/100 ml. Infuse slowly over 1 hour.
- FOSCAVIR injection.

PREGNANCY CATEGORY – C :

ADVERSE EFFECTS :

- Nephrotoxicity (typically occur in the 3rd week of treatment).
- In males, meatal irritation (about 2 weeks after the beginning of treatment).

KEY POINTS :

- Plenty of oral fluids are essential during foscarnet therapy to avoid nephrotoxicity and meatal irritation.
- Although it is expensive, this is the only effective antiviral for resistant herpes infections.
- Not used as a first line management due to toxicity.

CIDOFOVIR :

Antiviral agent effective against cytomegalovirus infections.

MECHANISM OF ACTION :

Cidofovir reaches the cell in a monophosphorylated form, and thus it is activated by cellular kinases. Cidofovir targets viral DNA polymerase and prevents transcription.

INDICATIONS :

CMV retinitis and disseminated CMV infections in AIDS or other immunosuppressed patients.

DOSES AND PREPARATIONS :

- CIDOFOVIR injection.
- Vial : 75 mg/ml.
- Induction dose of 5 mg/kg i.v. once weekly X 2 weeks followed by maintenance dose of 5 mg/kg i.v. every 2 weeks.
- Hydration with at least 1l of NS over 1 h, before dosing; the next 1l can be given during or after cidofovir dose. All doses must be given with probenecid (to block renal tubular secretion of cidofovir), 2 g p.o. 3 h before cidofovir, 1 g 2 h after dose, and 1 g 8 h after dose of cidofovir. Cidofovir must be diluted in at least 100 cc of NS and infused over 1 h.

PREGNANCY CATEGORY – C (Inadequate data) :

ADVERSE EFFECTS :

Nephrotoxicity, metabolic acidosis, nausea, vomiting, diarrhea, and asthenia.

KEY POINTS :

- Probenecid slows the excretion of ZDV and the doses of ZDV should be halved on cidofovir days. Also, increases the half-life of many drugs, including penicillins, oral hypoglycemics, rifampin, NSAIDs, ciprofloxacin, acetaminophen, acyclovir, ganciclovir, furosemide, and others.
- Monitoring of serum creatinine and urine protein, electrolytes, CBC, LFTs, is required during cidofovir therapy.
- Because cidofovir does not require activation by a viral kinase, it should theoretically have activity against acyclovir-resistant herpes simplex virus infections. However adequate data regarding clinical efficacy is lacking.

- Long-term topical application of cidofovir (1-3% cream) has been shown to be effective against molluscum contagiosum, viral warts, and herpes simplex infections.

GANCYCLOVIR :

Antiviral agent effective against cytomegalovirus infections.

MECHANISM OF ACTION :

Gancyclovir is a deoxynucleoside analogue cytomegalovirus (CMV) DNA polymerase inhibitor.

INDICATIONS :

CMV retinitis and disseminated CMV infections in AIDS or other immunosuppressed patients. Also used for prevention of CMV disease in adult transplant cases.

DOSES AND PREPARATIONS :

Induction :

5 mg/kg (iv at a constant rate over 1 hr) every 12 hours for 14-21 days.

Maintenance :

5 mg/kg (iv at a constant rate over 1 hr) every 24 hours for 7 days per week.

PREPARATIONS :

Cytovene IV TM 500 mg of Lyophilized Powder.

PREGNANCY CATEGORY :

Gancyclovir is not recommended during pregnancy.

ADVERSE EFFECTS :

Pyrexia, diarrhea, leukopenia, nausea, anemia, asthenia,

headache, cough, decreased appetite, dyspnea, abdominal pain, sepsis, hyperhidrosis.

KEY POINTS :

- Risk of seizures is reported when co administered with Imipenem.
- Risk of nephrotoxicity when administered with Amphotericin B and cyclosporine.
- Probenecid may increase gancyclovir levels.
- Adequate hydration and slow infusion is required for gancyclovir use.

x=x=x=x=x

4
Antiretroviral Drugs

Aniretroviral drugs are essential in the treatment of HIV-AIDS and antiretroviral therapy (ART) has been successful in saving lives of millions of people affected with HIV/AIDS all over the world. These drugs have been discussed in this chapter. Science of anti-HIV drugs and therapy has been continuously evolving with many newer safe and effective drugs being added.

CLASSIFICATION :

1. **Nucleoside/nucleotide reverse Transcriptase inhibitors (NRTI) :**
   - Zidovudine (AZT, ZDV).
   - Didanosine (ddl).
   - Zalcitabine (ddC).
   - Stavudine (d4T).
   - Lamivudine (3TC).
   - Abacavir
   - Tenofovir
   - Emtricitabine
2. **Nonnucleoside reverse transcriptase inhibitors (NNRTI) :**
   - Nevirapine
   - Efavirenz
   - Delaviridine
3. **Protease inhibitors (PI) :**
   - Indinavir

- Ritonavir
- Saquinavir
- Nelfinavir
- Amprenavir
- Fosarnprenavir
- Lopinavir
- Atazanavir

4. **Fusion inhibitors :**
   - Enfuvirtide

5. **Integrase inhibitors :**
   - Raltegravir, elvitegravir, daltegravir.

6. **CCR_5 Entry inhibitor :**
   - Maraviroc

7. **Miscellaneous :**
   - Hydroxyurea

NUCLEOSIDE/NUCLEOTIDE REVERSE TRANSCRIPTASE INHIBITORS (NRTI) :

MECHANISM OF ACTION :

Zidovudine and all other drugs in this class inhibit reverse transcriptase enzyme after getting phosphorylated by cellular enzymes.

INDICATIONS :

NRTI drugs are used in combination with either NNRTI or PI part of highly active antiretroviral therapy (HAART).

ZIDOVUDINE :

This is a prototype of the NRTIs.

INDICATIONS :

1. Zidovudine in combination with other NRTI like lamivudine + NNRTI (nevirapine or efavirenz) + Pl (*e.g.* ritonavir).
2. As a monotherapy to prevent perinatal transmission of HIV for infants with mothers previously exposed to NNRTI.

DOSES AND PREPARATIONS :

- 300 mg b.i.d., 2 mg/kg QDS, Syrup 5 mg/5 ml; IV infusion containing 10 mg/ml in 20 ml single-use vials.
- RETROVIR 100, 300 mg tab, ZIDOVIR 50 ml, 100 ml oral solution.

SIDE EFFECTS :

Systcmic :

Myelosuppression (directly related to dosage and duration occurs after 4-6 weeks of therapy), hepatotoxicity, lactic acidosis, myopathy, neurotoxicity, severe headache, insomnia, myalgia, and nausea.

Cutaneous :

Nail pigmentation and alopecia.

KEY POINTS :

- Zidovudine has good bioavailability (60-70%), good CSF penetration and distribution averages 60-68% of the plasma concentration. Drug also effectively crosses placental barrier.
- Resistance to zidovudine monotherapy develops within 9-12 months.

- Combination of zidovudine with stavudine is antagonistic because of limited phosphorylation of stavudine in presence of zidovudine.
- Other myelosuppressive drugs like dapsone, systemic pentamidine, pyrimethamine, co-trimoxazole, amphotericin flucytosine, ganciclovir, interferon, vincristine, vinblastine and doxorubicin are relatively contraindicated but may be used with caution.
- Zidovudine is relatively contraindicated in patients with anemia. For such patients a zidovudine-free regimen may be used.
- Zidovudine induced anemia can be managed by either zidovudine withdrawal or administering recombinant human erythropoietin.

LAMIVUDINE :

NRTI drug with mechanism of action similar to that of zidovudine.

Doses And Preparations :

- 150 mg b.i.d or 300 mg OD., 4 mg/kg b.i.d in children, 2 mg/kg b.i.d in neonates.
- LAMIVIR 150 mg, 300 mg tab.

Side Effects :

- Mild and uncommon.
- Lactic acidosis and severe hepatomegaly with steatosis have been reported.
- Pancreatitis, peripheral neuropathy, or splenomegaly (more commonly observed in pediatric patients than in adults).

Key Points :

- Least toxic NRTI because very low affinity for human DNA polymerase.

- Lamivudine should not be used alone. Resistance to mono therapy develops in 1-2 weeks.
- In both non-HIV infected and HIV-HBV co-infected patients-suffering from hepatitis B infections-on lamivudine therapy, discontinuation of lamivudine can cause exacerbations of infection. The causal relationship between discontinuation of lamivudine therapy and exacerbation of HBV infection is unknown.
- Drug interactions :
  - May inhibit the intracellular phosphorylation of zalcitabine.
  - Cotrimoxazole increases serum levels of lamivudine.

STAVUDINE (D_4T) :

NRTI drug with mechanism of action similar to that of zidovudine.

Doses And Preparations :

- 30 mg b.i.d., 1 mg/kg b.i.d. for patients with higher body weight 40 mg b.i.d.
- STAVIR 30 mg, 40 mg cap.

Side Effects :

- Common.
- Lactic acidosis, hepatotoxicity with steatosis, and peripheral neuropathy.
- Pancreatitis, arthralgia, hypersensitivity, myalgia, anorexia, chills and fever, rash, asthenia, gastrointestinal disturbances, headache, and insomnia.

Key Points :

- Stavudine crosses the blood-brain barrier with distribution being 55% of plasma concentration.

- Female gender, obesity, and prolonged exposure are risk factors for stavudine- or lamivudine-induced lactic acidosis.
- Lower dose of stavudine is to be used in renal failure.
- Important drug interactions :
  1. Didanosine or hydroxyurea may increase the risk of severe hepatotoxicity or pancreatitis if taken concurrently with stavudine.
  2. Caution should be used in co-administration of stavudine with other drugs that may cause peripheral neuropathy, such as chloramphenicol, cisplatin, dapsone, didanosine, ethambutol, ethionamide, hydralazine, isoniazid, lithium, metronidazole, nitrofurantoin, phenytoin, and zalcitabine. Stavudine-induced neuropathy may resolve completely if stavudine is withdrawn promptly.

DIDANOSINE (DDI) :

NRTI drug with mechanism of action similar to that of zidovudine.

Doses And Preparations :

- 125 mg b.i.d., 2-3 mg/kg b.i.d. on empty stomach.
- DINEX 100 mg, 250 mg, 400 mg tab.

Side Effects :

- Major side effect pancreatitis.
- Less common peripheral neuropathy, oral and esophageal ulcers, cardiomyopathy, malaise, and rash.

Key Points :

- Didanosine is used in patients intolerant or resistant to zidovudine.

- Didanosine is absorbed easily in a basic environment and is to be taken on empty stomach to avoid acidic environment after meal. Zalcitabine interferes with the absorption of didanosine.
- Drug interactions :
  - Didanosine hydroxyurea may increase the risk of severe hepatotoxicity or pancreatitis if taken concurrently with stavudine.
  - The concomitant use of other drugs like ketoconazole, itraconazole, and quinolone antibiotics that requires acidic environment for absorption should be avoided.

ZALCITABINE (DDC) :

NRTI drug with mechanism of action similar to that of zidovudine.

Doses And Preparations :

- 0.75 mg b.i.d. (750 μg tds), 10 μg/kg tds for children HIVID 0.75 mg tab.

Side Effects :

- Common.
- Pancreatitis, hepatotoxicity, peripheral neuropathy, and oral and esophageal ulcers.

Key Points :

- Zalcitabine has greatest effects when combined with zidovudine.
- Zalcitabine is indicated in advanced HIV infection or as an alternative to intolerant and failed regimens.
- Zalcitabine should not be given with lamivudine (inhibits zalcitabine), ddI and d4T (peripheral neuropathy).

ABACAVIR :

Most potent NRTI drug with mechanism of action similar to that of zidovudine.

Doses And Preparations :

- 300 mg b.i.d or 600 mg OD., 8 mg/kg b.i.d., no regard for meals.

Side Effects :

- Common.
- Nephrotoxicity, nausea, headache, diarrhea, and anorexia.
- Abacavir hypersensitivity syndrome (genotype studies with HLA-B* 5701 can help in preventing this syndrome).

Key Points :

- Abacavir is the most potent nucleoside analog.
- Resistance to zidovudine and lamivudine leads to cross resistance to abacavir.
- Alcohol increases abacavir blood levels by 41%.

TENOFOVIR (TENOFOVIR DISOPROXIL FUMARATE, TDF) :

It is a nucleotide analog (NRTI).

Mechanism Of Action :

It is similar to that of NRTIs. Before phosphorylation, tenofovir disoproxil fumarate is converted to tenofovir in the intestinal lumen and plasma by diester hydrolysis. Tenofovir is phosphorylated in the cells in sequential steps to tenofovir monophosphate and to its active metabolite, tenofovir diphosphate.

Dose :

- 300 mg once daily.
- TRUVADA 300 mg tab.

Side Effects :

Nausea, vomiting, renal insufficiency, hypophosphatemia, hypouricemia, proteinuria and normoglycemic glycosuria, bone demineralisation.

Key Points :

- Tenofovir alafenamide fumarate (TAF) is a new prodrug of tenofovir which is more stable and have more efficient penetration into the target cells than TDF. Tenofovir converted from TAF reaches plasma concentration which is 90% lower than that of TFV converted from TDF. Conversely, the active metabolite converted from TAF reaches a higher intracellular level in target cells than TFV from TDF. This allows a substantial reduction of its oral dose, decreasing the risk for renal and bone toxicity. Dose of TAF (available in India) is 25 mg once a day.

EMTRICITABINE :

Dose And Preparation :

- 200 mg once daily, no regard for meals.
- EMTRIVA 200 mg tab.

Side Effects :

Minimal toxic effects, rarely lactic acidosis, and hepatic steatosis can occur as with NRTI.

NONNUCLEOSIDE REVERSE TRANSCRIPTASE INHIBITORS (NNRTI) :

Include nevirapine, efavirenz, and delavirdine. Delavirdine is not available in India.

MECHANISM OF ACTION :

NNRTIs are noncompetitive inhibitors of reverse transcriptase (RT).

INDICATIONS :

NNRTI drugs are used in combination with either NRTI or PI as a part of ART. These drugs are not active against HIV-2.

NEVIRAPINE (NVP) :

Nevirapine is a nonnucleoside reverse transcriptase inhibitor.

INDICATIONS :

1. Nevirapine in combination with NRTI or PI as a part HAART regimen of antiretroviral therapy.
2. As a single-dose regimen to prevent perinatal transmission of HIV.

CONTRAINDICATIONS :

- Hypersensitivity to nevirapine.
- Severe hepatitis.
- Renal failure (or used with extreme caution).

DOSES AND PREPARATIONS :

- 200 mg tab o.d. for 14 days (training in period); then 200 mg b.i.d., 3-4 mg/kg b.i.d. in children.
- NEVIMUNE 200 mg tab.

ADVERSE EFFECTS :

Systemic :

Severe hepatotoxicity.

Cutaneous :

Maculopapular rash, erythema multiforme, Stevens-Johnson

syndrome, toxic epidermal necrolysis, drug hypersensitivity syndrome (within 6 weeks).

KEY POINTS :

- Nevirapine is more than 90% absorbed after oral administration.
- Nevirapine readily crosses the placenta and achieves neonatal blood concentrations comparable to those in the mother.
- Women with CD_4 cell counts greater than 250 cells/mm^3 are at considerably higher (12-fold) risk of serious hepatotoxicity.
- Mutations conferring resistance to nevirapine could be observed after a single dose, even with a low level of viral replication. Therefore, nevirapine should always be administered in combination with at least one other antiretroviral agent.
- Resistance to nevirapine usually confers class resistance to other NNRTIs (efavirenz and delavirdine). However, nevirapine-resistant isolates were susceptible to the nucleoside analogs zidovudine and didanosine.
- Patients who develop severe hepatic toxicity or skin reaction (those requiring hospitalisation) while on NVP should not be rechallenged.

EFAVIRENZ (EFV) :

Efavirenz is NNRTI.

INDICATIONS :

Efavirenz is used in combination with NRTI or PI as a part HAART regimen of antiretroviral therapy.

DOSES AND PREPARATIONS :

- 600 mg tab o.d. at bedtime, defer dosing with didanosine or antacids by 1 h.
- EFAVIR 200 mg, 600 mg tab.

ADVERSE EFFECTS :

Systemic :

Dizziness, vivid dreams, feeling of dissociation (symptoms appear within 1st or 2nd day of treatment and generally resolve after 2-4 weeks); teratogenicity.

Cutaneous :

Mild-to-moderate maculopapular rash (infrequent, occurs within first 2 weeks).

KEY POINTS :

- Meals with a high fat content, may greatly decrease absorption of EFV. EFV is excreted principally in the feces.
- Two contraceptive measures (a barrier and hormonal Contraceptive) should be used to avoid pregnancy by a woman taking EFV.
- **Drug interactions :**
  - Concurrent use of rifampicin but not rifabutin decreases EFV plasma concentrations. Higher doses of EFV may be required in such cases.
  - EFV decreases plasma concentration of protease inhibitors.

PROTEASE INHIBITORS :

PIs include drugs like saquinavir, indinavir, nelfinavir, ritonavir, etc.

MECHANISM OF ACTION :

Pls inhibit enzyme "Protease" of HIV, which is required for final processing of viral proteins. Unlike reverse transcriptase inhibitor-they inhibit viral replication in newly as well as Chronically infected cells.

INDICATIONS :

1. PI drugs are used in combination with either NRTI or NNRTI as a part of HAART. They are particularly used in patients with high viral load due to their greater efficacy in inhibiting viral replication.
2. Combination therapy for post exposure prophylaxis against HIV.

SAQUINAVIR :

First PI to be FDA approved for HIV patients.

DOSES AND PREPARATIONS :

- 1200 mg tablet t.i.d. (soft gel); 600 mg tablet t.i.d. (hard gel).

ADVERSE EFFECTS :

Systemic :

Diarrhea, nausea, abdominal discomfort, dyspepsia.

Cutaneous :

Lipodystrophy.

KEY POINTS :

- Oral availability of saquinavir is only 4% due to extensive first pass metabolism.
- Oral bioavailability is increased by taking the drug with softgel formulation, 2 h after food.

- Rifampicin and nevirapine should not be given with saquinavir due to fear of hepatotoxicity.

RITONAVIR :

Mechanism of Action is similar to the other Pls. Apart from that it reduces metabolism of other drugs leading to higher serum levels of other drugs including Pls. It is mainly used to boost other PI's

Doses And Preparations :

- 100 mg tab b.i.d., 6-8 mg/kg b.i.d. in children.
- 80 mg /ml oral solution.
- 100 mg oral powder.
- RITOVIR 100 mg cap/tablets (NORVIR).

Adverse Effects :

Systemic :

Nausea, vomiting, diarrhea, altered taste and perioral paraesthesia, and fatigue. Pancreatitis, increase in cholesterol and triglyceride levels, IRIS syndrome, lipodystrophy syndrome.

Key Points :

- Oral availability of ritonavir is good.
- Ritonavir is to be started on submaximal dose and then gradually increased to prevent resistance.
- Pls are boosted with ritonavir as the latter increases their levels.
- The capsule and solution formulation of ritonavir contains alcohol and should not be administered with disulfiram or metronidazole.

INDINAVIR :

Indinavir is a powerful protease inhibitor.

DOSES AND PREPARATIONS :

- 800 mg tab t.i.d., 10 mg/kg t.i.d. in children, on empty stomach with plenty of oral fluids.
- INDI VIR 400 mg cap.

ADVERSE EFFECTS :

Systemic :

Indinavir loin syndrome-nephrolithiasis due to precipitation of indinavir crystals in urine, insomnia, pharyngitis, asymptomatic hyperbilirubinemia.

Cutaneous :

Lipodystrophy (protease pouch), mild rash, dry skin.

KEY POINTS :

- Indinavir is best absorbed on empty stomach and absorption is decreased greatly in the presence of fat or proteins.
- Plenty of oral fluids should be taken during indinavir therapy to avoid nephrolithiasis. Risk of nephrolithiasis due to indinavir increases when doses of more than 2.4 g are used.
- Doses of indinavir should be reduced to 600 mg t.i.d. when given concurrently with itraconazole or ketoconazole or in patients with hepatic insufficiency.

NELFINAVIR :

Nelfinavir is a protease inhibitor used as a part of PI-based ART in patients with high viral loads.

Doses And Preparations :

- 750 mg tab t.i.d.
- NELVIR 250 mg tab.

Adverse Effects :

Systemic :

Diarrhea is the most common side effect (is controlled by antimotility agents).

Other adverse effects :

Asthenia, lack of concentration, and hypertension.

Cutaneous :

Lip dystrophy.

Key Points :

- Potential drug interactions of nelfinavir include dysrhythmias when taken with terfenadine, astemizole, or cisapride.
- Prolonged sedation when given in combination with benzodiazepines.
- Better tolerated and preferred over indinavir.

AMPRENAVIR :

Newest PI to receive FDA approval.

Doses And Preparations :

- AGENERASE Amprenavir 1200 mg single dose in soft gelatin capsule.

Adverse Effects :

Side effects are reported as mild.

Systemic :

Paraesthesias, diarrhea, nausea, vomiting, headache, hyperglycemia, and acute hemolytic anemia.

Cutaneous :

Maculopapular rash (28% of patients), Stevens-Johnson's syndrome (1%).

ATAZANAVIR :

Doses And Preparations :

- 400 mg tab once daily with foods, antacids to be avoided.
- 150 mg, 200 mg, 300 mg capsules, Oral powder (50 mg).

Adverse Effects :

Systemic :

Hyperglycemia, indirect hyperbilirubinemia, lipodystrophy, prolonged PR interval, increased bleeding in hemophilics.

Key Points :

- The only PI that contains sulfonamide moiety and hence propensity for drug eruptions.
- Advantage of reduced propensity to cause dyslipidemia and hyperglycemia.
- Fosamprenavir is a prodrug of amprenavir that has the advantage of improved oral bioavailability.

FUSION INHIBITORS :

ENFUVIRTIDE :

Enfuvirtide is a fusion inhibitor. It is a synthetic peptide.

MECHANISM OF ACTION :

Enfuvirtide; fusion inhibitor, 'inhibits one of the final steps viral entry : gp41-mediated fusion with the CD_4 cell membrane.

DOSES :

- It is approved for use only in treatment-experienced adults who have evidence of HIV replication despite ongoing HRT.
- 90 mg (1 ml) twice daily, subcutaneously.
- FUZEON vial containing 108 mg of enfurvirtide lyophilized powder to be reconstituted with 1.1 ml of sterile water.

ADVERSE EFFECTS :

- Local injection site reactions.
- Bacterial pneumonia.
- Hypersensitivity.
- Neuralgia.
- IRIS.

INTEGRASE INHIBITORS :

Currently there are three integrase inhibitors approved by USA FDA. These class of drugs include raltegravir and elvitegravir (first generation integrase inhibitors) and dolutagravir (second generation). The enzyme HIV-integrase helps in integration of viral DNA to host DNA. Integrase inhibitors inhibits this enzyme. These drugs are primarily used for third line ART in the national program.

DOLUTAGRAVIR :

MECHANISM OF ACTION :

Dolutagravir is a second generation viral integrase inhibitor that is currently a part of antiretroviral therapy in treatment naïve adults and adolescents. It is second generation Integrase Strand Transfer Inhibitor or INSTI.

INDICATIONS :

Dolutagravir in combination with two NRTI is indicated now-a-days in HIV/AIDS in following conditions.

1. Treatment naïve adults and adolescents
2. Postexposure prophylaxis
3. For achieving U=U (undetectable = untransmitable) status to reduce further risk of HIV transmission. Dolutagravir based regimens can achieve significant reduction of plasma viral load to undetectable levels (with less than 50 copies of virus) making viral transmission unlikely.

DOSE :

Dolutagravir 50 mg OD (INSTGRA 50 mg tablet).

SIDE EFFECTS :

- Headache, insomnia, diarrhea, rash, hepatotoxicity, raised creatinine (no clinical nephrotoxicity).

PREGNANCY PRESCRIBING CATEGORY-B :

DRUG INTERACTIONS :

- Dolutagravir is neither inducer nor inhibitor of CYP 45 enzyme, so chances of drug interactions are less with dolutagravir use.
- Dolutagravir inhibits renal organic cation transporter (OCT2) pathway. Hence dosages of drugs like dufitilide

(antiarrhythmetic) and metformin (antidiabetic) may need to be reduced as these drugs are eliminated by OCT2 pathway.

- Although rifampicin can reduce on levels of dolutagravir, dose adjustments with 50 mg twice daily administration of dolutagravir is not recommended as clinical efficacy of dolutagravir has not found to be altered.
- Dolutagravir should be taken 2 hours before or 6 hours after taking medications like antacids, laxatives or supplements containing polyvalent cations such as magnesium, aluminium, iron or calcium.

MISCELLANEOUS :

HYDROXYUREA :

Hydroxyurea was suggested as low-cost alternative antiretroviral drug several years ago when the cost of ART was unaffordable for a majority of patients in developing countries. However, it does not have a good antiretroviral activity and is not used routinely any more.

ART RESISTANCE :

Antiretroviral drug when used alone as monotherapy are likely to lead to resistance. Any patient who is not improving when on antiretroviral therapy should be asked about compliance either due to cost constraints or due to intolerance of medications before considering the possibility of drug resistance. There are two laboratory methods of detecting ART resistance :

- Phenotypic
- Genotypic

These methods are time-consuming, tedious, expensive, and yet-to-be standardized for Indian patients and hence not in routine practice.

HIGHLY ACTIVE ANTIRETROVIRAL THERAPY (HAART) :

ADVANTAGES OF HAART :

- Reduces the chances of infections with common and opportunistic infections.
- Improves CD_4 counts.
- Reduces the chances of malignancies or their progression.
- Improves constitutional symptoms.
- Reverses changes of HIV-induced encephalopathy, diarrhea wasting, thrombocytopenia, or bone marrow suppression.
- Adds to life expectancy.

DISADVANTAGES OF HAART :

- End point is not known.
- Relatively expensive therapy.
- Intolerance to drug can be a major limitation.
- Compliance to medications is difficult.
- Serious side effects of ART.

MONITORING SIDE EFFECTS OF ART :

- Liver function tests.
- Renal function tests.
- Serum amylase.
- For patients on PI :
  1. Serum lipids.
  2. Blood sugars.
  3. Serum sodium bicarbonate levels-to detect lactic acidosis.

Mild elevation of liver transaminases and ultrasonographic changes in patients on PI indicates fatty liver.

DIAGNOSIS OF PATIENTS WITH HIV :

- For clinically symptomatic cases : The sample should be reactive with 2 different kits.
- For clinically asymptomatic cases : The sample should be reactive with 3 different kits.

The testing strategy involves repeated testing of positive samples for the $2^{nd}/3^{rd}$ time based on different antigens using the same sample as that of the first test.

- For infants born to HIV positive mothers. DNA PCR on dried blood sample is done from 6 weeks to 18 months of age, as ELISA isn't reliable due to passive transfer of antibodies from the mother. After 6 months of age, DNA PCR is done only after screening for HIV antibodies.

NACO GUIDELINES FOR INITIATION OF ART : TREAT ALL!!!

All Laboratory confirmed cases are to be started on Anti-retroviral treatment irrespective of clinical stage and CD_4 count.

PREVENTIVE THERAPIES :

Cotrimoxazole Preventive Therapy :

Given for primary as well as secondary prevention of PCP (Pneumocystis Carinii pneumonia). One DS tablet of SMX-TMP (800/160) mg OD.

- Indicated in WHO stage 3/4.
- CD_4 count < 350 cells/mm^3.

In case of hypersensitivity to sulpha drugs, dapsone 100 mg OD can be used. In case of non severe hypersensitivity reaction, cotrimoxazole desensitization may be attempted after two weeks of resolution of symptoms.

DOSAGE FOR DESENSITIZATION :

Day 1 : 80 mg SMX + 16 mg TMP (2 ml oral suspension).

Day 2 : 160 mg SMX + 32 mg TMP (4 ml oral suspension).

Day 3 : 240 mg SMX + 48 mg TMP (6 ml oral suspension).

Day 4 : 320 mg SMX + 64 mg TMP (8 ml oral suspension).

Day 5 : 400 mg SMX + 80 mg TMP (One single-strength SMX-TMP tablet).

Day 6 : 800 mg SMZ + 160 mg TMP (Two single-strength SMX-TMP tablets or one double strength tablet).

Co-trimoxazole oral suspension contains 40 mg TMP + 200 mg SMX per 5 ml.

CPT can be stopped if CD_4 count > 350 cells/mm^3 (two reports atleast 6 months apart) and after ruling out WHO clinical stage 3/4 illnesses.

Isoniazid Preventive Therapy :

Given to all patients after ruling out active TB (Clinically and radiologically/microbiologically) to all patients on ART. It prevents progression of latent TB as well as prevents reinfection when exposed.

Prophylaxis for Cryptococcal Meningitis :

After successful treatment of cryptococcal meningitis, tablet fluconazole 200 mg/day is given as secondary prophylaxis till CD_4 count > 200 cells/mm^3 for 6 months. Primary prophylaxis is no longer recommended.

FIRST-LINE ART REGIMENS IN ADULTS AND ADOLESCENTS :

- First-line ART regimen for : All ARV naive PLHIV patients with HIV-1 infection, age > 10 years and body weight > 30 kg : Tenofovir + Lamivudine + Efavirenz.
- First-line ART regimen for all patients with abnormal serum creatinine values. All adults and adolescents with body weight less than 30 kg : Abacavir + Lamivudine + Efavirenz.

- First-line ART regimen for : All women with single dose Nevirapine exposure in a past pregnancy. All confirmed HIV-2 or HIV- 1 & HIV-2 co-infection : Tenofovir + Lamivudine + Lopinavir/ritonavir.
- Zidovudine + Lamivudine + Nevirapine OR Zidovudine + Lamivudine +Efavirenz : All patients who are on either of these first-line regimens initiated earlier in the programme need to be continued on the same regimen unless failing.

MONITORING GUIDELINES :

- CD_4 count done every 6 months.
- Virological monitoring done after 6 months and 12 months of ART initiation and yearly thereafter.

ART AND PREGNANCY AND PPTCT :

- Recommendations : To provide lifelong ART : TDF + 3TC + EFV to all pregnant and breastfeeding mothers regardless of CD_4 count and clinical stage for their own health and to prevent parent to child transfer of HIV during labour and breastfeeding. If they are already on AZT + 3TC + NVP/EFV, continue the same regimen. If the mother has previously been exposed to NVP/EFV for PPTCT, or coinfected with HIV 2, TDF + 3TC + LPV/r should be given.
- All infants born to HIV positive mothers should receive Nevirapine prophylaxis for 6 weeks. This duration may be extended to 12 weeks if mother has received ART for less than 4 weeks pre delivery or presented in Labour or after delivery with HIV. If the mother has been previously exposed to NVP, or if the mother is HIV 1 and 2 positive, zidovudine (AZT) is the drug of choice for prophylaxis in the infant.
  - Nevirapine 10-15 mg once daily (2 mg/kg).
  - Zidovudine 10-15 mg twice daily.

- Vaginal delivery should be encouraged. C section only for obstetric indications.
- DNA PCR to be done for the baby at 6 weeks of age. Antibody testing at 18 months of age : If DNA PCR is positive, the child should receive AZT/ABC + 3TC + LPV/r.

ART Toxicity :

Drug	Toxicity	Drug substitution
TDF	• Acute renal failure • Bone mineral density loss	• ABC • AZT if ABC not tolerated
ABC	Hypersensitivity reaction	• TDF • AZT if TDF not tolerated
NVP/EFV	Severe skin rash/hepatotoxicity/severe neuropsychiatric manifestations	ATV/r
Multiple NRTIs ABC/TDF/AZT	Toxicities	Raltegravir
ATV/r	Toxicity	LPV/r
LPV/r	Toxicity	ATV/r

ART RECOMMENDATIONS FOR INDIVIDUALS WITH TUBERCULOSIS (TB) AND HIV CO-INFECTION :

Tuberculosis is the commonest OI in India amongst HIV infected.

Intensified case finding approach for tuberculosis is followed. Isoniazid preventive therapy (IPT) for all patients without active TB (All suspicion regards to active TB is to be cleared before starting IPT). Any doubt regarding the activity of the disease, IPT should be delayed.

Dose : 300 mg OD for adults for 6 months.

IPT is safe in pregnancy and lactation.

For treatment of TB, daily regimen is preferred for HIV positive patients over alternate day regime.

Case scenarios :

- If a patient is not on ART and presents with HIV and Tb at the same time, AKT should be started first followed by initiation of ART (TDF + 3TC + EFV) between 2 weeks and 2 months of initiation of AKT.
- If patient is on NVP based regimen, substitute NVP by EFV and continue EFV even after TB treatment is completed.
- If patient is on PI based regimen, substitute rifampicin in AKT by Rifabutin (150 mg daily).
- If the patient is on Raltegravir based regimen, substitute rifampicin in AKT by Rifabutin OR Increase the dose of raltegravir from 400 BD to 800 BD if rifampicin is continued.

Development of Pulmonary TB/single Lymph node TB or uncomplicated pleural effusion within the first 6 months of ART initiation should not be considered as ART failure. Extrapulmonary Tb may be considered under failure of ART.

COEXISTENT HEPATITIS B WITH HIV :

- Serum SGPT, Hepatitis HBeAg levels and HBV DNA levels may have to be checked for Hepatitis B activity. ART regime should have atleast two drugs active against Hep B.
- ART regimen of choice : TDF + 3TC + EFV.
- TDF and 3TC are active against hepatitis B.
- Lamivudine should never be given alone as increase chances of HBV to become resistant to 3TC. So if tenofovir may have to be discontinued i/v/o toxicity, other drugs like entecavir may have to be added after consulting a gastroenterologist.

- All hepatitis B HIV positive patients should be vaccinated against hep B. Dose 4 doses 40 microg intramuscular (as against conventional 3 doses of 20 microg).
- All infants born to HbsAg positive mothers have to be immunized with 10 microg of HBV vaccine i.m at birth within 12 hours, 1, 2, 6 months and HBIG 0.5 ml i.m.

ART FAILURE :

Causes of ART failure can be :

- Poor compliance of patients (socioeconomic failure).
- Intolerance of antiretroviral medications (pharmacologic failure).
- Monotherapy.
- Drug resistance.

In general, ART failure is suspected in the presence of decreasing CD_4 counts and increasing viral load. The viral load is expected to fall to less than 1000 copies/ml at 6 months of ART initiation and CD_4 count is expected to rise by 50-100 cells/year of ART.

Failure to achieve 70% reduction in plasma viral load after a 1 month period is termed as virologic failure. Decreasing viral load but CD_4 counts failing to rise despite ART is termed as immunologic failure. Decreasing viral load and increasing CD_4 counts in a patient on ART but without the expected clinical improvement is termed as clinical failure. Out of these, virological failure is the most important in determining the shift to Second line ART.

SECOND LINE ART :

Viral load is recommended for monitoring and diagnosing treatment failure for patients on ART. The decision to switch to second or third line ART is taken by the SACEP.

Regimen	Substitution
AZT + 3TC + NVP/EFV	TDF + 3TC + ATV/r
TDF/ABC + 3TC + NVP/EFV	AZT + 3TC + ATV/r
TDF/ABC + 3TC + NVP/EFV if anemic Hb < 9	RAL + LPV/r (3TC and TDF to be continued if HbsAg +).
All other cases of first-line failure and exposure to more than 1 NRTI (multi-NRTIs - AZT/d4T, TDF, ABC).	RAL + LPV/r (3TC and TDF to be continued if HbsAg +).

IMMUNE RECONSTITUTION INFLAMMATORY SYNDROME (IRIS OR HAART ATTACK) :

Immune reconstitution inflammatory syndrome is an unusual inflammatory reaction to an opportunistic infection that occurs in late HIV infection ($CD_4 < 200/\mu l$) during the reconstitution of immune system in the initial months of HAART. It usually occurs after 4-8 weeks of ART initiation but late IRIS can occur for upto 6 months.

Manifestations of IRIS syndrome include unmasking of dormant infections, mainly pulmonary and extrapulmonary tuberculosis or manifestations, due to altered immunological reactivity like psoriasis or Reiter's disease. Typically patients having CMV infection (known to occur at very low CD_4 counts) may develop infections occurring at relatively higher CD_4 counts like toxoplasmosis or cryptococcosis.

IRIS has to be differentiated from ART failure by finding of increasing CD_4 counts and decreasing viral load.

Treatment of IRIS syndrome includes treatment of manifestations due to underlying diseases and continuation of antiretroviral therapy. Short term therapy with anti-inflammatory agents like prednisolone may help. Temporary stoppage of ART may be required if life threatening forms of IRIS develop.

POST EXPOSURE PROPHYLAXIS :

Exposure route HIV transmission rate :

Blood transfusion	90-95%
Perinatal (without any intervention)	15-40%
Sexual intercourse	0.1 to 10%
Vaginal	0.05-0.1%
Anal	0.065-0.5%
Oral	0.005-0.01%
Injecting drugs use	0.67%
Needle stick exposure	0.3%
Mucous membrane splash to eye, oro-nasal	0.09%

Comparative risk after needle-stick injury for HBV is 9-30% and for HCV is 1-1.8%

ART regimen for PEP : TDF + 3TC + LPV/r for 4 weeks after counselling and testing.

x=x=x=x=x

5

Systemic Antiparasitic Agents

Systemic antiparasitic agents are frequently prescribed by pediatricians for treatment of protozoal and worm infestations in children. Dermatologists in their day-to-day practice also come across various skin infections caused due to protozoa or parasites. Drugs used for protozoal and parasitic infestations are summarized in the following Table 5.1 :

MEBENDAZOLE :

Broad-spectrum benzimidazole antihelminthic.

MECHANISM OF ACTION :

It causes depletion of glycogen stores and blocks glucose uptake in the parasite.

It binds to beta-tubulin of susceptible worms and inhibits polymerization of the cells of the worm.

TABLE 5.2 : **Indications and doses of mebendazole**

Round worm/hook worm/trichuriasis	200 mg b.i.d. 3 days
Enterobius vermicularis	100 mg single dose, repeat after 2 weeks
Tape worms	200 mg b.i.d. 4 days (less effective).
Trichinella sprilaris	200 mg b.i.d. 4 days (less effective).

DOSES AND PREPARATIONS :

- 200 mg b.i.d./t.i.d.

TABLE 5.1 : **Antiparasitic agents : drugs and doses**

	Drugs and doses
Protozoal infestations :	
Amebiasis cutis	Metronidazole 750 mg t.i.d. 10 days.
Trichomoniasis	Metronidazole 500 mg b.i.d. 7 days.
Toxoplasmosis	Sulfadoxine 120 mg/kg/day 15 days with pyrimethamine 2 mg/kg 2 days followed by 1 mg/kg 15 days.
Leishmaniasis	Described below.
Endo-Parasitic infestations :	
Schistosomiasis	Praziquantel 20 mg/kg b.i.d. for one day only.
Cysticercosis cutis	Praziquantel 10 mg/kg, single dose.
Echinococcosis	Albendazole 400 mg.
Enterobiasis (Pinworm)	Mebendazole 100 mg, repeated in 2 weeks, Pyrantel pamoate 11 mg/kg PO once.
Ankylostomiasis (Hook worm infestation)	Albendazole 400 mg once, mebendazole 100 mg b.i.d. 3 days.
Cutaneous larva migrans	Ivermectin 150 µg/kg single dose, albendazole 200 mg b.i.d. 3 days.
Larva currens (strongyloidiasis)	Albendazole 400 mg/day 3 days, Thiabendazole 25 mg/kg b.i.d. 7 days, Ivermectin 200 µg/kg/day for 2 days.
Filariasis	Diethylcarbamazine (DEC) 6 mg/kg/day 12 days, ivermectin 100-400 µg/kg one dose.
Dracunculosis	Metronidazole 30-40 mg/kg tds for 3 days in two divided doses, thiabendazole 50 mg/kg/day in two divided doses for 3 days (drugs allows natural extrusion of worm but do not kill parasite or larvae).
Ecto-Parasitic infestations :	
Scabies and Pediculosis	Ivermectin 12 mg single dose or 200 µg/kg single dose.

- MEBEX 100 mg chewable tablet, 100 mg/5 ml suspension.
- Doses and duration is same for children above 2 years and adults, half dose is required for children less than 2 years of age.

PREGNANCY CATEGORY – C :

ADVERSE EFFECTS :

Systemic :

Well tolerated, GIT disturbances can occur.

Cutaneous :

Allergic reaction, alopecia with high doses.

KEY POINTS :

- Minimal absorption; 75-90% of oral mebendazole passes in feces. Fatty food increases absorption.
- Complete clearance of the parasite from GI tract may take up to 3 days.
- More effective than albendazole for trichuriasis.
- Though used extensively for mass treatment, a 3-day dosage schedule is a potential drawback as far as compliance is concerned.

ALBENDAZOLE :

Broad-spectrum anthelmintic is a congener of mebendazole.

MECHANISM OF ACTION :

Similar to that of mebendazole.

DOSES AND PREPARATIONS :

- 400 mg single dose, 10-14 mg/kg in children.
- ZENTEL 400 mg chewable tablet, 200 mg/5 ml suspension.

PREGNANCY CATEGORY – C :

TABLE 5.3 : **Indications and doses of albendazole**

Round worm/hook worm/*Trichuris*/ *Enterobius* infestations	400 mg single dose.
Tape worm/strongyloidosis	400 mg daily for 3 days.
Neurocysticercosis	15 mg/kg for 1 month (as efficacious as praziquantel).
Larva migrans/larva currens	200 mg b.i.d. 3 days.

Adverse Effects :

Systemic :

Well tolerated, GIT disturbances can occur.

Cutaneous :

Alopecia is reported.

Key Points :

- Inconsistent absorption, widespread distribution and good CSF penetration.
- Less effective than mebendazole for trichuriasis.

THIABENDAZOLE :

Thiabendazole is a broad-spectrum antihelminthic agent.

Mechanism Of Action :

It inhibits helminth-specific fumarate reductase.

Indications :

1. Cutaneous larva migrans (Ankylostoma braziliense, Necator americans).
2. Larva currens (Strongyloides stercoralis).
3. Visceral larva migrans (Toxocara canis).

4. Trichinosis.
5. Guinea worm infestation (allows the worm to extrude).

DOSES AND PREPARATIONS :

- 1.5 g for two successive days, 25 mg/kg b.i.d.
- MINTEZOL 500 mg chewable tab, 500 mg/5 ml suspension.

PREGNANCY CATEGORY – C :

ADVERSE EFFECTS :

Systemic :

Nausea, vomiting, and diarrhea.

Cutaneous :

Local irritation with topical preparation.

REMARKS :

- Thiabendazole tablet should be first chewed and then swallowed.
- May increase plasma levels of theophylline.

PYRANTEL PAMOATE :

Pyrantel pamoate broad-spectrum antihelminthic agent.

MECHANISM OF ACTION :

It is a neuromuscular blocker causing spastic paralysis of helminths.

INDICATIONS :

1. Ascariasis and Hookworm infestations (11 mg (base)/kg PO q/Day for 3 days).
2. Pinworm infestation (11 mg/kg Single dose).

DOSES AND PREPARATIONS :

- Cap NEMOCID 180 mg; 180 mg is equivalent to 62.5 mg of base.
- 11 mg (base)/kg PO q/Day for 3 days.

PREGNANCY CATEGORY – C :

ADVERSE EFFECTS :

Systemic :

Dizziness, Insomnia, hepatic dysfunction.

PRAZIQANTEL :

Praziqantel is an antihelminthic agent used for schistosomiasis, cysticercosis and hydatid disease and other flukes.

MECHANISM OF ACTION :

It increases permeability of schistosomes cells towards calcium ions thereby inducing contraction of parasite muscles leading to paralysis.

Vacuolation and blebbing of worm tegumental and subtegumental structures leading to its destruction and parasite's antigenic, exposure to immune cells.

DOSES AND PREPARATIONS :

- Tab CYSTICIDE, PRAZIN 600 mg.
- 20 mg/kg/day in 3 divided dosages in a day completes the therapy.

PREGNANCY CATEGORY – B :

ADVERSE EFFECTS :

Systemic :

Malaise, headache, dizziness, abdominal discomfort.

DIETHYLCARBAMAZINE (DEC) :

Diethylcarbamazine is an antifilarial agent.

Mechanism Of Action :

It modifies microfilariae so that they are engulfed by phagocytes but do not have direct microfilaricidal action.

Doses And Preparations :

- Filariasis - 6 mg/kg/day in three divided doses after meals for 2 weeks.
- Loaiasis - 50 mg t.i.d. on day 1 and 2, 100 mg t.i.d. on day 3, and 2 mg/kg t.i.d. from day 4-21.
- HETRAZAN 100 mg tab, BANOCIDE 50, 100 mg tab, 60 ml syrup 50 mg/5 ml.

Adverse Effects :

Systemic :

Nausea, vomiting, diarrhea, headache, and giddiness.

Key Points :

- Adequate data not available for safety in pregnancy, advisable to defer use until delivery.
- Frequent courses of DEC may be required as microfilariae can reappear.
- DEC has no effect on the adult parasite.
- Brugian filariasis is more susceptible to treatment than Bancroftian filariasis.

IVERMECTIN :

Ivermectin is an avermectin derivative and is a macrocylic lactone antibiotic isolated from fermentation products of *Streptomyces avermitilis.*

MECHANISM OF ACTION :

GABA-nergic action, blocks chloride channels leading to tonic paralysis of parasites.

INDICATIONS :

- Scabies
- Pediculosis
- Onchocerciasis (drug of choice).
- Filariasis
- Larva currens
- Strongyloidiasis

DOSES AND PREPARATIONS :

- 12 mg single dose to be repeated after 2 weeks, 200 μg/kg single dose in children.
- SCAVISTA 6 mg tablet, IVERMECTOL 12 mg tablet.

PREGNANCY CATEGORY – C :

ADVERSE EFFECTS :

Systemic :

Headache and giddiness.

Cutaneous :

Local irritation with topical preparation.

REMARKS :

- Ivermectin has an advantage of single dosing in all the conditions for which it is used (Table 5.1). Safety profile of ivermectin is good making attractive option for treatment of scabies in mass population in non-pregnant women and children of all ages including infants.
- Cure rates of 60-70% are observed with a single dose of

ivermectin in scabies. An additional dose of ivermectin after 2 weeks improves cure rates upto 100%.

- As ivermectin is adulticidal for scabies mite but does not have ovicidal activity, repeat dose after 2 weeks is essential to ensure that newly hatched mites are killed. Repeat dosages of 3 times/week or 5 times/2 weeks or 7 times/4 weeks are required to be used in crusted scabies where mite population is extremely high.

ANTILEISHMANIAL AGENTS :

Antileishmanial agents include sodium stibogluconate, pentamidine, amphotericin-B, ketoconazole, allopurinol, and paromomycin sulphate and miltefosine.

SODIUM STIBOGLUCONATE : (SODIUM ANTIMONY GLUCONATE)

It is a water-soluble pentavalent antimonial.

Mechanism Of Action :

It inhibits SH-dependent enzymes of the parasite and bio-energetics of the parasite is interfered.

Blocks glycolytic and fatty acid oxidation pathways.

Doses And Preparations :

- 20 mg/kg (max : 850 mg) daily by i.m. (in the buttocks) or i.v. injection for 28 days for mucocutaneous and visceral disease, for 20 days for cutaneous leishmaniasis.
- ABANTE, STIBAMINE, PENTOSTAM 100 mg (antimony)/ml in 30 ml vial.
- No adequate data available for safety in pregnancy.

Side Effects :

Nausea, vomiting, metallic taste, cough, abdominal pain, pain and stiffness of injected muscle, sterile abscesses, and liver and kidney damage.

KEY POINTS :

- Drug of choice for *kala azar;* also better tolerated than other antimonials.
- Rapidly absorbed from the site of i.m. injection. It is excreted unchanged in urine.
- Repeated doses are cumulative, increasing efficacy as well as risk of liver and renal toxicity.
- Liver and renal function tests should be done at the baseline and after 10 days of therapy.
- Susceptibility to both sodium stibogluconate and meglumine antimoniate was found to be stage specific and parasite intrinsic. Amastigotes were found to be 73-271 times more susceptible to sodium stibogluconate than were promastigotes.
- Resistance to antimonials is not uncommon in India. Stepwise mutation is the postulated mechanism of resistance to sodium stibogluconate. Interestingly, there is no cross-resistance between sodium stibogluconate and trivalent antimony compounds.

PENTAMIDINE :

Pentamidine isethionate is an antiprotozoal agent.

MECHANISM OF ACTION :

Probably interacts with kinetoplast DNA or inhibits aerobic glycolysis.

DOSES AND PREPARATIONS :

- 4 mg/kg i.m. or slow i.v. injection on alternate days : total 12-15 injections.

- Dry powder in 300 mg vial.
- PENTACARINAT 300 mg/vial.

PREGNANCY CATEGORY – C :

ADVERSE EFFECTS :

Acute reaction :

Sharp fall in BP, palpitations, fainting, vomiting, rigor, and fever (with i.v. injection, less frequent with i.m.).

Others :

Rashes, ECG changes, liver and kidney damage, rarely cardiac arrhythmias.

KEY POINTS :

- Should be used only as salvage therapy after antimonial failure.
- It initially causes cytolysis of pancreatic B cells—release of insulin—hypoglycemia and later permanent diabetes.

AMPHOTERICIN B :

Amphotericin is a broad-spectrum systemic antifungal drug, and also used for disseminated and visceral leishmaniasis including leishmaniasis resistant to antimonials.

MECHANISM OF ACTION :

Like fungi, leishmania have a high percentage of ergosterol and hence are susceptible to amphotericin B.

DOSES AND PREPARATION :

- 0.5 mg/kg by slow intravenous infusion for leishmaniasis, total dose of 7-20 mg/kg is usually required.

- AMFOTEX, AMFOCAN 50 mg vial. AMBISOME (Liposomal amphoterisin is preferred due to its favourable efficacy and safety.)

PREGNANCY CATEGORY – B :

KEY POINTS :

- Reserved for patients not responding to both antimonials and pentamidine.
- Useful in mucocutaneous and disseminated leishmaniasis.
- Look under "Antifungal agents" for more details.

KETOCONAZOLE :

Ketoconazole is a broad-spectrum antifungal drug, which is also used for leishmaniasis for its mild antileishmanial activity.

DOSES AND PREPARATIONS :

- 600 mg/day for 4 weeks for leishmaniasis.
- PHYTORAL, NIZRAL 200 mg tablet.

PREGNANCY CATEGORY – C :

- Effective in post-*kala azar* dermal leishmaniasis and cutaneous leishmaniasis, but being rapidly replaced by fluconazole.
- Look under "Antifungal agents" for more details.

FLUCONAZOLE :

4 triazole antifungal, it has also shown good efficacy in treatment of cutaneous leishmaniasis. At a dose of 5 mg/kg/day for 4 weeks, it has 75% efficacy but at a higher dose of 8 mg/kg/day, it is claimed to have 100% efficacy in treating cutaneous leishmaniasis. Due to its favourable safety profile & once daily dosing, it has the potential of becoming the first-line therapy in cutaneous leishmaniasis.

ALLOPURINOL :

Allopurinol is a xanthine oxidase inhibitor, that has been also used in leishmaniasis.

MECHANISM OF ACTION :
It inhibits protein synthesis. Purine salvage pathway in leishmania metabolizes allopurinol into corresponding nucleotides, which are incorporated in RNA resulting in interference with protein synthesis.

DOSES AND PREPARATIONS :

- 4-12 mg/kg t.i.d. for 3-4 weeks.
- ZYLORIC 100 mg tablet.

PREGNANCY CATEGORY – C :

KEY POINTS :

- Failure rate has been high.
- Used as a companion drug to antimonials in cases which do not respond to the latter alone.

RIFAMPICIN :

Rifampicin, the main antituberculous agent, is also used for leishmaniasis.

DOSES AND PREPARATIONS :

- 600-900 mg daily for 4 weeks for cutaneous leishmaniasis and post kala azar dermal leishmaniasis (PKDL).
- R-CIN 150, 300, 450, 600 mg cap, 200 ml sus 100 mg/5 ml.

PREGNANCY CATEGORY – C :

KEY POINT :

- Rifampicin may not be co-administered with ketoconazole for leishmaniasis, as it induces cytochrome P450 enzyme while ketoconazole inhibits the same, leading to inefficacy.

MILTEFOSINE :

Miltefosine is a broad spectrum antimicrobial phospholipid drug that is also effective in majority of patients of leishmaniasis including those with antimonial resistant disease. The drug was originally developed as an anticancer agent but is found to be useful in visceral, cutaneous and mucocutaneous leishmaniasis.

> **MECHANISM OF ACTION :**
>
> The drug acts by disturbing the lipid dependant cell signalling pathways of the parasites. It also causes mitochondrial dysfunction in the parasites.

INDICATIONS :

1. It is effective against all the strains of leishmania. Hence, it is effective in all forms of leishmaniasis, cutaneous, mucocutaneous and visceral (including post-kala azar dermal leishmaniasis). Most studies are small but demonstrate about 95% efficacy.
2. It is also effective against brain infections caused by free living amoebae Acanthamoeba and Naegleria.
3. Miltefosine is also used in trypanosomiasis of South American (Chagas) and African type including resistant strains.

DOSE AND PREPARATIONS :

Available as 50 mg tablet (IMPAVIDO). The usual adult dose in cutaneous leishmaniasis is 50 mg 3 times daily. For persons 25 to 45 kg weight 50 mg twice daily whereas 50 mg once daily is adequate if the weight is enough.

CONTRAINDICATIONS :

Miltefosine is teratogenic and should be avoided in pregnancy, except in life threatening situations. Miltefocine is contraindicated in children below 10 years and during lactation.

Side Effects :

Most frequent side effects are due to gastrointestinal intolerance nausea, vomiting, anorexia and diarrhoea in up to 40 per cent of patients but they are rarely severe enough to stop the drug. Renal toxicity (elevated serum creatinine) and liver toxicity (elevated transaminases) are not so common but require supervision.

x=x=x=x=x

6
Antileprosy Drugs

Multidrug therapy (MDT) or chemotherapy has drastically improved cure rates of leprosy. Drugs used for the treatment of leprosy are listed below :

TABLE 6.1 : **Antileprosy drugs**

Drugs	Doses	MIC (μg/ml)
Primary drugs :		
Dapsone	Tablet 100 mg o.d.	0.003
Clofazimine	Capsule 50 mg o.d.	Unknown
Rifampicin	Tablet 600 mg once monthly	0.3
Secondary drugs :		
Ethionamide/prothionamide	250-500 mg daily, 4-5 mg/kg	0.05
Thiacetazone	150 mg daily, 2 mg/kg/day	0.2
Thiambutosinc	1500 mg daily	0.5
Sulfamethoxypyridazine	1000 mg daily	30
Aminoglycosides (streptomycin)	Injection 1 g thrice weekly	Unknown
Newer drugs :		
Ofloxacin (fluoroquinolones)	400 mg tablet o.d.	1.5 microgram/ml
Minocycline (tetracyclines)	Capsule/Tablet 100 mg o.d.	0.2 microgram/ml
Clarithromycin (macrolides)	500 mg tablet o.d.	1.2 microgram/ml
Ancient drugs :		
Hydnocarpus oil	—	—
Arsenic	—	—

TABLE 6.2 : **WHO-MDT : fixed duration therapy (FDT) in leprosy (WHO Expert Committee 2018)**

Type of leprosy	Doses	Duration
Paucibacillary leprosy	Same 3 drug regimen for both paucibacillary and multibacillary cases.	6 months of therapy to be completed
Multibacillary leprosy	Dapsone 100 mg daily self-administered + clofazimine 50 mg daily self-administered plus 300 mg once monthly supervised and Rifampicin 600 mg once monthly supervised.	12 months of therapy to be completed

The practice of single-dose therapy with ROM (rifampicin 600 mg, ofloxacin 400 mg, and minocycline 100 mg) for treatment of single skin lesion (SSL) leprosy, has been stopped.

DAPSONE (4, 4'-DIAMINODIPHENYL SULFONE, DDS) :

Bacteriostatic drug used for leprosy as a part of multidrug therapy.

MECHANISM OF ACTION :

Competitive antagonist of *para*-aminobenzoic acid (PABA) for enzyme dihydropteroate reductase enzyme of *M. leprae*.

SIDE EFFECTS :

Systemic :

Hematological :

- Hemolysis in G6PD deficient patients (common).
- Methemoglobinemia (not common).
- Agranulocytosis (rare).
- Thrombocytopenia (rare).

Neurological :

- Wooly headache or "light-headedness".
- Psychosis.
- Peripheral neuropathy (distal axonal, motor, dose-related and reversible).

Renal :

- Nephrotic syndrome.

Hepatic :

- Hepatitis (uncommon but common with dapsone hypersensitivity syndrome).
- Cholestatic jaundice (uncommon).

Cutaneous :

- Maculopapular rash.
- Fixed drug eruption.
- Stevens-Johnson syndrome/Toxic epidermal necrolysis.
- Dapsone hypersensitivity syndrome ("Dapsone syndrome").

DRUG INTERACTIONS :

1. Hematologic adverse reactions may increase with folic acid antagonists, *e.g.*, pyrimethamine (monitor for agranulocytosis during second and third month of therapy).
2. Probenecid increases dapsone toxicity.
3. Dapsone levels may significantly decrease when administered concurrently with rifampicin.

KEY POINTS :

1. Dapsone is completely (more than 90%) absorbed when taken orally. It is excreted freely in bile with enterohepatic

recirculation so that it is mainly lost from the body through urine as the glucuronide.

2. Dapsone monotherapy (widely used in the past) leads to resistance. It has been combined with other antileprosy drugs to increase efficacy, decrease side effects, and to decrease development of resistance. Resistance is mainly due to the selection of mutant strains and dominance of mutant population over a period of time (secondary dapsone resistance).
3. Dapsone is preferably taken at night as it causes 'lightheadedness'.
4. Intramuscular dapsone (DADDS, 220 mg every 11 weeks) is not indicated as it releases very small amount of dapsone unable to kill *M. leprae* even in paucibacillary leprosy.
5. Dapsone, like other antileprosy drugs, can precipitate type II lepra reaction.
6. Dapsone had been given in pregnancy or lactation in the past without teratogenic side effects. In fact, it has the advantage of killing viable bacilli in the breast milk during lactation.
7. Urine spot test for detection of dapsone was used in the past for checking the compliance of patients. A drop of the patient's urine is put onto a filter paper and then a drop of Ehrlich's reagent is added. The filter paper shows the formation of an orange ring, which indicates the presence of dapsone in urine.
8. G6PD (Glucose-6-phosphate dehydrogenase) enzyme is required for the synthesis of glutathione that maintains integrity of RBCs. In G6PD deficient individuals, RBCs become susceptible to oxidant drugs like dapsone thereby precipitating hemolysis. In G6PD deficient individuals, dapsone should be started as a low dose (25 mg twice weekly) and gradually increased to 50-100 mg daily over 3-4 weeks if no severe hemolysis occurs.

9. Dapsone-induced methemoglobinemia is one of the rare side effects of dapsone. Both hydroxylamine derivates of dapsone are equipotent in their methemoglobin (MetHb) forming ability. Inside the erythrocytes, hydroxylamine derivatives deliver a severe oxidative stress to Hb in the red blood cells superceding the compensatory physiologic reductive capacity. Oxidative damage converts Fe^{2+} in the heme to Fe^{3+} (MetHb) with poor affinity for oxygen thereby making Hb an inadequate oxygen transporter. It does not produce signs and symptoms if methemoglobin levels are below 20%. A peculiar chocolate-brown color blood rather than the dark red of deoxygenated venous blood or bright red oxygenated arterial blood suggests MetHb above 20%. Levels above 70% are usually fatal. Treatment includes intravenous infusion of 1% methylene blue 1-2 mg/kg of body weight every 5 minutes. Within red blood cells, methylene blue activates NADPH-MR to form leukomethylene blue, which acts as a reducing agent (electron donor) of oxidized Hb, converting the ferric ion (Fe^{3+}) back to its oxygen-carrying ferrous (Fe^{2+}) state. Dosages of more than 7 mg/kg can paradoxically worsen methemoglobinemia. Non-enzymatic antioxidants like ascorbic acid and glutathione are also recommended. The addition of cimetidine to dapsone reduces the likelihood of methemoglobinemia.

10. "Dapsone syndrome" or "sulfone hypersensitivity syndrome" develops between 2 and 6 weeks after dapsone is started ("6 weeks syndrome") and is characterized by :
   - Fever and constitutional symptoms.
   - Generalized lymphadenopathy.
   - Hepatitis with elevated liver enzymes, hepatomegaly.
   - Facial edema and skin rash, which may begin as maculopapular rash and may progress to exfoliative dermatitis.

- Eosinophilia and atypical lymphocytes in peripheral smear.

Management consists of immediate stoppage of the drug and, if required, oral steroids for 4–6 weeks with slow tapering dosages. If allowed to progress without omission of dapsone, the condition can be fatal with the risk of multiorgan involvement especially of fulminant hepatic failure due to en-mass hepatic necrosis. Hence, rechallenge with dapsone is not advocated.

Paucibacillary leprosy cases with dapsone syndrome may be treated with daily clofazimine and monthly rifampicin or even clofazimine monotherapy. Multibacillary cases with dapsone syndrome may require replacement of dapsone by either minocycline or ofloxacin or clarithromycin in the regimen.

Other indications of dapsone are discussed in the chapter "Antiinflammatory Agents".

CLOFAZIMINE :

Riminophenazine dye is used as a part of multidrug therapy for multibacillary leprosy.

Mechanism Of Action :

Exact mechanism is unknown. It supposedly inhibits aerobic respiration of *M. leprae,* stimulates the release of oxygen radicals and phagocytic activity and inhibits function of DNA.

Side Effects :

Systemic :

- When used in higher doses, the drug gets deposited in mesenteric lymph nodes and causes a syndrome of acute abdomen that may mimic appendicitis. Pain may be accompanied by vomiting, diarrhea, and GI hemorrhage.
- Eosinophilic enteritis.

- Renal failure.
- Splenic infarct.

Cutaneous :

- Brown pigmentation of the infiltrated skin initially as "Mahogany red" followed by "Charcoal black".
- Ichthyosis.
- Phototoxicity (rare).

KEY POINTS :

- Severity of skin discoloration due to clofazimine depends upon the dose and the degree of skin infiltration by the leprosy. Due to the discoloration, clofazimine may be avoided in fair-colored individuals. Alternative drugs may be used in such patients.
- Pigmentation is blotchy and more pronounced in photo-exposed areas. It requires 6-12 months for clearance after discontinuation of the drug. It can also be seen in the cornea and conjunctiva.
- Due to anticholinergic action, clofazimine can cause diminished sweating and tear formation (leads to more dryness of skin and eyes).

Other indications of clofazimine in dermatology are discussed in the chapter "Antiinflammatory Agents".

RIFAMPICIN :

Rifampicin is the most effective bactericidal drug used for leprosy.

MECHANISM OF ACTION :

It inhibits bacterial RNA synthesis by inhibiting DNA-dependent RNA polymerase of *M. leprae.*

SIDE EFFECTS :

Systemic :

- GI disturbances.
- Hepatotoxicity.
- Fatigue, lethargy, and headache.
- Red discoloration of urine, feces, sweat, sputum, saliva, and tears. Cutaneous discoloration from high doses of rifampicin can give rise to a "red man" appearance in fair-skinned persons.

Cutaneous :

- Urticaria.
- Maculopapular rash.
- Stevens-Johnson syndrome/Toxic epidermal necrolysis.

KEY POINTS :

- Rifampicin is the fastest acting and most effective antileprosy drug that renders patients noninfectious within 5 weeks of starting MDT.
- Single dose (600 mg) of rifampicin kills 99.9% of non-dormant (dividing) *M. Leprae.*
- Being lipid soluble, rifampicin can kill both intracellular and extracellular bacteria.
- Rifampicin is ultimately excreted through the gastrointestinal tract requiring no dosage adjustments in impaired renal functions.
- Rifampicin induces liver microsomal enzymes thereby reducing drug levels of dapsone, steroids, and OC pills reducing their efficacy. Reduction in levels of dapsone is insignificant in patients taking 100 mg of dapsone per day.
- Autoimmune side effects of rifampicin (thrombocytopenia, flu-like syndrome, nephritis, abdominal pain) seen with

intermittent therapy, as practiced for tuberculosis, are not encountered (or very unlikely) with once-monthly doses in antileprosy therapy.

- Newer derivative of rifampicin *i.e.* rifapentin (900 mg as against 600 mg of rifampicin) has higher peak serum concentration and longer half life making it more effective drug for leprosy in animal studies.

ETHIONAMIDE/PROTHIONAMIDE :

Bactericidal drug but less effective than rifampicin.

Mechanism Of Action :

It may inhibit protein synthesis of *M. leprae.*

Dosages :

250 mg or 500 mg OD.

Side Effects :

Metallic taste, nausea, vomiting, abdominal pain, anorexia, hepatotoxicity, postural hypotension, mental depression, drowsiness, peripheral neuropathy, and asthenia.

Key Points :

1. Chemically, the drug is related to isoniazid.
2. It was used in sulfone-resistant cases in combination with other drugs like clofazimine. However, with advent of newer and better drugs for leprosy, it is no longer used by dermatologists.
3. ISOPRODIAN is a preparation that contains isonicotinic acid hydrazide, prothionamide and dapsone. This was used by German group of investigators in patients of leprosy.

THIACETAZONE :

Bactericidal drug but less effective than rifampicin.

MECHANISM OF ACTION :

Not known.

SIDE EFFECTS :

Systemic :

Agranulocytosis, nausea, vomiting, abdominal pain, anorexia, vertigo, blurred vision, and hepatotoxicity.

Cutaneous :

Erythema multiforme, skin rash.

THIAMBUTOSINE :

Thiourea bacteriostatic drug.

MECHANISM OF ACTION :

Not known.

KEY POINT :

- Should be used in combination to avoid resistance.

INSTRUCTIONS TO PATIENTS STARTED ON MDT :

TIMINGS OF ANTILEPROSY MEDICATIONS :

- Dapsone should be taken at night as it causes "lightheadedness".
- Rifampicin is taken on an empty stomach before breakfast for better absorption.

MEDICATIONS :

- Medications like rifampicin cause red discoloration of urine, tears, or other secretions. Patient should be told about it as patient may confuse it with hematuria or blood in tears or secretions.

- Clofazimine causes red discoloration of skin and fish-like skin.
- Clofazimine-induced discoloration of skin is likely to subside within 6 months to 1 year after its discontinuation.

DURATION :

Duration of treatment of multi-bacillary leprosy (MB-MDT) is 12 months while that of paucibacillary leprosy (PB-MDT) is 6 months. In cases of default, patient should be restarted on MDT for scheduled duration.

FOLLOW-UP :

Follow-up is usually required after 2-4 weeks especially to look for drug hypersensitivity syndromes due to dapsone or rifampicin or type I lepra reaction in paucibacillary leprosy. In case of reactions, immediate consultation with the doctor is necessary.

TABLE 6.3 : **Doses of MDT in children**

Dose compared to adult dose	Weight
	< 15 kg
½	15-30 kg
	30-45 kg
Adult dose	> 45 kg

TABLE 6.4 : **MDT for leprosy in a patient of tuberculosis**

For paucibacillary leprosy	Initial phase of ATT no new drug added Maintenance phase of ATT dapsone is added to tuberculosis regimen
For multibacillary leprosy	Initial phase-dapsone is added Maintenance phase-dapsone and clofazimine is added to tuberculosis regimen

ATT : Antituberculosis treatment

Tests :

Tests for leprosy include tests for diagnosis of leprosy like skin biopsy or slit-skin smears. Tests for initiating treatment and follow-up include G6PD estimation, hemoglobin and complete blood counts, and liver function tests.

Reactions :

Redness or pain of existing leprosy plaques or nerve pains are the signs of leprosy reaction in paucibacillary leprosy and not because of "worsening" of leprosy due to treatment. Treatment should not be stopped and consultation with the treating doctor is important. Severe nerve pain, muscle weakness, loss of grip, paralysis, numbness, painless blisters in areas of anesthesia are warning signs of leprosy reaction and treatment should be sought immediately. Certain medicines are required to control severe reaction. In multibacillary leprosy, Type II lepra reaction usually occurs late, 6 months to 2 years after the initiation of treatment.

Signs of Neurological Worsening (Silent Neuritis) :

The loss of muscle power or paralysis can occur even in the absence of nerve pain. This is called silent neuritis and treatment with steroids is required for this. A typical case with no contraindication for steroids should receive 40 mg/day prednisolone with weekly taper of 5 mg/day.

Pregnancy :

Female patients on antileprosy treatment need not stop treatment if they become pregnant during therapy. Adequate data are available on benefits exceeding side effects as far as antileprosy medications are concerned. Reactions and neurological worsening are common in pregnancy. Leprosy organisms can be transferred to neonates or infants through breastfeeding in untreated cases.

NEWER DRUGS IN LEPROSY :

Newer drugs currently in use for leprosy include ofloxacin, minocycline, and clarithromycin. Other drugs are experimental and their actions against *M. leprae* are being investigated. Currently, they are not in use in India.

DRUG RESISTANT LEPROSY :

Rifampicin resistant leprosy is rare. WHO recommended treatment of rifampicin-resistant leprosy is to administer at least two second-line drugs (clarithromycin, minocycline or ofloxacin) plus clofazimine daily for 6 months, followed by clofazimine plus one of these drugs for an additional 18 months.

NEWER REGIMENS FOR LEPROSY :

There are many experimental regimens for the treatment of leprosy. Data on their long-term efficacy are not yet available, and therefore, they are not recommended for regular use. (Table 6.5)

MONTHLY ROM :

MONTHLY ADMINISTERED ROM FOR MB AND PB LEPROSY

Rifampicin 600 mg, **O**floxacin 400 mg, and **M**inocycline 100 mg (ROM). Administered monthly (monthly ROM).

For paucibacillary leprosy – monthly ROM for 6 months.

For multibacillary leprosy – monthly ROM for 12 months.

Trials evaluating the efficacy of the above regimen are being currently conducted in Myanmar, Guinea and Senegal.

ANCIENT MEDICATIONS :

CHAULMOOGRA OIL (HYDROCARPUS OIL) :

Burmese prince got cured of leprosy accidentally by eating

TABLE 6.5 : **Newer drugs in leprosy**

Newer drugs	Remarks
Fluoroquinolones	Pefloxacin, ofloxacin, and sparfloxacin are used; kill 99-99.99% bacilli in less than 1 month of therapy. Less effective than rifampicin.
Tetracyclines	Only minocycline has marked bactericidal action against *M. leprae.*
Macrolides	Only clarithromycin has marked bactericidal action against *M. Leprae.* Kills 99% bacilli in 28 days while 99.9% in 56 days of clarithromycin 500 mg OD.
Aminoglycosides	Streptomycin is found to be synergistic. Amikacin and kanamycin require high doses to exert action
Ansamycins	Rifabutin and rifapentine
Sulfonamide derivatives	Brodimoprim 20 mg + DDS 25 mg combination is tried, which has better penetration in mycobacterial cell wall.
Fusidic acid	Inhibits protein synthesis by inhibiting elongation factor G; dose 500-750 mg/day, highly lipophilic, safe and high serum concentrations, and long shelf life.
Beta-lactam antibiotics	Cephaloridine, cephaloglycin (oral agent), cefuroxine and cefoxitin. Not practical for use in leprosy.
Amoxicillin plus clavulanic acid	Found to be bactericidal.
Derivatives of thiacetazone	PH22 and PQ22 are derivatives of thiacetazone.
Desoxyfructo-serotonin	Human metabolite, immunological actions are being explored (NAL-Nutritional Antileprosy diet).
Diuciphon	Pyrimidine sulfone derivative.

fruits and seeds of Chaulmoogra. Also known as 'kalaw' in Burma and 'tuvaraka' in Southern/Eastern India, its fruits contain numerous seeds in a moist flesh inside a shell. Suggested mechanism of action is activation of host lipases that helps in destroying foreign lipids including the cell wall of *M. leprae.* It is suggested to be given in very large doses (15 ml per week) both orally and intradermally.

UNIFORM MDT (U-MDT) :

The MB MDT regimen as a uniform regimen for both PB and MB patients is termed as uniform MDT. This is being contemplated and evaluated, though not yet recommended for general use.

Merits :

- Low chances of relapse and resistance to *M. leprae.*
- Easier logistics support and information system.
- Reduced training requirements and better integration is possible.

Demerits :

- Will overtreat PB leprosy patients and undertreat MB patients, especially those with a high initial BI.

ACCOMPANIED MDT (A-MDT) :

A-MDT means providing patients with a full course of treatment on their first visit to the leprosy clinic after diagnosis. The term accompanied is chosen because someone close to or important to the patient takes responsibility for helping the patient to complete the therapy. This therapy is in the evaluation stage and not yet in widespread use.

Merits :

- Valuable aid to mobile populations, and patients living in remote areas.
- Will increase patient compliance and decrease default.

Demerits :

- Advantage of supervision of MDT will be lost and thus may lead to irregularity of treatment and resistance.

OTHER REGIMENS :

- Clofazimine 50 mg plus any two of ofloxacin 400 mg/

minocycline 100 mg/clarithromycin 500 mg daily for 6 months and clofazimine 50 mg plus any one of ofloxacin 400 mg/minocycline 100 mg daily for another 18 months.

INDICATIONS :

This regimen is used when standard MDT regimen cannot be employed due to severe side effects, or in case of rifampicin or dapsone resistance (very rare).

- Rifampicin 600 mg, ofloxacin 400 mg, and clarithromycin 500 mg daily for 1 year for multibacillary leprosy.

TREATMENT OF BACTERIOLOGICAL RELAPSE IN LEPROSY :

This tends to occur in patients with high bacterial load (BI $\geq$ 4 +) after a period of 3-5 years after completion of therapy. These cases respond to the standard WHO MB-MDT as they do not represent drug resistance but reactivation due to persisters.

PROPHYLAXIS IN LEPROSY :

CHEMOPROPHYLAXIS IN CONTACTS OF LEPROSY PATIENTS :

Chemoprophylaxis of contacts older than 2 years is now recommended by WHO. The 2018 guidelines recommend the use of single-dose rifampicin after excluding leprosy and tuberculosis (TB) disease and in the absence of other contraindications. The $COLEP_2$ randomized controlled trial (RCT) reported a 57% reduction in the risk of contracting leprosy amongst contacts after 2 years though the protection reduced to 30% after 5-7 years.

x=x=x=x=x

7
Antituberculosis Agents

Antituberculous agents can be classified as first-line and second-line drugs. First-line drugs have high efficacy, low toxicity, and are used routinely by dermatologists for the treatment of cutaneous tuberculosis. Second-line drugs have low efficacy, high toxicity, and are used in resistant cases only. However, second line drugs are generally not required to be used by dermatologists except in cases of tuberculosis in HIV/AIDS (Table 7.1).

Antituberculous therapy (ATT) is indicated in the following conditions in dermatology :

1. Lupus vulgaris.
2. Tuberculosis verrucosa cutis (TBVC).
3. Primary inoculation tuberculosis (tuberculous chancre).
4. Scrofuloderma.
5. Tuberculosis cutis orificialis.
6. Disseminated tuberculosis affecting skin.
7. Tuberculids like lichen scrofulosorum, papulonecrotic tuberculid (PNT), erythema nodosum (EN), and erythema induratum due to tuberculosis (Bazin's disease).
8. Tuberculosis associated with HIV infection.

INH (ISONIAZID) :

Isoniazid is an inexpensive, easily administered, bactericidal, and first-line antituberculous agent.

INH (ISONIAZID)

TABLE 7.1 : **Antituberculous drugs**

	Adult doses	Pediatric dosages
First-line drugs :		
Isoniazid	300 mg/day PO	5 mg/kg/day PO (usually 300 mg/day).
Rifampicin	450 mg/day PO	10-20 mg/kg/day PO not to exceed 600 mg/day.
Pyrazinamide	1.5 g/day	15-30 mg/kg PO.
Ethambutol	800 mg/day or 15 mg/kg/day PO	Not recommended in children less than 6 years of age.
Streptomycin	1 g i.m. daily; 2 times/week dosing : 15 mg/kg/day i.m.; not to exceed 1 g/day; 3 times/week dosing : 25-30 mg/kg/day i.m.; not to exceed 1.5 g/day	2 times/week dosing : 20-40 mg/kg/day i.m.; not to exceed 1 g/day; 3 times/week dosing : 25-30 mg/kg/day i.m.; not toexceed 1.5 g/day.
Second-line drugs :		
Thiacetazone	150 mg/day PO	2-3 mg/kg/day
Para-amino salicylic acid	12 g/day PO in 2 or 3 divided dosages	150 mg/kg/day PO in 3 or 4 divided dosages
Ethionamide	0.5-1 g/day PO in 4 divided doses	15-20 mg/kg/day PO in 3 or 4 divided dosages
Cycloserine	0.5-1 g/day PO in divided doses	10-20 mg/kg/day; not to exceed 0.75-1 g/day
Kanamycin	15 mg/kg/day i.m.	15 mg/kg/day i.m.
Amikacin	750 mg/day i.m.	15 mg/kg/day in 3 divided doses
Capreomycin	1 g i.m. daily for 60-120 day, followed by 1 g i.m. b.i.d./t.i.d.	15 mg/kg/day i.m.
Second-line newer drugs :		
Ciprofloxacin	750 mg PO b.i.d.	Not recommended in less than 18 years of age
Ofloxacin	400-800 mg/day PO 2 divided dosages	Not recommended in less than 18 years of age
Levofloxacin	0.5-1 g PO in 2 divided dosages	Not recommended in less than 18 years of age
Clarithromycin	500 mg b.i.d.	7.5 mg b.i.d.
Rifabutin	300-600 mg/day PO	10-20 mg/kg/day PO
Bedaquiline	weight > 30 kg 400 mg once daily for 2 weeks and then 200 thrice a week for 22 weeks	

> MECHANISM OF ACTION :
>
> Tuberculocidal agent inhibits mycolic acid synthesis. Mycolic acid is an essential component of mycobacterial cell wall.

MECHANISM OF RESISTANCE :

INH resistance occurs principally due to the mutation of catalase peroxidase genes.

SIDE EFFECTS :

Systemic :

- Hepatotoxicity.
- Peripheral neuropathy (less common with 5 mg/kg dose and occurs due to increased urinary excretion of pyridoxine).

Cutaneous :

Acneiform eruptions, hypersensitivity reactions, erythema multiforme, Stevens-Johnson syndrome/toxic epidermal necrolysis, erythroderma, pellagroid dermatitis, drug-induced LE, and lichenoid drug reactions.

KEY POINTS :

- Isoniazid acts on fast multipliers, extracellular as well as intracellular mycobacteria and inhibits the quiescent stage of mycobacterium. It has no effect on atypical mycobacteria. Also isoniazid is not effective against non-replicating or slow metabolizing bacteria or under anaerobic conditions.
- It is completely absorbed from the gastrointestinal tract. Penetration into all body fluids and cavities is good. It is metabolized in the liver by both slow and fast acetylators.

- Pyridoxine should be supplemented to isoniazid containing antituberculous regimen in chronic alcoholics, pregnant women, and those having seizure disorders.
- **Drug interactions :**
  1. Aluminium hydroxide inhibits INH absorption from GI tract.
  2. PAS inhibits INH metabolism increasing their blood levels.
  3. INH is inhibitor of hepatic cytochrome P450 enzyme thereby increasing serum levels of phenytoin, barbiturates, carbamazepine, and warfarin sodium.

RIFAMPICIN :

Rifampicin is the most effective bactericidal drug used for tuberculosis.

Mechanism Of Action :

It inhibits bacterial RNA synthesis by inhibiting DNA-dependent RNA polymerase of M. tuberculosis.

Side Effects :

Systemic :

- GI disturbances.
- Hepatotoxicity.
- Fatigue, lethargy and headache.
- Red discoloration of urine, feces, sweat, sputum, saliva and tears.

Cutaneous :

- Urticaria
- Maculopapular rash.

- Stevens-Johnson syndrome/Toxic epidermal necrolysis.
- Cutaneous discoloration from high doses of rifampicin can give rise to a "red man" appearance in fair-skinned persons.

KEY POINTS :

- Being lipid soluble, rifampicin can kill both intracellular and extracellular mycobacteria. It is effective against multiplying and inactive organisms. It is also effective against atypical mycobacteria.
- Orange discoloration of secretions, body fluids or urine may occur during rifampicin therapy. Staining of contact lenses can also occur.
- Rifampicin is ultimately excreted through the gastrointestinal tract requiring no dosage adjustments in impaired renal functions.
- Rifampicin induces hepatic microsomal enzymes and thus reduces drug levels of dapsone, steroids, sulfonylurea, OC pills, phenytoin, cyclosporine, beta-blockers, enalapril, etc., reducing their efficacy. Co-administration with isoniazid or pyrazinamide may result in a higher rate of hepatotoxicity than with either agent alone. In cases of drug-drug interactions due to rifampicin, rifabutin may be preferred.
- Autoimmune side effects of rifampicin like thrombocytopenia, hemolytic anemia, flu-like syndrome and acute renal failure are seen with intermittent administration of rifampicin.

PYRAZINAMIDE :

Pyrazinamide is an analog of nicotinamide. It is prodrug that is converted to its active form pyrazinoic acid the enzyme pyrizinamidase.

MECHANISM OF ACTION :

Mechanism of action is unknown. Bacteriostatic or bactericidal against *M. tuberculosis,* depending on the concentration of the drug attained at the site of infection. It is highly effective against organisms in macrophages and against semi-dormant bacilli in acidic environment.

SIDE EFFECTS :

Systemic :

Hypersensitivity, hepatotoxicity and acute gout.

Cutaneous :

Uncommon.

KEY POINTS :

- Inhibits renal excretion of urates; may result in hyperuricemia (usually asymptomatic).
- **Drug interactions :**
  1. Concurrent administration of PZA with rifampicin has more risk of hepatotoxicity.

ETHAMBUTOL (ETB) :

MECHANISM OF ACTION :

Diffuses into tubercle bacilli and impairs cell metabolism by inhibiting synthesis of one or more metabolites, causing cell death.

SIDE EFFECTS :

Systemic :

Optic neuritis and hypersensitivity.

Cutaneous :

None is reported.

KEY POINTS :

- Optic neuritis is a well-known side effect of ethambutol therapy. It is dose-dependent with incidence of 1% when given in the dosage of 15 mg/kg/day. Visual acuity and color vision needs to be monitored. Administration in children is avoided, if vision cannot be tested. Ethambutol is generally not recommended in children less than 6 years of age.
- *Drug interactions :* Aluminium salts may reduce absorption of ethambutol.

STREPTOMYCIN :

Streptomycin, an aminoglycoside antibiotic, is effectively used as a component of first-line antituberculous therapy. However with increasing resistance to streptomycin in some countries and significant side effects, it is not commonly used as first line anti-tuberculous drug. In Treatment of MDR Kochs, it is used as a substitute to Amikacin. Please refer to the chapter "Antibacterials" for further details of streptomycin.

SECOND-LINE ANTITUBERCULOUS AGENTS :

Second line antituberculous drugs are indicated in patients where first line antitubercular drugs have failed to control the disease mostly because of drug resistance. Occurrence of multi-drug resistant TB (MDR-TB) is a concern especially when resistance develops to isoniazid and rifampicin. Second line antituberculous drugs are therefore required.

Most effective second line antituberculous drugs are oral fluoroquinolones (ciprofloxacin, levofloxacin, ofloxacin and moxifloxacin) and injectable aminoglycosides (amikacin and kanamycin). Drugs like ethionamide/propionamide, para-amino salicyclic acid (PAS), clofazimine and cyclosporine are also used. Please refer the chapter on 'systemic antibacterials" for more pharmacologic details of fluoroquinolones and aminoglycosides.

Extensively drug resistant TB (XDR-TB) is MDR-TB with additional resistance to any fluoroquinolone or one second line injectable aminoglycoside. Drugs like Linezolid, bedaquiline and delamanid/pretomanid are evolving and promising for XDR-TB.

Group A (highly effective, strongly recommended, included in regimens unless contraindicated)	Group B (Agents of second choice)	Group C (weigh balance V/s benefit)
Levofloxacin/Moxifloxacin	Clofazimine	Ethambutol
Bedaquiline	Cycloserine/Terizidone	Delamanid
Linezolid		Pyrazinamide
		Imipenem/Cilastin
		Meropenem
		Amikacin (Streptomycin)
		Ethionamide/Protionamide
		PAS

CYCLOSERINE :

MECHANISM OF ACTION :

Inhibits cell wall synthesis in *M. tuberculosis*. It is a structural analog of D-alanine, which antagonizes the role of D-alanine in bacterial cell wall synthesis and inhibits growth.

SIDE EFFECTS :

- *Systemic* : CNS toxicity, *i.e.*, convulsions, headache, tremor, depression, confusion, psychosis, somnolence, vertigo, paresis, dysarthria.
- Megaloblastic anemia.

KEY POINTS :

- **Drug interactions :**
  1. Alcohol consumption may increase the risk of convulsions in patients of cycloserine therapy.
  2. INH in combination with cycloserine may cause dizziness.

ETHIONAMIDE :

MECHANISM OF ACTION :

Bacteriostatic against *M. tuberculosis,* it inhibits mycolic acid synthesis like isoniazid.

SIDE EFFECTS :

May cause hypersensitivity and hepatotoxicity.

PARA-AMINOSALICYLIC ACID (PAS) :

MECHANISM OF ACTION :

Bacteriostatic against *M. tuberculosis,* it inhibits dihydropteroate synthetase enzyme.

KEY POINTS :

- Gastrointestinal toxicity is the main side effect.
- Inhibits onset of bacterial resistance to streptomycin and INH.
- **Drug interactions :**
  1. Oral absorption of digoxin may be reduced. So, increase in digoxin dosage may be necessary in patients of congestive heart failure.
  2. PAS interferes with GI absorption of vitamin B_{12}. Parenteral vitamin B_{12} supplementation may be required.

CAPREOMYCIN, AMIKACIN, AND KANAMYCIN :

Capreomycin, amikacin, and kanamycin are aminoglycoside antibiotics used as second-line drug for the treatment of tuberculosis.

KEY POINTS :

- The adverse reactions or side effects profile is similar to other aminoglycosides.
- Please refer to the chapter "Antibacterials" for further details.

NEWER ANTITUBERCULOUS DRUGS :

CIPROFLOXACIN, LEVOFLOXACIN AND OFLOXACIN :

Ciprofloxacin, levofloxacin, and ofloxacin are now also used for the treatment of mycobacterial infections.

KEY POINT :

- Please refer to the chapter "Antibacterials" for further details.

AZITHROMYCIN AND CLARITHROMYCIN :

Azithromycin and clarithromycin are newer macrolide antibiotics for the treatment of mycobacterial infections.

KEY POINT :

- Please refer to the chapter "Antibacterials" for further details.

REGIMENS FOR TREATMENT OF TUBERCULOSIS :

First-line antituberculous therapy (2EHRZ/4HR) in immunocompetent adult.

Isoniazid (H), rifampicin (R), pyrazinamide (Z), ethambutol (E) for *initial 2 months* followed by isoniazid and rifampicin for 4 (or 4-7) *months*, streptomycin can also be used in place of ethambutol.

OR **2(HRZE)$_3$**/4(HR)$_3$

administer isoniazid (H), rifampicin (R), pyrazinamide (Z), and ethambutol (E) in higher doses *thrice weekly for 2 months* followed by isoniazid (H) and rifampicin (R) *for 4 months* (by directly observed treatment-DOTS only).

The 7-month continuation phase is recommended only for :

- Patients with cavitary or extensive pulmonary TB disease caused by drug-susceptible organisms and with sputum culture positivity at the time of completion of 2 months of initiation treatment
- Patients whose initial phase of treatment did not include PZA; or
- Patients being treated with once-weekly INH and RPT and whose sputum culture at the time of completion of the initial phase (*i.e.*, after 2 months) is positive.

The earlier alternate day regimen has been replaced by a daily fixed drug combination regimen.

In Children :

Similar regimen of 2EHRZ/4HR is used in children with doses adjusted according to weight. Hepatotoxicity is less common in children, but monitoring for ocular side effects of ethambutol is difficult.

In Pregnancy :

Because of the risk of fetal ototoxicity and nephrotoxicity, aminoglycosides should not be used. Regimen remains the same except streptomycin. The safety of pyrazinamide in pregnancy is still not sufficiently documented.

IN LACTATION :

Lactating women who are under treatment can continue to breastfeed. A lactating mother should breastfeed before taking medication. Bottle-feeding should be done for the first feeding after taking the dose.

IN IMMUNOCOMPROMISED INDIVIDUALS :

The response to therapy is generally as favorable as in immunocompetent individuals. But side effects and drug interactions are more common in HIV-infected patients. For patients on PI-based antiretroviral therapy, rifabutin (5 mg/kg) is given instead of rifampicin. Nevirapine is also contraindicated during rifampicin-based ATT due to the risk of severe hepatotoxicity and drug interactions. The duration of ATT in HIV positive individuals may be required to be longer than the usual 6 months.

Under revised national tuberculosis control program (RNTCP), following regimens are practiced as second line therapy.

Isoniazid (H) resistant tuberculosis (no rifampicin resistance).	(6) Lfx R E Z
Rifampicin (R) resistant MDR Tuberculosis (MDR RR TB).	
Shorter MDR TB regimen	**Intensive** : (4-6) Mfx Km/Am EtoCfz Z H E **Continuation** : (5) MfxCfz Z E
All oral longer MDR TB regimen	(18-20) Bdq (6) LfxCfz Cs

Lfx-Levofloxacin, **R**-Rifampicin, **E**-Ethambutol, **Z**-Pyrizinamide, **Km**-Kanamycin, **Am**-Amikacin, **Eto**-Ethionamide, **Cfz**-Clofazimine, **Bdq**-Bedaquiline, **Cs**-Cycloserine, **Mfx**-Maxifloxicin.

N.B. : Figures in brackets indicates months (for duration of therapy).

The shorter MDR TB regimen : When the patient has not been exposed previously > 1 month to second line agents, without resistance to FQ + a second line agent, a shorter regime of 9-12 months may be used.

Before start of shorter MDR Tb regime, DST to FQ and second line injectable agents should be done.

The all oral longer MDR regimen includes at least four drugs:

- Three group A + one group B
- Two group A + two group B
- If regimen can't be completed with group A and B, group C is to be used.

This oral long regimen is usually preferred by patient and physician, in pregnancy, disseminated, CNS TB, Extrapulmonary Tb in PLHIV, confirmed resistance or suspected ineffectiveness in the shorter MDR regimen, exposure to short MDR regime drugs > 1 month in absence of susceptibility data.

In patients with MDR/RR TB, elective lung partial resection may be used alongside a recommended MDR-TB regimen.

BEDAQUILINE :

It belongs to a new class of antibiotics viz. diarylquinolines that is bactericidal to mycobacteria. It is a wonder drug for patients with multidrug resistant tuberculosis. It has also kindled hope of a cure for XDR-TB though the outcome in such patient is also dependent on severity of disease and host immunity.

MECHANISM OF ACTION :

It inhibits the proton pump of mycobacterial ATP synthase, needed for generation of energy in mycobacteria.

INDICATIONS :

1. Bedaquiline is extremely effective in MDR-TB (multi-drug-resistant tuberculosis) and
2. It is also effective for XDR-TB (Extensively drug resistant tuberculosis).

DOSE AND PREPARATION :

100 mg tablet (SIRTURO). Typical adult dose is 400 mg once daily for the first two weeks followed by 200 mg three days a week for the next 22 weeks. The dose should be taken at a fixed time after food and there should be a minimum 48 hour interval between these doses.

SIDE EFFECTS :

Gastrointestinal intolerance (anorexia, nausea, vomiting, diarrhea) and otovestibular toxicity. Prolongation of QT interval and elevation of transaminases.

REGIMENS FOR ATYPICAL MYCOBACTERIAL INFECTIONS :

Atypical mycobacterial infections are not as responsive to antituberculous therapy as infections caused by *M. tuberculosis.* Surgical intervention is required at times, for treatment of skin infections caused by atypical mycobacterial infections like swimming pool granuloma, scrofuloderma due to M. scrofulaceum, or Buruli's ulcer.

TABLE 7.2 : **Regimens for atypical mycobacterial infections**

Atypical mycobacterial infection	Antituberculous therapy
M. marinum infection	Cotrimoxazole 2 tablets b.i.d. for 8-16 weeks or minocycline 100 mg b.i.d. for 8-16 weeks or rifampicin plus ethambutol
M. kansasii infection	Combination therapy (2 or 3) out of the drugs like rifampicin, ethambutol, isoniazid, cotrimoxazole, azithromycin, clarithromycin, ciprofloxacin, minocycline for 18 months
Infections caused by *Mycobacterium* avium complex (MAC).	Clarithromycin 500 mg b.i.d. or azithromycin 500 mg/day plus ethambutol 800 mg ± rifabutin. In resistant cases, add amikacin or levofloxacin
Infection caused by *M. ulcerans*	Rifampicin 600 mg/day PO is effective in small ulcers or preulcerative lesions only

DIRECTLY OBSERVED TREATMENT-SHORT COURSE CHEMOTHERAPY (DOTS) :

Noncompliance is a major problem with antituberculous therapy and is seen mainly in drug addicts, HIV-infected patients, the homeless, and in patients who failed to respond to previous therapy. This gives rise not only to increased mortality in patients, but also leads to transmission of more severe multi-drug resistant tuberculosis (MDR-TB) in the community. This has led to the concept of directly observed therapy (DOTS) in which the patient swallows tablets in the presence of medical personnel (under direct supervision or observation).

This therapy applies to patients who are on daily treatment dosages or those on twice or thrice weekly therapy. DOTS program implemented at primary health care level has drastically improved cure rates of tuberculosis in India.

x=x=x=x=x

8

Oral and Injectable Steroids

Immunosuppressives and immunomodulatory drugs are widely used in dermatology for inflammatory, autoimmune, allergic, and other dermatoses. Immunosuppressives that are used extensively for dermatological indications can be classified as follows :

1. *Steroidal :* include corticosteroids which have stronger anti inflammatory effects.
2. *Nonsteroidal :* include cyclophosphamide, azathioprine, mycophenolate mofetil, leflunomide, cyclosporine etc.

Corticosteroids have dramatically improved the management of various dermatological conditions of varying etiologies as they possess diverse therapeutic effects.

CORTICOSTEROIDS :

Corticosteroids are antiinflammatory and immunosuppressive agents (Table 8.1).

MECHANISM OF ACTION :

Corticosteroids exert their *antiinflammatory* effects through the following mechanisms :

1. Stabilization of lysosomal membranes.
2. Inhibition of prostaglandins and leukotrienes synthesis by blocking phospholipases.
3. Decreased chemotaxis of proinflammatory cells at the sites of inflammation by exerting vasoconstriction effect of dermal vasculature.

Corticosteroids exert their *immunosuppressive* effects through the following mechanisms :

1. Induction of lymphocyte and eosinophil apoptosis.
2. Depletion of Langerhans cells in epidermis and dermis.
3. Decreased immunoglobulin synthesis by B-cells.
4. Decreased IL-2 production by T-cells.

Corticosteroids bind to cytosolic receptors in the cell and GC-receptor complex enters nucleus to bind with genomic DNA to influence or inhibit production of pro-inflammatory cytokines through trans-activation and trans-repression.

TABLE 8.1 Classification of corticosteroids

Drug	Duration of action (in hours)	Relative mineralocorticoid (MC) activity	Relative glucocorticoid (GC) activity
Short acting :			
Cortisone	8-12h	0.8	0.8
Hydrocortisone	8-12 h	1	1
Intermediate acting :			
Prednisone	24-36 h	0.8	4
Prednisolone	24-36 h	0.8	4
Deflazacort	24-36 h	—	—
Triamcinolone	24-36 h	0	5
Methyl prednisolone	—	Minimal	5
Long acting :			
Betamethasone	36-54 h	Negligible	30
Dexamethasone	36-54 h	Minimal	30
Fludrocortisone	12-36 h	125-150	10-15

INDICATIONS :

1. Immunobullous disorders, *e.g.* pemphigus vulgaris, bullous pemphigoid, cicatricial pemphigoid, linear IgA dermatosis, acquired epidermolysis bullosa.
2. Autoimmune connective tissue disorders, *e.g.* systemic lupus erythematosus, dermatomyositis.

3. Systemic vasculitis, *e.g.* Small vessel leukocytoclastic vasculitis, Wegener's granulomatosis, periarteritis nodosa, etc.
4. Neutrophilic dermatoses, *e.g.* Sweet's syndrome, pyoderma gangrenosum, etc.
5. Allergic disorders, *e.g.* severe urticaria, angioedema.
6. Widespread and recalcitrant eczemas, *e.g.* atopic eczema.
7. Erythroderma with life-threatening systemic complications.
8. Severe Type-I lepra reactions and Type-II lepra reactions especially in the presence of neuritis, iridocyclitis, or epididymoorchitis.

OPTIONAL INDICATIONS OF STEROIDS INCLUDE :

9. Acute widespread lichen planus.
10. Severe drug eruptions including drug hypersensitivity syndrome, erythroderma, widespread erythema multiforme bullous fixed drug eruption.
11. Sarcoidosis.
12. Generalized pustular psoriasis including impetigo herpetiformis though other drugs are now preferred.
13. Graft versus host disease.
14. Acne conglobata and acne fulminans.
15. Addisonian pigmentation due to adrenal insufficiency and recalcitrant acne vulgaris/hirsutism due to elevated androgen levels (*Low dose :* 0.125-0.325 mg dexamethasone at night).
16. Low dose steroids are frequently used in autoimmune diseases like vitiligo alopecia areata but their efficacy is variable.

Indications where use of steroids is controversial :

1. Stevens-Johnson syndrome and toxic epidermal necrolysis.
2. Herpes zoster for prevention of postherpetic neuralgia (PHN).

3. Hemangioma in infants.
4. Systemic sclerosis.

There are different classes of steroids available in the market with different half lives and potency. Also requirement of steroid dosages is different for different indications. For the sake of having uniformity of steroid dosage across different classes, the concept of steroid equivalence has been in vogue and is practiced since long time by dermatologists in selecting a corticosteroid for a given dermatological disorder. This has been depicted in the following Table.

TABLE 8.2 : **Steroid equivalence, doses, and preparations**

Drug	Steroid equivalence Doses	Doses	Preparations in the market
Hydrocortisone	20 mg	100 mg i.v.	EFFCORLIN 100 mg vial
Prednisolone	5 mg	1 mg/kg/day (2 mg/kg for pemphigus vulgaris)	OMNACORTIL 10, 20, 40 mg tablets
Deflazacort	6 mg	1 mg/kg/day	DEFCORT 1, 6, 30 mg tablets
Triamcinolone	4 mg	Equivalent doses to prednisolone	KENACORT 4 mg tab, Injection 10 and 40 mg/ml (Depot preparation)
Methyl prednisolone	4 mg	500-1000 mg i.v. x 3 consecutive days for pulse; equivalent doses to prednisolone for others	PREDNIMET 4, 16 tablets; SOLUMEDROL 500 mg/vial injection
Betamethasone	0.75 mg	0.1 mg/kg for oral mini pulse (OMP); equivalent doses to prednisolone for others	BETNESOL 0.5; BETNESOL 1 mg FORTE
Dexamethasone	0.75 mg	100 mg iv. x 3 consecutive days for pulse; equivalent doses to prednisolone for others	DECADEK 4 mg tablet, 2 mg/ml Injection

TABLE 8.3 : **Adverse effects of systemic steroids**

Side effects	Precipitating/risk factors	Prevention/management
Acute	**IV intermediate/long-acting steroids**	
Anaphylaxis	None	Secure "ABC," Inj. Epinephrine 0.3 cc s.c. stat. Intradermal tests at later dates
Electrolyte disturbances	Hypokalemia due to other causes	Oral/i.v. K^+ supplementation
Psychosis	Psychiatric illness	Antipsychotic drugs
Hyperglycemia	Diabetes mellitus	Inj PI (plain insulin) 10 U i.v. in 500 ml NS
Chronic	**Long term use of steroids**	
Osteoporosis/ Osteopenia	Thin built, female, menopause, increased age, inactive patients	DEXA Scan Calcium 500 mg t.i.d. + Vit. D_3 800 IU, Alendronate or riseodronate 70 mg-35 mg/week, moderate exercises
Avascular necrosis	Trauma, smoking, alcohol, hyper-coagulable states	Prompt referral, MRI, core decompression, joint replacement
Gastric/duodenal ulceration	Acid peptic disease, NSAIDs	Proton pump inhibitors, H_2-antihistamines, sucralfate suspension
Steroid induced diabetes	DM, obesity, family history	Diabetic diet, oral hypoglycemics, insulin
Steroid-induced hypertension	Hypertension, elderly patients, steroid treatment with MC action	Salt-restricted diet, antihypertensives like amlodipine, atenolol, etc.
Weight gain	Obesity, steroids with MC action	Avoid steroids with potent MC action
HPA axis suppression	High dose CS, longer acting CS, divided doses, evening dosages, dosages more than 3-4 weeks parenteral CS preparations	Morning single dose, avoid i.m. preparation, and potent steroids, basal cortisol estimation for tapering of steroids
Infections	High dose CS, other immunodeficiency states including HIV, chemotherapeutic drugs, concomitant immunosuppressives	Anti-infective agents, rapid tapering of steroids, control of sugars and other co-morbidities
Agitation/ psychosis	CS above 80 mg/day, previous psychiatric illness, females	Antipsychiatric drugs, psychotherapy

Of the above, steroids that are frequently used or found convenient by majority of dermatologists in India in their day-to-day practice include prednisolone, betamethasone and dexamethasone. However, use of oral methyprednisolone and deflazacort have increased over a period of time due to some advantages that have been claimed. As mentioned earlier, although there are differences in effects and side effects, most of the steroids when used for a longer duration of time and in high dosages can result into various adverse effects which are mentioned in the following Table (Table 8.3).

While prescribing steroids, patients need to be educated about possible side effects of oral or injectable corticosteroids. Following are general instructions to the patient, especially when long-term high dose steroid therapy is planned.

Dos :

1. Moderate exercise.
2. Take a potassium rich diet (banana, pineapple juice, coconut water etc) and calcium rich diet (ragi, green leafy vegetables, milk and milk products like cheese, butter milk).
3. Inform your doctor/specialist regarding the doses of steroids taken or missed.
4. Maintain a steroid card.
5. Take adjuvant medications regularly for the prevention of steroid side effects.
6. Get your body weight and blood investigations done as per your doctor's advice.
7. If fever, cough or hemoptysis develop, please inform or visit doctor to rule out possibility of pulmonary tuberculosis.

Don'ts

1. Do not miss your daily doses of steroids.

2. Do not share your tablets with other patients, friends, or relatives.
3. Do not visit overcrowded places.

PREGNANCY CATEGORY – C :

REMARKS :

- Cortisol-binding globulin (CBG) is decreased in hypothyroidism, kidney and liver disease, and obesity with increased free CS, while hyperthyroidism, pregnancy, and estrogen therapy increase CBG and subsequently decrease free CS.
- Corticosteroids in the free form are water insoluble and thus used as tablets and not for parenteral use. Chemically bound CS to ester (acetate and acetonide) form has limited water solubility but is lipid soluble and is used for oral, intramuscular, intralesional and intraarticular administration. Chemically bound CS to succinate and phosphate salts is readily soluble in water and ideal for intravenous use.
- HPA axis suppression occurs when the duration of therapy exceeds 3-4 weeks or when long-acting preparations like betamethasone or dexamethasone are used. In such cases, the sudden withdrawal of steroids or a sudden increase in body requirements for steroids (trauma, surgery, infections, etc.) may precipitate adrenal crisis.
- Morning single dose of steroids, and if appropriate, alternate day therapy is ideal as they minimize risk of HPA suppression.
- For steroid responsive acute dermatoses, 30-60 mg of prednisolone tapered over 10-14 days is effective.
- Oral methylprednisolone has faster onset of action, shorter biological half life and slightly higher potency as compared to prednisolone (4 mg of it is equivalent to 5 mg of prednisolone). It is claimed to have lesser musculoskeletal side effects but the evidence is weak.

- Deflazacort is the newer derivative of prednisolone with minimum mineralocorticoid action and supposedly lesser frequency of side effects like osteoporosis, hyperglycemia, acid-peptic disease. However, deflazacort is relatively expensive and side effects still occur.
- Oral minipulse therapy (OMP) consisting of oral betamethasone or dexamethasone is widely used by Indian dermatologists in patients of spreading vitiligo, alopecia areata, lichen planus etc. especially in children with good efficacy. However exact studies on concentration achieved by drugs used in OMP and its subsequent effects on efficacy and safety in patients remains unknown. Also with higher dose of CS as used in pulse form only results in modest increase in duration of action. In spite of this, oral mini-pulse therapy is popular due to its lesser frequency and severity of side effects. It is especially suited in chronic autoimmune diseases like vitiligo and alopecia areata which commonly respond to lower doses of steroids and where it has been successful in reducing the cumulative dose of steroids needed.

INJECTABLE CORTICOSTEROIDS :

Injectable corticosteroids have specific place in the management of various acute and chronic dermatological disorders.

Indications of injectable steroids :

1. Severe autoimmune disorders like pemphigus vulgaris or acute SLE or acute dermatomyositis with poor oral intake or patients with altered consciousness.
2. Acute urticaria, angioedema and anaphylactic shock (hydrocortisone).
3. Adrenal shock in Type II lepra reaction in lepromatous leprosy (hydrocortisone).
4. Life-threatening generalized pustular psoriasis.

5. Patients who cannot tolerate oral steroids or have developed gastrointestinal side effects of oral steroids.

ADVANTAGES OF INJECTABLE STEROIDS :

- Excellent bioavailability.
- Rapid action.
- Minimum GI side effects of steroids.
- Can be used in patients with altered consciousness.

DISADVANTAGES OF INJECTABLE STEROIDS :

- Pain and injection site reactions, abscesses.
- Tapering difficult for depot steroids like triamcinolone acetonide.
- Difficult for use in children.

Some of the preparations and dosages of injectable steroids are described below in the following ***Table 8.4.***

SIDE EFFECTS **of injectable corticosteroids :**

- Electrolyte disturbances
- Anaphylaxis
- Seizures
- Psychosis.
- Suppression of HPA axis when long-acting injectable steroids are used.
- All other side effects of oral steroids may appear if the number of days of therapy extends beyond 2 weeks.

KEY POINTS :

- Intramuscular administration of steroids has disadvantages of unpredictable or variable absorption despite guaranteed dose, difficult tapering, and HPA axis suppression.

TABLE 8.4 : **Injectable steroids**

Drug	Steroid equivalence	Doses	Preparations
Hydrocortisone	20 mg	100 mg i.v.	EFCORLIN 100 mg/vial
Methyl prednisolone	4 mg	500-1000 mg i.v. X 3 consecutive days for pulse; equivalent doses to prednisolone for others	SOLUMEDROL 500 mg injection
Triamcinolone acetonide	4 mg	Equivalent doses to prednisolone	KENACORT 10, 40 mg/ml injection
Betamethasone	0.75 mg	Equivalent doses to prednisolone	BETNESOL 4 mg/ml injection
Dexamethasone	0.75 mg	100 mg i.v. x 3 consecutive days for pulse; equivalent doses to prednisolone for others	DECADEK 4 mg tablets, 2 mg/ml injection
Hydrocortisone (depot preparation)	20 mg	25 mg IL every 4 weeks	WCORT 25 mg/ml vial IL Inj (IL-Intralesional)
Triamcinolone acetonide(depot preparation)	4 mg	10 mg IL, 40 mg i.m. every 4-8 weeks (dose and frequency of dosing depends upon clinical response and side effects)	KENACORT 10 mg/ml or 40 mg/ml i.m./IL use (IL-intralesional)
Methyl prednisolone acetate (depot preparation)	4 mg	10 mg IL, 40-160 mg i.m. every 4-8 weeks (dose and frequency of dosing depends upon clinical response and side effects)	DEPOMEDROL 10 mg/ml, 40 mg/ml i.m/IL use (IL-injection).

- Injectable steroids especially long acting do not permit diurnal variations of cortisol levels unlike single dose morning oral CS thereby increasing chances of HPA suppression.
- Methylprednisolone pulse is mostly preferred by rheumatologists for early and effective control of acute SLE, acute dermatomyositis or other acute autoimmune disorders.

- Injectable steroids are an essential part of DC/DCP pulse therapy (described in the following paragraphs).

DC/DCP PULSE THERAPY :

Pulse therapy with steroids is either intravenous dexamethasone pulse (DC) or more commonly dexamethasone-cyclophosphamide pulse (DCP) therapy regimen. It consists of giving 100 mg dexamethasone for an average adult dissolved in 500 ml of normal saline/5% dextrose as a slow intravenous drip over 2 h on 3 consecutive days. On the second day, 500 mg of cyclophosphamide is added in the same drip but dexamethasone and cyclophosphomide is added exclusively to 5% dextrose solution. This constitutes one DCP. Such DCPs are repeated at exactly 28-day intervals, counted from the first day of the pulse. In between the DCPs, the patient may receive only 50 mg cyclophosphamide orally per day. In children under 12 years, whenever indicated half of the adult doses are given. Indications of intravenous dexamethasone (with or without cyclophosphamide) pulse therapy :

1. Pemphigus vulgaris, bullous pemphigoid, acquired epidermolysis bullosa.
2. Systemic lupus erythematosus, dermatomyositis, systemic sclerosis.
3. Pyoderma gangrenosum, Behcet's syndrome.
4. Rapidly spreading and extensive alopecia areata (experimental).

Situations where DC pulse is preferred :

1. Patients who cannot tolerate high doses of daily steroids.
2. Patients who have developed side effects of daily corticosteroids.
3. Patients who are in clinical remission but have to take maintenance doses of corticosteroids/immunosuppressive drugs.

4. However, some dermatologists prefer to use DCP therapy as the first-line therapy for the above indications due to its lower side effects profile and higher patient compliance. Introduction of rituximab has provided an additional option in pemphigus patients.

CONTRAINDICATIONS :

Pregnancy and lactation :

- DCP therapy can be given in children when benefits overweigh the risk involved.
- DCP therapy can also be given to patients having diabetes mellitus, hypertension, hyperacidity, osteoporosis, tuberculosis, etc., but each patient must receive additional appropriate treatment for the concomitant disease as required.

SIDE EFFECTS :

Side effects include weakness and tiredness due to corticosteroid withdrawal for days after the pulse, bad taste in the mouth, and loose motions coinciding with or immediately after the pulses. Occasional patients may develop hypertension or sudden shifts in electrolytes, especially if the dexamethasone is given rapidly. This may lead to hyperkalemia and arrhythmias. Patients with any cardiac problems may also be given DCP therapy under cardiac monitoring with due diligence. Additional possibility of cardiotoxicity due to cyclophosphamide should be kept in mind and cardiology opinion should be sought.

PASRICHA'S REGIMEN (MODIFIED) FOR THE TREATMENT OF PEMPHIGUS :

Phase I :

DCP therapy at 28-day intervals with daily cyclophosphamide 50 mg orally till all lesions heal and no new lesions appear.

Phase II :

DCP therapy at 28-day intervals with daily cyclophosphamide 50 mg orally for up to 9 months after Phase I.

Phase III :

Daily cyclophosphamide only for 9 months after Phase II.

Phase IV :

Observe for 1 year with no therapy.

If any new lesions appear during Phases II-IV, the patient goes back to Phase I.

MONITORING NEEDED DURING PULSE THERAPY :

Intrapulse Monitoring :

- Monitor pulse and BP every 15 min for 1st I h, then for every 30 min.
- Give infusion slowly over 2 h (60-65 drops/min).
- Once pulse is over, send post-pulse investigations (serum electrolytes, random blood sugar, and BUN) and prompt collection of the reports.

Interpulse Monitoring :

- Hb, CBC (10 days after pulse initially, every month for 3-6 months, if no complications then every 3 months).
- LFT, RET.
- Blood sugars (if patient is on daily oral steroids or diabetic).
- Serum electrolytes.
- Urine routine microscopy.
- X-ray chest (only if patient is symptomatic otherwise once in 6 months).
- Urine cytology.

With the advent of rituximab, anti-CD20 monoclonal antibody which inhibits synthesis of pemphigus causing anti-desmoglein antibodies, use of DC pulse has declined over the last few years. However, DC pulse remains an effective and less expensive therapy for the treatment of pemphigus vulgaris in resource limited set ups in many parts of India.

x=x=x=x=x

9

Non-steroidal Immunosuppressive Drugs

Non-steroidal immunosuppressive agents are used either alone or as steroid sparing agents for various dermatoses requiring long term immunosuppression. Commonly used non-steroidal immunosuppresive agents are :

1. Methotrexate
2. Cyclophosphamide
3. Azathioprine
4. Cyclosporine and tacrolimus
5. Mycophenolate mofetil
6. Leflunomide

METHOTREXATE :

Antimetabolite agent with antiinflammatory properties and immunosuppressive effect.

MECHANISM OF ACTION :

Inhibits DNA synthesis by competitively and irreversibly inhibiting enzyme, dihydrofolate reductase (DHFR), which converts dihydrofolate to tetrahydrofolate essential for DNA synthesis.

Methotrexate increases local concentration of adenosine antiinflammatory mediator, by blocking AICART enzyme.

It decreases the concentration of S-adenyl methionine (SAM proinflammatory mediator) by blocking methionine synthetase.

It causes immunosuppression by lymphocyte inhibition.

INDICATIONS :

1. Psoriasis including non-responsive or disabling plaque psoriasis of more than 20% BSA, psoriatic arthritis, pustular psoriasis, and psoriatic erythroderma.
2. Reiter's disease (for cutaneous and rheumatologic manifestations).
3. Dermatomyositis (useful predominantly for muscle involvement).
4. Vasculitis and SLE.
5. Atopic dermatitis, Disabling allergic contact dermatitis, Vitiligo, LP, Alopecia areata, Autoimmune urticaria.
6. Generalised morphea and systemic sclerosis.
7. Sarcoidosis (with systemic involvement).
8. Mycosis fungoides (patch and plaque stage).
9. Pemphigus vulgaris.
10. Pityriasis rubra pilaris (higher doses as compared to psoriasis).
11. Crusted scabies (MTX rarely required these days).

DOSES AND PREPARATIONS :

- 7.5-15 mg/week.
- NEOTREXATE, ONCOTREX, FOLITRAX 2.5-15 mg tablet.
- IMUTREX 15 mg/ml (2 ml injection), FOLITRAX 25/50 mg/2 ml, given i.m./s.c. especially in patients with GI side effects.

PREGNANCY CATEGORY – X :

ADVERSE EFFECTS :

Systemic :

Mucositis, nausea, vomiting, abdominal pain, hepatotoxicity, including liver cirrhosis (long term), pancytopenia, nephrotoxicity (with high doses), stress fractures, hypersensitivity pneumonitis (Idiosyncratic immune reaction), pulmonary fibrosis.

Cutaneous :

Aphthous stomatitis, alopecia, hyperpigmentation, toxic epidermal necrolysis, ulceration in psoriatic plaques with acute methotrexate toxicity, erythema recall after discontinuation of PUVA therapy.

ACUTE METHOTREXATE TOXICITY :

Most cases of acute methotrexate toxicity are due to medication error and are completely preventable. Prescritpions should be carefully and clearly written and explained and re-explained to patients and relatives in their local dialect. The most common mistake is to accidentally consume the tablet daily and patients, especially the elderly should be cautioned against it.

Signs and Symptoms :

- Nausea, vomiting, diarrhea (earliest).
- Fever, arthralgias.
- Mucositis, painful skin ulceration, erythema and ulceration of psoriasis plaques.
- Photosensitivity.
- Bone marrow suppression.
- Multiorgan failure.

Management :

- Adequate hydration : 2-3 L/m^2/ day. Urine output should be maintained at 100 ml/ hour.
- Alkalinization of urine to prevent crystallization, 40-50 mEq of sodabicarbonate per litre of IV fluid.
- Leucovorin (Folinic acid) replenishes the intracellular stores of tetra hydrofolate given 10-30 mg iv bolus (or higher than the last dose of methotrexate) followed by 20-30 mg given every 6 hours. After the crises subsides, it is to be continued for several days orally 20 mg BD.
- In cases of neutropenia, GM-CSF is given 300 mg s.c for 3 consecutive days.
- Inj Glucarpidase 50 U/Kg bolus brings down the blood levels of methotrexate within 15 mins. It is helpful when given within 48 hours. It prevents renal shut down caused by methotrexate. Leucovorin should not be given 2 hours before or after glucarpidase.

KEY POINTS :

- Various studies have shown that a single dose of methotrexate on one fixed day of every week is as effective as three divided doses 12 hours apart.
- Folic acid supplementation (5 mg/day except on methotrexate days) prevents gastrointestinal side effects of methotrexate and reduces severity of acute methotrexate toxicity due to hypersensitivity.
- Although estimation of liver enzymes, ultrasonography, procollagen peptide CIII assay are recommended for the diagnosis of MTX hepatotoxicity, liver biopsy is considered by some to be the "goldstandard". However, recent reports indicate that aminoterminal peptide of procollagen III (levels more than 4.2 ng ml in Orion assay indicate hepatotoxicity) may emerge as a noninvasive and reliable indicator for monitoring of livertoxicity. It may be falsely high in psoriatic arthritis patients.

Of late, fibroscan has emerged as a non-invasive, recordable and reproducible test. Fibrotest is a composite serum marker using the values of GGT, Haptoglobulin, APO A1, bilirubin, a2 macroglobulin to predict liver fibrosis. Fibroscan *i.e.* transient elastography is an ultrasonic assessment of the tissue stiffness as an indirect measure of fibrosis (ultrasonic or magnetic resonance elastographic imaging). Abnormalities in at least two of the above tests may guide decision making for liver biopsy.

- Methotrexate-induced cirrhosis has less aggressive course.
- Methotrexate is to be avoided if creatinine clearance is < 30 ml/min.
- The combination of dyspnea, a history of MTX intake, upper lobe infiltrates on imaging studies and eosinophilia should arouse suspicion of MTX-induced lung toxicity.

TABLE 9.1 : **Monitoring guidelines for methotrexate therapy**

Test	Frequency
Complete blood count	Every 2-4 weeks for 1 month followed by once in 3 months, lymphocyte count of less than 3500/cu mm and platelet count of less than 100,000/cu mm indicate toxicity.
Liver enzymes (SGOT, SGPT)	Levels two times that of the baseline indicate hepatotoxicity.
Chest X-ray	At baseline and after 6 months.
Liver biopsy	After cumulative dose of 4g.

TABLE 9.2 : **Methotrexate therapy and liver biopsy**

Biopsy grade	Liver histopathology	Remarks
I	Normal, mild fatty infiltration, and portal inflammation	MTX can be given
II	Moderate-to-severe fatty infiltration and portal inflammation	MTX can be given
IIIA	Mild fibrosis	MTX can be given, but another liver biopsy after 6 months
IIIB	Moderate-to-severe fibrosis	MTX cannot be given
IV	Cirrhosis	MTX cannot be given

- Risk factors for methotrexate-induced cirrhosis are :
  - Alcoholism.
  - Past history of hepatitis.
  - Obesity.
  - Diabetes mellitus.
  - Daily methotrexate regimens.
  - Cumulative dose exceeding 4 g.
  - Impaired kidney function.

Contraception should be followed during methotrexate therapy and 3 months after its discontinuation.

CYCLOPHOSPHAMIDE :

This alkylating agent is a potent immunosuppressive drug.

> **Mechanism Of Action :**
> Inhibits DNA synthesis by causing intrastrand and interstrand cross-linking of DNA base pairs (cell cycle nonspecific). Effect on B cells is considered to be more pronounced than T cells.

Indications :

1. Immunobullous disorders like pemphigus, bullous pemphigoid, acquired epidermolysis bullosa, etc.
2. Autoimmune connective tissue disorders like systemic lupus erythematosus, dermatomyositis or systemic sclerosis.
3. Systemic vasculitis (as a steroid sparing agent) including Wegener's granulomatosis, microscopic polyangiitis, and polyarteritis nodosa.
4. Pyoderma gangrenosum.
5. Graft versus host disease.

DOSES AND PREPARATIONS :

- Oral 50 mg/day, 1-2 mg/kg/day.
- ENDOXAN, CYTOXAN 50 mg tablet.
- Intravenous : 500 mg/vial in powdered form to be dissolved in distilled water given monthly alone or along with dexamethasone pulse.

PREGNANCY CATEGORY – D :

TABLE 9.3 : **Monitoring guidelines for cyclophosphamide therapy**

Test	Frequency
Complete blood count	Weekly for a month and biweekly thereafter Leukocyte count of less than 4000-4500/cu mm and platelet count of less than 100,000/cu mm an indication for discontinuing therapy or at least reducing dose.
Urinalysis for red cells	Weekly (biweekly after 2-3 months of therapy).
Liver enzymes	Monthly (after 3-6 months, every 3 months).
Chest X-ray	At least every 6 months.
Urine cytology	At least every 6 months.

ADVERSE EFFECTS :

Systemic :

Nausea, vomiting, pancytopenia, hemorrhagic cystitis, cardiac toxicity including arrhythmias, pericardial effusion and cardiac failure, reactivation of tuberculosis, gonadal failure (amenorrhea and azoospermia), increased risk of carcinogenesis. Can also cause deafness, tinnitus.

Cutaneous :

Skin and nail hyperpigmentation, anagen effluvium, and pigmented bands over teeth.

KEY POINTS :

- Adequate hydration with plenty of oral/i.v. fluids are

required during cyclophosphamide administration to avoid hemorrhagic cystitis.

- Acute hemorrhagic cystitis usually manifests in first 24-48 hours of administration of high dose cyclophosphamide and is characterized by dysuria, increased frequency of micturition and hematuria. It usually resolves in 5-7 days of drug discontinuation. Sodium 2-mercaptoethane sulfonate (MESNA) prevents hemorrhagic cystitis by binding to acrolein, toxic metabolite of cyclophosphamide, which causes bladder toxicity. In severe cases, MESNA can be administered for therapeutic purpose.

  'Dose is usually 60-160% of dose of cyclophosphomide in case of toxicity and prophylactic dose is 20% of cyclophosphomide dose when injected, 4 and 8 hours after each dose (100 mg/ml injection and 400 mg tablet). As high dose intravenous cyclophosphomide is rarely used in dermatological indications (except in DC pulse), bladder toxicity is rarely seen.'

- Cyclophosphamide has propensity to cause bladder carcinoma and other malignancies on long-term use.

AZATHIOPRINE :

Anticancer agent is a potent immunosuppressive drug.

Mechanism Of Action :
Prodrug of 6-mercaptopurine inhibits purine synthesis.

Indications :

1. Immunobullous disorders.
2. Autoimmune connective tissue disorders.
3. Vasculitis (as a steroid sparing agent).
4. Pyoderma gangrenosum.

5. Atopic dermatitis, LP, vitiligo, progressive and recalcitrant alopecia areata.
6. Chronic actinic dermatitis (including persistent photoallergic contact dermatitis, persistent light reactors, and actinic reticuloid).
7. Graft versus host disease.

DOSES AND PREPARATIONS :

- 50 mg/day, 1-2 mg/kg
- AZORAN, AZR, NUZARINE 50 mg tablet.
- For patients who tolerate Azathioprine, it can be used in higher doses in once/twice weekly regimens.

PREGNANCY CATEGORY – D :

TABLE 9.4 : **Monitoring guidelines for azathioprine therapy**

Test	Frequency
Complete blood count	Weekly for first month, monthly for next 3 months and bimonthly thereafter
Liver function test	Monthly for first 3 months and bimonthly thereafter

Note : TPMT levels before initiating azathioprine is recommended in order to prevent the dreaded bone marrow suppression due to azathioprine usually seen in the initial few weeks.

ADVERSE EFFECTS :

Systemic :

Leukopenia, thrombocytopenia, weakness, sore throat, fever, nausea, vomiting, nephrotoxicity, hepatotoxicity, and reactivation of tuberculosis, rarely pancreatitis.

Cutaneous :

Alopecia, hyperpigmentation of skin and nails, allergic rash, pellagroid dermatitis.

Key Points :

- Azathioprine should not be given with drugs like 6-mercaptopurine and mycophenolate mofetil as all of them inhibits purine synthesis and enhances toxicity.
- Azathioprine does not cause gonadal dysfunction and hence can be used in young unmarried individuals unlike cyclophosphamide and methotrexate.
- Deficiency of enzyme hypoxanthine guanine phosphoribosyl transferase (HGPRT) as in Lesch-Nyhan syndrome, makes azathioprine ineffective, as the enzyme is required for the activation of azathioprine.
- Azathioprine should not be given with allopurinol, which inhibits enzyme xanthine oxidase required for metabolism or deactivation of azathioprine.
- Patients with low levels of thiopurine methyl transferase (TPMT), catabolic enzyme for azathioprine, have more chances of azathioprine bone marrow toxicity. Measurement of enzyme activity in red blood cells is the predictor for azathioprine toxicity and is recommended by FDA before starting azathioprine. However in most of the centers in India, genotypic studies to detect TPMT polymorphism are being done. This is said to have good correlation with phenotypic estimations. In resource poor settings where facilities for TPMT estimation is not available or in non-affording patients, serial estimation of complete blood counts is mandatory. In rare instances, inspite of doing TPMT levels, bone marrow toxicity has been reported.

CYCLOSPORINE :

Cyclosporine is a calcineurin-inhibitor, used as immunomodulatory agent in dermatology.

MECHANISM OF ACTION :

It modulates immune cell function by inhibiting calcineurin dependent dephosphorylation-activation of specific nuclear factors, thus preventing transcription of pro-inflammatory cytokines.

- It inhibits activation of T-cells by suppressing IL-2 production. This calcineurin inhibitors act specifically against antigen activated T-cells and thus is a specific immunosuppressive unlike other immunosuppressives like cyclophosphomide, azathioprine or methotrexate.
- It inhibits antigen presentation by Langerhan's cells and neutrophil chemotaxis.

INDICATIONS :

1. Recalcitrant psoriasis. Severe generalized pustular psoriasis, erythrodermic psoriasis, impetigo herpetiformis.
2. Atopic dermatitis and disabling contact allergic dermatitis.
3. Stevens Johnson syndrome/Toxic epidermal necrolysis.
4. Behcet's disease.
5. Epidermolysis bullosa acquisita.
6. Lichen planus, alopecia areata, Vitiligo, autoimmune urticaria.
7. Pyoderma gangrenosum.

DOSES AND PREPARATIONS :

NEORAL, PSORID 2-5 mg/kg/day, increments should not be more than 0.5-1 mg/kg/day at 2-4 week intervals. *Dose for psoriasis :* Cyclosporine can be started at 5 mg/kg till adequate response is attained and gradually tapered by 0.5-1 mg/kg every 2-4 weeks till maintenance dose is reached OR it can be started at 2-3 mg/kg and dose increased by 0.5-1 mg/kg every 2-4 weeks according to patients tolerance.

PREGNANCY CATEGORY – C :

TABLE 9.5 : **Monitoring guidelines for cyclosporine therapy**

Test	Frequency
Blood pressure	Weekly for the first 6 weeks, and then monthly
CBC, electrolytes, BUN	Every 2 weeks for 2 months, then monthly or every 2-3 months once stable
Creatinine, and uric acid	Every 6 months in patients on long-term therapy
Creatinine clearance estimation	If needed
Hyperlipidemia	Monthly for first 3 months
Weight gain	Monthly for first 3 months, then 3 monthly for next 6 months

ADVERSE EFFECTS :

Systemic :

Nephrotoxicity, hypertension, hyperkalemia, hypertriglyceridemia, hyperuricemia, hyperglycemia, hypomagnesaemia, worsening of pre-existing infections or occurrence of new infections.

Intolerance, nausea, vomiting, gastritis, diarrhea, dizziness, headache, flushing, tingling, tremors, cramps, edema feet.

Cutaneous :

Acneiform eruptions, hirsutism and hypertrichosis, gingival hyperplasia, cutaneous infections, cutaneous malignancies.

KEY POINTS :

- The main systemic side effects of cyclosporine, namely hypertension and nephrotoxicity, appear to be related to drug-induced endothelin release independent of calcineurin inhibition.
- Cyclosporine trough levels (wholeblood concentration

before next dosing) greater than 200-300 ng/ml are associated with toxicity.

- Nephropathy can be reduced by avoiding doses greater than 5 mg/kg/day and by avoiding elevation in serum creatinine 30% above baseline. Acute toxicity is reversible while chronic toxicity is irreversible.
- If the serum creatinine level rises more than 30% above baseline, repeat measurements are required within 2 weeks. If persistent, cyclosporine dose is reduced by at least 1 mg/kg/day (for 1 month). If serum creatinine remains more than 30% above baseline even after 1 month then cyclosporine should be stopped.
- Hypertension (mean diastolic pressure > 95 mm Hg) on two consecutive occasions requires a decreased dose of cyclosporine or introduction of antihypertensives like calcium channel blockers, *i.e.* nifedipine and amlodipine and withdrawal of nonsteroidal antiinflammatory drugs if given concurrently.
- New onset hypertriglyceridemia (400-500 mg/dl) may require dose reduction.
- A combination of cyclosporine with retinoids is not only efficacious, but also protective against development of cutaneous malignancies.
- Contraindications for cyclosporine include renal disease, uncontrolled hypertension, gout, active infections and past or family history of skin cancers.

TACROLIMUS :

Mechanism Of Action :

It inhibits release of IL-2 from lymphocytes.

Dose :

0.05-0.1 mg/kg/day.

INDICATIONS :

1. Psoriasis.
2. Atopic dermatitis.

SIDE EFFECTS :

1. Nephrotoxicity.
2. Hypertension (lesser than that with cyclosporine).

PREGNANCY CATEGORY – 'C' :

MYCOPHENOLATE MOFETIL (MMF) :

Mycophenolate mofetil is the ester of mycophenolic acid (MPA).

MECHANISM OF ACTION : MMF blocks purine synthesis by inhibiting the enzyme Inosine Monophosphate Dehydrogenase (IMPDH).

- It induces apoptosis of activated T cells.
- It decreases the recruitment of lymphocytes and induces immune tolerance.

INDICATIONS :

1. Autoimmune bullous disorders.
2. Atopic dermatitis.
3. Psoriasis.
4. Pyoderma gangrenosum.
5. Hypertrophic and recalcitrant lichen planus.
6. Graft versus host disease.
7. Childhood vitiligo.

MMF is best suited for individuals in whom other systemic therapies are contraindicated because of hypertension, impaired renal function, or liver disease.

DOSES AND PREPARATIONS :

- 1 g twice daily, 30-40 mg/kg/day.
- CELLIMMUNE, CELLCEPT, MMF 500 mg tablet.
- A sodium salt of mycophenolate is now available and is associated with lesser gestrointenstinal side effects. The equivalent dose of this is 360 mg.

PREGNANCY CATEGORY – C :

ADVERSE EFFECTS :

Systemic :

Nausea, cramps, vomiting, and diarrhea are the most frequent side effects, leukopenia, and anemia are uncommon. Systemic infections are common.

Cutaneous :

Infections including candidiasis are frequent.

KEY POINTS :

- The mofetil ester provides the advantage of increased bioavailability with less side effects. Cost is the limiting factor.
- After oral administration, MMF is rapidly hydrolyzed to its active acid form, MPA. After oral administration, 93% of MMF is eliminated in the urine primarily as MPA glucuronide.
- Concurrent administration of salicylates and furosemide may lead to an accelerated elimination of MMF as MMF competes with these drugs for plasma albumin binding.
- MMF should not be used in combination with azathioprine as both block purine synthesis by the same pathway.

LEFLUNOMIDE :

Leflunomide is a newer immunomodulatory agent.

MECHANISM OF ACTION :

It inhibits pyrimidine synthesis of reversibly by inhibiting the mitochondrial dihydroorotate dehydrogenase. It inhibits T-cell proliferation and production of autoantibodies by B-cells.

INDICATIONS :

1. Psoriasis vulgaris and psoriatic arthropathy.
2. Bullous autoimmune disorders.
3. Wegener's granulomatosis and systemic vasculitis.
4. Dermatomyositis, Subacute cutaneous LE.

DOSES AND PREPARATIONS :

- 100 mg once daily for 3 days and then continue with 10-25 mg daily used to be practised before. However, this practice of using a loading dose is now out of favour due to higher changes of serious adverse cutaneous drug eruptions including DRESS syndrome, Stevens Johnson Syndrome and toxic epidermal necrolysis. Hence, currently 10 to maximum of 20 mg daily doses are commonly used.
- ARAVA, LEFNO 10, 20 mg tablets.

PREGNANCY CATEGORY – X :

ADVERSE EFFECTS :

Systemic :

Gastrointestinal disturbances, anemia, hepatotoxicity.

Cutaneous :

Drug hypersensitivity syndrome, SJ syndrome, 'TEN, erythroderma, exacerbation of SCLE.

x=x=x=x=x

10
Oral Retinoids

Retinoids are naturally occurring and synthetic compounds related to vitamin A but with enhanced biologic activities. Hence they are predominantly used for acne, psoriasis and disorders of keratinization.

MECHANISM OF ACTION :
Normalizes keratinization (regulates cell growth, differentiation and morphogenesis of keratinocytes).
Decreases cell cohesiveness ("antikeratinizing" and comedolytic effect) useful in acne vulgaris.
Prevents tumorigenesis and carcinogenesis.
Immunomodulatory action.

INDICATIONS OF ORAL RETINOIDS :

1. Pustular psoriasis, erythrodermic psoriasis, severe and recalcitrant psoriasis including palmo plantar psoriasis.
2. Acne vulgaris.
3. Rosacea, pyoderma faciale.
4. Keratinization disorders, *e.g.* ichthyoses, Darier's disease, keratoderma, pityriasis rubra pilaris, porokeratosis.
5. Epithelial cancers and precancerous conditions, *e.g.* Nevoidbasal cell carcinoma syndrome (Gorlin's syndrome), multiple actinic keratoses, epidermodysplasia verruciformis, xeroderma pigmentosum, leukoplakia.
6. Lichen planus (oral, erosive and hypertrophic), lichen sclerosus et atrophicus.

7. Non-epithelial malignancies *e.g.* mycosis fungoides' AIDS related Kaposi's sarcoma.
8. Recalcitrant hand eczema.
9. Granulomatous disease, *e.g.* sarcoidosis, granuloma annulare.
10. Extracellular matrix alterations, *e.g.* scleromyxedema, follicular mucinosis.
11. Miscellaneous, *e.g.* graft versus host disease, TAD (transient acantholytic dermatosis).

FDA approval :

Acitretin for psoriasis, Isotretinoin for acne, Bexarotene for mycoses fungoides. Alitretinoin for Kaposi's sarcoma in AIDS.

CONTRAINDICATIONS :

Absolute :

Pregnancy and lactation (Category – X).

Relative :

Hyperlipidemia, children, diabetes mellitus, liver disease, raised intracranial pressure, suicidal ideations.

MONITORING GUIDELINES :

KEY POINTS :

- Retinoids act through family of nuclear receptors RAR and RXR with their subtypes α, β, and γ Receptor drug complex affect transcription and translation of the genes involved in the process of keratinization.
- Vitamin A and its derivatives like tretinoin and isotretinoin act on all the retinoid receptors and hence are associated with more side effects. Selective retinoids act on specific retinoid receptor bringing down the possibility of side effects. (Tables 10.1, 10.2 & 10.3)

TABLE 10.1 : **Classification of oral retinoids**

Classification	Chemical structure	Retinoid	Half life
First-generation retinoids	Monoaromatic	Isotretinoin, tretinoin alitretinoin	Isotretinoin - 10-20 hours Tretinoin - 40-60 mins
Second-generation retinoids	Monoaromatic with replaced rings	Etretinate acitretin	80-160 days 50 hours
Third-generation retinoids	Polyaromatic (arotenoids)	Bexarotene, alitretinoin	

TABLE 10.2 : **Side effects of oral retinoids**

Side effects	Prevention/management
Cutaneous and mucosa/ (type l)	
Skin	Dryness, palmoplantar peeling, exfoliative dermatitis (bexarotene), photosensitivity, facial dermatitis, skin infections, pyogenic granuloma like lesions.
Oral mucosa	Cheilitis.
Nasal mucosa	Dryness.
Ocular mucosa	Dry eyes, blepharoconjunctivitis.
Hair	Telogen effluvium, hair thinning.
Nail	Fragile nails, onycholysis, paronychia.
Retinoid dermatitis	Ill-defined skin eruptions with retinoids uncommon).
Systemic (type II)	
Teratogenicity	Retinoid embryopathy.
Ocular	Delayed dark adaptation, photophobia, blurring of vision.
Gastrointestinal	Nausea, diarrhea, abdominal pain, elevated liver enzymes and bilirubin.
Neurologic	Headache (pseudotumor cerebri), depression, seizures, altered mood.
Metabolic	Hypertriglyceridemia, hypothyroidism (bexarotene).
Musculoskeletal system	Premature epiphyseal closure, diffuse interstitial skeletal hyperostosis (DISH), tendon and ligament calcification, myopathy.
Hematological system	Leukopenia and agranulocytosis (bexarotene), thrombocytopenia.

TABLE 10.3 : **Monitoring guidelines for oral retinoids**

At baseline, monthly for first 3-6 months and then every 3 months
Clinical examination
Liver function tests
Urine pregnancy test
Lipid profile
CBC with platelets (with bexarotene).
Renal function test (optional)

1. Absolutely contraindicated during pregnancy and lactation and those willing for conception.
2. Malformations known to occur with retinoid therapy include external ear abnormalities, hydrocephalus, microcephaly, dysmorphism, microphthalmia, cardiovascular, craniofacial, acral (more with etretinate), and axial skeletal abnormalities occur in almost 50% cases with first trimester isotretinoin exposure. Abortions occur in one third of patients.
3. Less frequent use of etretinate and acitretin as compared to isotretinoin and use in older population may be the reason for less teratogenicity observed with etretinate or acitretin.

- *Hypertriglyceridemia :*
  1. Reversible hypertriglyceridemia and hypercholesterolemia occurs more with isotretinoin and bexarotene therapy.
  2. "Statins" are preferred (though less effective) over gemfibrozil because of the drug interaction. Omega 3 fatty acids, diet such as fish, nuts also helps to reduce triglyceride levels.
  3. Hypertriglyceridemia is probably due to the displacement of triglyceride from albumin by retinoids and increased levels of circulating lipoproteins.

- *Drug Interactions :*
  1. Vitamin A, tetracyclines, gemfibrozil, macrolides, andazoles increases serum retinoid levels potentiating toxicity.
  2. Rifampicin, rifabutin, and aromatic anticonvulsants decrease serum levels.
  3. Retinoids potentiate toxicity of cyclosporine.
  4. Reduces efficacy of mini (progesterone) pills.
  5. Should not be given concurrently with other agents like vitamin A, tetracyclines, and steroids, which cause raised intracranial pressure.

- Retinoids and PUVA therapy are combined (Re-PUVA) to minimize doses of both retinoids and PUVA, to decrease the side effects and increase efficacy. Retinoids decrease the potential risk of malignancy associated with ultraviolet exposure.

ISOTRETINOIN :

Isotretinoin is a first-generation retinoid used for acne disorders.

Mechanism Of Action :

In addition to the mechanisms mentioned earlier, isotretinoin works in acne as follows :

1. Inhibits sebum production by inhibiting sebaceous proliferation, differentiation, decreasing sebaceous gland size and skin dihydrotestosterone and down regulation of androgen receptors in skin.
2. Antibacterial action : indirect action due to the reduction of follicular space and nutrient supply of *Propioni bacterium acnes.*
3. Antiinflammatory action.

INDICATIONS :

1. Severe nodulocystic acne, acne fulminans, and acne conglobate.
2. Moderate acne (Pillsbury grade II/III) that may produce scars or that is not responding to long-term (3 months) antibiotics therapy (to be used with discretion).
3. Gram-negative folliculitis.
4. Rosacea and pyoderma faciale.
5. Hidradenitis suppurativa (limited efficacy).

DOSES AND PREPARATIONS :

- 0.5 mg kg/day.
- ISOTRET, ACUTRET 10 mg, 20 mg tablet.

INSTRUCTIONS TO THE PATIENT :

1. Do not give/share tablets with other patients.
2. Isotretinoin can cause mucosal dryness (in 75% cases). It marks the onset of action. Vaseline can be applied to prevent and treat mucosal and skin dryness.
3. Avoid photoexposure; use sunscreens. Take tablets at night to avoid phototoxicity.
4. Initial flare up is possible. Report to the treating dermatologist.
5. Avoid pregnancy by atleast two methods of effective contraception.
6. Report if severe headache; inability to concentrate or alteration in mood occur.
7. Avoid certain drugs that are not advised by the dematologist/physician.
8. Avoid surgery/traumatic procedures on the face for 3-6 months (skin may become fragile after isotretinoin).
9. Do not donate blood or semen during or up to 1 month after therapy.

KEY POINTS :

1. Retinoid is the drug of choice for acne treatment as it affects all etiological factors in the pathogenesis of acne. Only isotretinoin possesses sebo-suppressive action among retinoids.
2. Lag period of 1-3 months may exist before the onset of therapeutic effect of isotretinoin.
3. Initial flare of the disease can be avoided by a course of systemic steroids 4 weeks prior to isotretinoin therapy tapered within next 4 weeks. Flare up may occur due to an impaired cutaneous barrier with secondary staphylococcal colonization.
4. Isotretinoin may alter expression of vascular endothelial growth factor (VEGF), thereby leading to increased incidence of pyogenic granulomas.
5. Treatment with isotretinoin need not be continued till clearance of all acne lesions as improvement in acne lesions continues even after the stoppage of isotretinoin.
6. Higher doses of isotretinoin for a longer duration are required for the treatment of truncal acne. Acne secondary to hyperandrogenism is also resistant to isotretinoin.
7. The commonest cause of isotretinoin failure is microcystic acne and closed comedones.
8. Contraceptive precautions are advocated during isotretinoin therapy and for 1 month after its stoppage as blood levels of isotretinoin return to physiologic levels within 10 days of treatment completion.
9. The chance of relapse after an isotretinoin course is related to the total cumulative dose of isotretinoin (120 mg/kg, with no further benefits more than 150 mg/kg) received during the course in question.

ETRETINATE AND ACITRETIN :

Etretinate and acitretin are second-generation retinoids.

MECHANISM OF ACTION :

Similar to other retinoids.

INDICATIONS :

Same as that with retinoids but less useful for acne disorders as compared to isotretinoin.

They are more useful for psoriatic erythroderma and generalized pustular psoriasis. An initial dose of 25 mg/day followed by a maintenance dose 20-50 mg/day is indicated for psoriasis.

DOSES AND PREPARATIONS :

- 0.25-1 mg/kg/day.
- ACITRIN, ACROTAC 10, 25 mg tablet.

KEY POINTS :

1. Acitretin is the acid metabolite of etretinate (etretinate is prodrug). Etretinate is lipophilic and is stored in the fat cells for up to 2 years after its stoppage. Hence, due to its teratogenicity, a woman treated with etretinate should not get pregnant for 2 years. Etretinate is no more available commercially.
2. Acitretin is rapidly eliminated from the body (elimination half life 2 days) as it is 50 times less lipophilic than etretinate. Some of the acitretin gets re-esterified into etretinate in the body. This necessitates that pregnancy should be avoided in women up to 2 years after stoppage of acitretin.
3. Alcohol should be avoided as it not only causes hepatotoxicity, but also convert acitretin to more toxic etretinate. Attention should be given to the use of cough syrups as they have high alcohol content.

BEXAROTENE :

Bexarotene is the specific RXR-selective retinoid (rexinoid).

Mechanism Of Action :
Induction of apoptosis of malignant cells.

Indications :

Cutaneous T-cell lymphoma.

Doses And Preparations :

TARGRETIN (not available in India) 150-300 mg/day for cutaneous T-cell lymphoma.

Key Points :

1. Absorption of bexarotene is increased with fatty meals. Excretion occurs primarily through the hepatobiliary system.
2. Clearance profile of bexarotene is similar to isotretinoin.
3. Bexarotene has higher chances of metabolic and hematological abnormalities, central hypothyroidism, and exfoliative dermatitis.

Alitretinoin :

Oral Alitretinoin has been approved in United States for AIDS related Kaposi's sarcoma and in Europe for treatment of chronic hand eczema. Availability is an issue in other parts of the world.

Alitretinoin is a first generation retinoid that has side effects similar to isotretinoin. Topical 0.1% gel alitretinoin gel has been found useful for recalcitrant hand eczema.

x=x=x=x=x

11

Systemic Photoprotective Agents

ANTIMALARIALS :

Antimalarials used in dermatology include :

- Chloroquine
- Hydroxychloroquine
- Quinine
- Quinacrine

TABLE 11.1 : **Comparison of chloroquine and hydroxychloroquine**

	Chloroquine (CQ)	**Hydroxychloroquine (HCQ)**
Salt	Phosphate (CQP)	Sulphate (HCQS)
Dosage	250-500 mg/day	200-400 mg/day
Ocular safety limit	3.5 mg/kg/day (for 6 months)	6.5 mg/kg/day (for 6 months)
Bioavailability	50%	Better
Protein binding	50-65%	Less common
GI tolerance	Poor	Good
Ocular toxicity	More common	Less common
Excretion	Mainly in urine	Mainly in bile
Renal failure	Should not be given	can be given but dose adjustment is required.

CHLOROQUINE AND HYDROXYCHLOROQUINE :

MECHANISM OF ACTION :

Antiinflammatory/immunomodulatory actions :

1. Stabilizes lysosomal membrane.

2. Reduces chemotaxis and phagocytosis of lymphocytes and macrophages.
3. Decrease in the T-cell pro-inflammatory cytokines like ILI, IL2, IL6 and TNF
4. Inhibits production of phospholipases leading to decreased leukotrienes and bradykinins.

Photoprotection (systemic sunscreen) :

1. Ability to bind to melanin, antioxidant effect, and blockage of a cascade of immunological actions that follow light exposure.
2. Bind to porphyrins and facilitate their clearance in urine.
3. Solubilization and mobilization of hepatic porphyrins and their clearance.

OTHER EFFECTS :

1. Hydroxychloroquine lowers triglycerides, cholesterol and glucose levels and thus HbA1c.
2. It inhibits platelet aggregation.
3. Membrane stabilization leading to antioxidant effect.

INDICATIONS IN DERMATOLOGY :

1. Lupus erythematosus and other photosensitivity dermatoses like :
   a. Polymorphous light eruption.
   b. Hutchinson's summer prurigo.
   c. Hydroa vacciniforme.
   d. Solar urticaria.
   e. Senear-Usher syndrome.
   f. Reticular erythematous mucinosis.
   g. Porphyria cutanea tarda.

2. Sarcoidosis.
3. Lepra reactions Type I and II.
4. Dermatomyositis.
5. Rheumatoid arthritis.

ANTIMALARIALS IN LE :

INDICATIONS :

1. CCLE (including tumid LE and lupus panniculitis) not responding to :
    - Avoidance of sunlight.
    - Topical sunscreens.
    - Topical/intralesional steroids.
2. Subacute and acute LE with cutaneous lesions, photosensitivity and arthritis.
3. Prevention of flare-ups in SLE.
4. Antiphospholipid antibody syndrome.

ANTIMALARIALS IN PORPHYRIA CUTANEA TARDA :

Hydroxychloroquine 100 mg thrice a week for 1 month followed by 200 mg thrice a week for 1 month and then 200 mg daily for 6-18 months or till the urinary uroporphyrin level falls below 100 μg/day

LESS COMMON INDICATIONS :

- Pemphigus foliaceus and vulgaris.
- Psoriatic arthritis.
- Recurrent/persistent erythema nodosum.
- Sjögren's syndrome.
- Actinic lichen planus.
- Rosacea.

EXPERIMENTAL INDICATIONS :

- Urticarial vasculitis.
- Generalized granuloma annulare.
- Lymphocytoma cutis.
- Necrobiosis lipoidica.
- Multicentric reticulohistiocytosis.

SIDE EFFECTS :

Gastrointestinal :

Nausea, vomiting, diarrhea (10% GI intolerability with chloroquine), raised transaminases.

Nervous System :

Irritability, nervousness, altered mood, psychosis, headache, vertigo, tinnitus, nystagmus, myopathy.

OCULAR (DOSE DEPENDENT) :

Reversible :

- Corneal deposits.
- Loss of accommodation (chloroquine).
- Retinal : premaculopathy field defects but vision intact.
- Retinal pigmentation.

Irreversible :

- Central scotoma and bull's eye retinopathy.
- Maculopathy loss of vision.
- Generalized pigmented retinopathy.

Prevention of ocular side effects : Though the ocular side effects are much less common with hydroxychloroquine, it is preferable to do baseline retinal examination. Informing the patient to report any eye problems and keeping communication channels open are helpful to detect early side effects. Amsler grid is a practical way of checking field defects in the clinic.

CUTANEOUS SIDE EFFECTS :

Rashes (maximum with quinacrine, up to 30%) :

- Urticaria.
- Lichenoid drug eruption.
- Morbilliform rash.
- Erythroderma.
- Purpura.
- Acute generalized exanthematous pustulosis (AGEP).

Pigmentary :

- Blue - black pretibial, face and palate (chloroquine binds with melanin pigment in dermis).
- Bleaching of hairs.
- Pigmentary bands over nails.

Exacerbation or induction of psoriasis :

- Fewer flare-ups with chloroquine (less than 10%) and fewer still with Hydroxychloroquine.

PREGNANCY CATEGORY – C :

MONITORING GUIDELINES :

TABLE 11.2 : **Monitoring guidelines for antimalarials**

Test	Frequency
Vision, perimetry, slit lamp examination, fundoscopy	Baseline and every 6 months for a year and then yearly.
Serum transaminases	At 1 month, 3 months, and 6 months.

KEY POINTS :

- The onset of action for chloroquine and

hydroxychloroquine is 2-8 weeks and an adequate response is usually achieved after 1-3 months.

- Less useful for hypertrophic and verrucous CCLE or for CCLE lesions in patients with SLE.
- The maximum ocular toxicity of antimalarials is seen with quinacrine and the minimum with hydroxychloroquine. Intermittent therapy can be given to prevent ocular toxicity.
- If there is no adequate response to HCQ at 1-3 months, change to chloroquine or to quinacrine 100 mg daily (monitoring of blood counts is required for quinacrine). Other immunosuppressives may be added.
- Hydroxychloroquine, when used for psoriatic arthritis, is not associated with any exacerbation of psoriasis (unlike chloroquine). However, it should be used with caution for psoriatic arthritis only for unresponsive cases.
- **Interactions :**
    1. Chloroquine and hydroxychloroquine are not combined for fear of additive retinal toxicity.
    2. Chloroquine and hydroxychloroquine increase levels of digoxin, D-penicillamine, methotrexate and cyclosporine.
    3. Kaolin and magnesium trisilicate decrease chloroquine absorption.
    4. Reduces bioavailabilitiy of ampicillin.
    5. Smoking decreases efficacy of antimalarials.

OTHER PHOTOPROTECTIVE AGENTS :

BETA-CAROTENE :

The photoprotective action of beta-carotene is at best mild and hence it should not be used as a substitute for antimalarials in photosensitive dermatoses.

Mechanism of Action :

1. Scavenging free radicals and reactive oxygen species (ROS) (antioxidant effect).
2. Preservation of Langerhans cells (immunopotentiation effect).

Indications In Dermatology :

1. Erythropoietic protoporphyria.
2. Congenital erythropoietic porphyria.
3. Hydroa vacciniforme.
4. Polymorphic light eruption.
5. Prevention against cancers.

Doses :

- 60-180 mg/day; children < 12 years of age mg/day.

Side Effects :

Yellowing of palms, soles, hands and feet, and to a lesser extent the face (carotenoderma), diarrhea, dizziness, joint pain, bruising (rare).

Key Points :

1. Serum levels of more than 600-800 μg/ml are required for therapeutic effect. These levels are achieved in 1-2 of therapeutic doses of beta-carotene.
2. Beta-carotene is known to interact with cholestyramine and vitamin A.

x=x=x=x=x

12
Psoralens, PUVA and Phototherapy

PSORALENS :

Psoralens are naturally occurring or synthetic photosensitizing agents widely used in dermatology for PUVA (Psoralen + UVA) therapy.

MECHANISM OF ACTION :

Inhibition of DNA, RNA, and protein synthesis :

1. Forms bifunctional adducts with cellular DNA inhibiting DNA synthesis.
2. Generates O_2 reactive species, which bind to RNA and cellular proteins.

Immunosuppressive effect :

1. Depletion of Langerhans cells.
2. Induces apoptosis of CD_4 lymphocytes.

Stimulation of melanogenesis :

1. Psoralens stimulate mitosis and proliferation of melanocyte on photoconjugation.
2. Increased melanization of melanosomes.
3. Increased transfer of melanosomes to keratinocytes.
4. Increased synthesis and activation of tyrosine.

TABLE 12.1 : **Psoralens and other photosensitizers**

Psoralen	Source	Remarks
8-methoxypsoralen (8-MOP)	Natural	More phototoxic after oral administration.
5-methoxypsoralen (5-MOP)	Natural	Less erythemogenic, does not induce intolerance reactions.
Trimethylpsoralen (Trioxsalen)	Synthetic	Less phototoxic after oral administration, more phototoxic when used topically
Khellin	Natural	No phototoxicity

INDICATIONS :

1. *Inflammatory autoimmune disorders :*
   - Psoriasis.
   - Pityriasis lichenoides chronica.
   - Pityriasis rosea.
   - Alopecia areata.
   - Lichen planus.
   - Morphea (high-dose UVA_1 therapy is more effective).
   - Graft versus host disease.

2. *Depigmenting disorders :*
   - Vitiligo.
   - Acquired leukoderma.
   - Pityriasis versicolor (not routinely advocated).

3. *Photosensitive dermatoses (to induce tolerance or "hardening") :*
   - Polymorphic light eruption.
   - Solar urticarial.
   - Photoallergic dermatitis.
   - Persistent light reaction and actinic reticuloid.

4. *Neoplastic/proliferative disorders :*
   - Patch and plaque stage of mycoses fungoides.
   - Hypopigmented mycosis fungoides.
   - Histiocytosis X.

5. *Pruritic dermatoses :*
   - Atopic dermatitis.
   - Urticaria pigmentosa.
   - Prurigo nodularis.
   - Pruritus associated with polycythemia vera.
   - Pruritic papular exanthem of HIV.

DOSES AND PREPARATIONS :

- 8-methoxypsoralen (8-MOP) 0.4-0.6 mg/kg OCTAMOP tablet 10 mg.
- 5-methoxypsoralen (5-MOP) – 1.2-1.8 mg/kg (better tolerated but not available in India).
- Trimethoxypsoralen (Trioxsalen) – 0.6 mg/kg TRIMOP tablet 5 mg, 25 mg.
- Khellin 100 mg PO daily, 2% khellin solution (less phototoxic but not available in India).

A liquid formulation of 8-MOP, available in soft capsule form (Oxsoralen-Ultra), in doses of 0.25-0.5 mg/kg, enhances bioavailability. However, liquid 8-MOP is associated with an increased incidence of nausea.

PREGNANCY CATEGORY – C :

Psoralens are contraindicated in pregnancy because of their effect on DNA.

SIDE EFFECTS :

1. *Due to psoralens :*
   - Gastrointestinal disturbances nausea and vomiting are most common during the first 2 weeks.

- Hepatotoxicity, elevation of transaminases.
- Pruritus and maculopapular rash.
- CNS disturbances like headache, vertigo, tinnitus, etc.

2. *Psoralens and ultraviolet A therapy (PUVA) :*

   a. *Acute (short term) :*

   - Tanning is the most common side effect of PUVA therapy.
   - PUVA-induced acute phototoxicity : presents as burning pain within an hour of exposure followed by blistering with or without erythema in 1-3 days. Delayed phototoxic reaction in the dark skinned occurs after 48 h without preceding erythema or burning.
   - Photo-onycholysis affects nails.
   - Photokoebnerization : Occurrence of new lesions of a pre-existing disease over sites of PUVA therapy.
   - Exacerbation of photosensitive dermatoses like herpes labialis, seborrheic dermatitis, pemphigus vulgaris, pemphigus foliaceous, etc.
   - Exacerbation of psoriasis or precipitation of pustular psoriasis in psoriatics.
   - Precipitation of a secondary attack of herpes simplex or rarely herpes zoster.

   b. *Chronic (long term) :*

   - Photoaging of skin (heliosis).
   - PUVA lentigines.
   - Pigmentation of skin (tanning) and nails.
   - Melanoma and nonmelanoma cancers (especially SCC) seen in white skinned except when another confounding factor is present in Indians like arsenic poisoning or immunosuppression.

- Cataract (anterior cortical) and corneal opacities (when eye protection is not strict).

CONTRAINDICATIONS :

Absolute :

- Hypersensitivity to psoralens.

Relative :

- Pregnancy and lactation.
- Children below 12 years of age.
- Lupus erythematosus and other photosensitive dermatoses including porphyrias.
- Hepatic or renal disease.
- Cataract.
- Pemphigus and bullous pemphigoid (as PUVA causes exacerbation).
- Immunosuppression (including HIV).
- Concomitant intake of phototoxic drugs (like doxycycline, sparfloxacin, etc.).
- Past history of skin cancer.
- Aphakia due to risk of retinal damage.

PRINCIPLES OF PUVA THERAPY :

1. Psoralen tablets need to be ingested 1½ to 2 h prior to exposure to either, natural sunlight (PUVASOL therapy), or UVunit chamber (PUVA therapy). For PUVASOL therapy, exposure between 9.0-11.30 am and 2.30-3.30 pm is ideal with maximum proportion of UVA rays.
2. Exposure is either twice or thrice a week and not every day as PUVA-induced erythema takes minimum 48 h to subside and also to assess erythema due to previous exposures.
3. Eyes should be protected during 6 to 8 h after PUVA therapy by wearing UV-blocking glasses. Genitals also

need to be protected by genital shields, undergarments, or other appropriate measures during exposure.

4. Increments of exposure doses should be done at every alternate sitting. This may be modified, depending upon the clinical response and side effects. For psoriasis : the final dose that maintains the clearance is held constant and then gradually reduced in frequency up to once in 2 weeks.
5. Minimum phototoxic dose (MPD) is the minimum dose of ultra violet light that produces perceptible and well-defined erythema. MPD testing is carried on covered sites such as the buttocks and read 72 h after light exposure. Ideally, MPD should be determined before the initiation of PUVA therapy and erythemogenic doses used for vitiligo and suberythemogenic doses (70% of dose causing minimum perceptible erythema) for psoriasis. Doses can be increased relatively rapidly in psoriasis (increment of 10-20% at every sitting) as compared to vitiligo (increment of 10-20% every week).

COMBINATION TREATMENTS FOR PSORIASIS :

1. *PUVA + Acitretin (RePUVA) :*
   - The required dose of both therapies is reduced, thereby reducing their toxicity.
   - Acitretin 1 mg/kg, started 2 weeks prior to PUVA.
   - PUVA added until clearance.
   - Acitretin stopped and PUVA is continued (Table 12.2).
2. *PUVA + Methotrexate :*
   - Methotrexate 7.5 mg started 3 weeks prior to PUVA.
   - PUVA added until clearance.
   - Methotrexate stopped and PUVA is continued.
   - Initiating methotrexate immediately after the stoppage of PUVA therapy may cause PUVA-induced erythema to worsen (erythema recall).

TABLE 12.2 : **Light sources for the various phototherapies**

Phototherapy type	Light source
Ultraviolet A	Fluorescent lamps, high-pressure halide lamp
KUVA (Khellin + UVA)	Fluorescent lamps, high-pressure halide lamp
Broadband UVB	Philips T L-12 fluorescent lamp
Narrowband UVB	Philips T 1-01 fluorescent bulbs, Sylvania UV21
Extracorporeal photopheresis	Fluorescent lamps (same as that used for UVA)
Photodynamic therapy	Visible light
Blue light therapy	Blue light

3. *PUVA + UVB :*

   PUVA with UVB (75% of MED with increments).

4. *PUVA + Calcipotriol*

5. *PUVA + Tazarotene*

6. *PUVA + Cyclosporin*

UVB PHOTOTHERAPY :

Ultraviolet B therapy is an important option in therapeutic photomedicine, which involves the use of ultraviolet B rays (290-320 nm) the treatment of skin diseases particularly psoriasis and vitiligo. It comprises the use of broadband (290-320 nm) UVB therapy and narrowband (311 nm) UVB therapy. Narrowband is much more effective than broadband UVB therapy as it more effectively depletes Langerhans cells of the epidermis and similarly functioning dermal dendritic cells, leading to more immunosuppression. It involves the use of light sources like the Philips TL-OI fluorescent lamp. Generally, first exposure is 70% of minimum erythema dose (MED) followed by increments of 20% in each sitting if no phototoxicity occurs.

ADVANTAGES OF UVB OVER PUVA THERAPY :

1. No need for intake of psoralens. Hence, side effects of psoralens can be avoided.
2. Useful in children under 12 years of age when psoralens are contraindicated.
3. Can be used in pregnancy and lactation where psoralens are contraindicated.
4. Can be used in the elderly or those with poor hepatic or renal function where psoralens may be contraindicated.
5. Since no coordination with drug intake is required, it is more convenient or patient-friendly.
6. No eye protection is necessary outside the chamber.
7. Shorter exposure times as compared to PUVA therapy.

DISADVANTAGES :

1. Expensive.
2. Since exposure times are in seconds, the chance of sunburn due to accidental over exposure is higher unless a timer is used.
3. Requires more supervision since every exposure dose needs to be adjusted.
4. More carcinogenic than PUVA therapy.

INDICATIONS OF UVB THERAPY :

- Psoriasis.
- Vitiligo.
- Atopic dermatitis.

EXPERIMENTAL INDICATIONS :

- Pruritus - generalised.
- Photosensitivity dermatoses like polymorphic light eruption, actinic prurigo, hydroa vacciniforme, and the

cutaneous porphyrias (hardening effect or tolerance), may cause flares more frequently.

- Lichen planus.
- Mycosis fungoides (patch and plaque stage).
- Pityriasis lichenoides chronica.
- Pityriasis rubra pilaris.
- Prurigo nodularis.
- Scleroderma.
- Seborrheic dermatitis.

COMBINATION THERAPY WITH UVB :

- UVB + Calcipotriol (UVA + calcipotriol is not advisable as UVA degrades calcipotriol).
- UVB + Topical tazarotene.
- UVB + Saltwater bath (Balneotherapy).
- UVB + Systemic retinoids.

In responsive patients NB-UVB can be given for a maximum of 24 months. After I year, a resting period of 3 months is recommended to minimize the annual cumulative dose of U VB. In children, the maximum duration allowed is 12 months.

TARGETED UVB PHOTOTHERAPY :

NB-UVB is delivered via a portable unit with ultraviolet exposure limited only to the affected areas (targeted) like psoriatic plaques or vitiliginous macules. Advantage over conventional NB-UVB light sources is that one is able to deliver large doses of UVB to the target site without the limitation of causing phototoxicity in the surrounding normal skin. Hence, incremental higher doses can be delivered leading to rapid results.

EXCIMER LASER AND EXCIMER LASER LAMPS :

Excimer lasers are named after the formation of "excised

dimers" in their technology Excimer lasers use a specific wavelength of 309 nm that is found to be extremely effective for the treatment of psoriasis and vitiligo. Excimer lasers (309 nm) closely resemble narrowband UVB therapy (311 nm) in terms of wavelength used for treatment. However, they deliver monochromatic light and hence are more effective.

INDICATIONS :

Same as narrowband UVB phototherapy; however, due to the limited spot size localized lesions are more amenable to therapy with this machine.

ADVANTAGES :

1. Effective therapy.
2. Specific wavelength is used.

DISADVANTAGES :

1. Costly.
2. Side effects of laser; chance of burning.
3. Treatment of larger areas is impractical with this instrument.

The above disadvantages of excimer laser are overcome by using excimer laser lamps which have become popular in the last 5-10 years. Excimer laser lamps are less expensive, provide larger treatment area (spot size) and equally good results. Due to their ease of use and lower maintenance costs they have become popular though the peak of wavelength is slightly different *i.e.* 308 nm.

EXTRACORPOREAL PHOTOCHEMOTHERAPY (ECP, PHOTOPHERESIS) :

Peripheral blood is withdrawn by the machine from a patient who has ingested 0.6-0.8 mg/kg of 8-MOP, 1.5-2 h earlier is separated of its cell constituents, namely red blood cells and white blood cells (mainly lymphocyte buffy coat) by extracorporeal pheresis machine. Red blood cells are returned into circulation while lymphocyte buffy coat is irradiated by ultraviolet light. Irradiated white blood cells are then returned into the patient's circulation.

The mechanism of action is T-lymphocyte apoptosis and enhancement of anti-T-cell immunological responses. Volume shifts during extracorporeal photochemotherapy may cause hypotension, congestive cardiac failure, flushing, and palpitations. Extracorporea photochemotherapy is contraindicated in pregnancy, lactation, low hematocrit (less than 23%), low diastolic BP (less than 70 mm Hg), and congestive heart failure.

INDICATIONS OF EXTRACORPOREAL PHOTOCHEMOTHERAPY :

- Cutaneous T-cell lymphoma.
- Autoimmune bullous disorders.
- Connective tissue disorders.
- Graft versus host disease.

ADVANTAGES :

1. Effective therapy.
2. Less frequent visits are required.

DISADVANTAGES :

1. Invasive.
2. High rates of infection (in the inexperienced hands).
3. Expensive (requires special medicine).
4. Requires skills.

PHOTODYNAMIC THERAPY (PDT) (SYSTEMIC?)

In the presence of oxygen, photosensitizers like porphyrins-upon exposure to visible light-generate free oxygen radicals (singlet oxygen) causing cytotoxic effects, vascular damage, and immunological reactions. Photodynamic therapy can be either systemic or topical. Systemic PDT involves the use of hematoporphyrin X derivative. Topical PDT uses 20% aminolevulinic acid cream (ALA-PDT) under occlusion, followed by visible light (red light is commonly used) exposure after minimum 6 h. It is one of the safest phototherapies as no ultraviolet rays are used.

INDICATIONS :

- Actinic keratosis (FDA approved).
- Cutaneous T-cell lymphoma.
- Superficial basal cell carcinoma.
- Bowen's disease.

ARSENIC KERATOSES BLUE LIGHT (417 NM) :

Unlike ultraviolet rays, blue light therapy is a photodynamic therapy, which uses visible light in blue light range thereby avoiding side effects of ultraviolet exposure. However, unlike photodynamic therapy, it does not involve the use of synthetic photosensitizers like hematoporphyrin X derivative (HpD-X) or aminolevulinic acid (ALA). Blue light therapy is popularly used in patients of noninflammatory acne vulgaris based on the principle that organisms *Propionibacterium acnes* produce porphyrin that acts as a natural photosensitizer.

HIGH-DOSE UVAI THERAPY :

High-dose ultraviolet A1 therapy (340-400 nm) is mainly used in the following conditions. It has an advantage of not using oral or topical psoralens prior to the exposure similar to UV-B therapy. Longer wavelength rays penetrate deeper in dermis and are therefore useful for dermal as well as epidermal affections.

INDICATIONS :

- Morphea and systemic sclerosis.

- Vitiligo
- Atopic dermatitis.
- Polymorphic light eruptions and solar urticarial.
- Mastocytosis.
- Cutaneous (low dose)

LOW LEVEL RED LIGHT THERAPY :

It uses non thermal effects of low intensity light at red or near infrared wave length.

MECHANISM OF ACTION :

It works on the principle of photobiomodulation. Cytochrome c is the main chromophore. The absorbed photons release nitrous oxide which increases the blood flow around the hair follicles stimulating the telogen hair follicles to reenter the anagen phase, prolong duration of anagen phase, increase anagen proliferation and prevent premature catagen development. It is also claimed to modulate the activity of 5-alpha reductase enzyme and inflammation.

Modes : LASER (wavelength around 60 nm) and LED. LASER is better as LED dose is more variable and light is divergent.

INDICATIONS :

- AGA and FPHL.
- Alopecia areata.
- Chemotherapy induced alopecia.

DEVICES :

- Hoods
- Combs

- Bands
- Helmet

Hairmax lasercomb has been approved safe by FDA for AGA in males in 2007 and females in 2011.

Dosage :

Three times a week for 15 mins each session for 1st 3 months has supplementary beneficial effects in alopecia but can be used alone depending on patient preference for the treatment.

SIDE EFFECTS :

Temporary onset of telogen effluvium in first 1-2 months after commencing treatment. It disappears on continued treatment.

x=x=x=x=x

13 Immunobiologicals

Immunobiologicals are the biologically active agents with immunological actions that are useful for the management of immunologically mediated diseases. A prototype of such diseases is psoriasis, which is now considered a T-cell-mediated disease with a complex immunopathogenesis that is simplified in Figs. 13.1 & 13.2.

The skin is a large immune organ. It consists of keratinocytes that play a key role in immune recognition by producing a variety of cytokines. It also contains antigen-presenting cells (Langerhan's cells) that communicate with immune T-cells in the dermis to elicit immune reactivity. Several cutaneous disorders occur due to immunological imbalance.

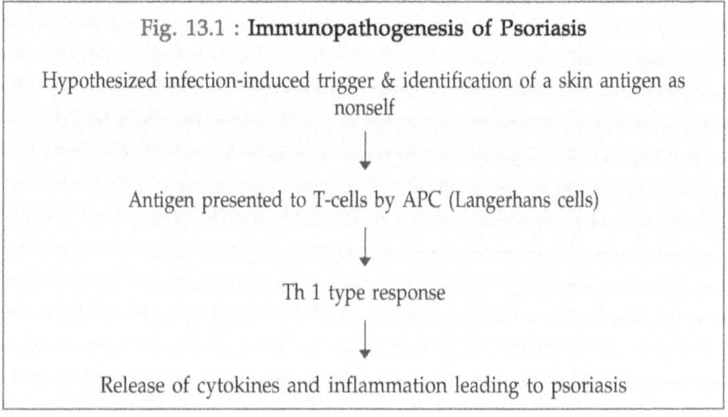

Fig. 13.1 : **Immunopathogenesis of Psoriasis**

Biologicals are the molecules that modify the cascade of immunologic processes leading to inflammation. Principal immunobiologicals are monoclonal antibodies (Mab), fusion

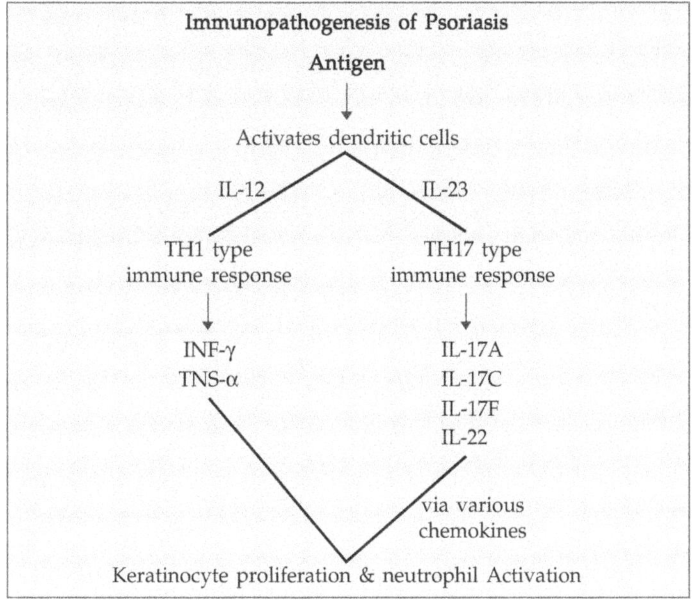

inhibitors and interferons (IFN). Monoclonal antibodies may be classified according to the decreasing order of antigenicity of their components into murine, chimeric, primatized and humanized.

MONOCLONAL ANTIBODIES (MAB) :

Commonly used monoclonal antibodies that have been tried in clinical trials and approved for the use in some dermatological conditions or in diseases mediated by T-lymphocytes are described later. The expense of treatment, lack of proven efficacy, and a limited follow-up currently prohibits the use of many of these agents for the management of skin or other disorders (Table 13.1). Moreover, it is important to realize that immunobiologicals rarely cure autoimmune disorders. At best, they control them or put them in remission.

TABLE 13.1 : **Immunobiologicals of clinical relevance**

	Target	Type
Cytokine blocking agents :		
Infliximab	Anti-TNF-α	Chimeric
Adalimumab	Anti TNF-α	Humanized
Ustekinumab	IL12 and IL23	Human
Secukinumab	IL17A blocker	Human
Etarnacept	TNF-α and TNF-β receptor blocker	Fusion protein
Omalizumab	IgE	Humanized
Lanadelumab	Kallikrenin	Human
Dupilumab	IL4	Human
Agents targeting cell surface epitopes		
Alefacept (in psoriasis poor efficacy)	CD_2-LFA-3	Fusion protein
Itolizumab	CD-6	Humanized
Siplizumab	CD_2	Humanized Mab
Rituximab	CD_{20}	Chimeric
Efalizumab (not used due to serious side effects - PML caused by JC virus)	CD_{11a}/CD_{18}	Humanized Mab
Denileukin Diftitox	CD_{25}/Ib_2	Fusion toxin

PRE TREATMENT EVALUATION :

1. *For organ function :* CBC, urine R/M, liver and kidney function tests.
2. *For preexisting infections :* Hep B Surface antigens, Hep B core IgM antibody, Antibodies to HCV, HIV, History of tuberculosis, Chest X-ray, Mantoux test, IGRA assay.
3. *For preexisting immune phenomenon :* ANA titres.

Note :

1. Tuberculosis : Screening for active tuberculosis is mandatory. If active infection is found (chest X-ray or CT scan), the biological should be administered after completion of treatment. In cases with latent infection

(mantoux or IGRA positivity) after ruling out active TB, the patient can be given the biological after two months of initiation of two drug antituberculosis prophylaxis with Rifampicin and Isoniazid for 3-4 months.

2. Live vaccines should not be administered 2 weeks before and 3-6 months after biological therapy. The immune response of inactivated or recombinant vaccines is also questionable with certain drugs when given in this duration. Pneumococcal, Influenza and hepatitis B vaccination is recommended, safe and effective for patients on immunobiological treatment in India.

INFLIXIMAB :

Infliximab is a chimeric (fused segments of mouse and human antibodies) monoclonal antibody that has been used in many disorders with variable success.

Mechanism Of Action :

Chimeric Mab; inhibits cytokine tumor necrosis factor alpha (TNF-α) and not TNF-β by binding to them.

Indications :

1. Psoriasis and psoriatic arthritis.
2. Reactive arthritis.
3. Rheumatoid arthritis.
4. Behcet's disease.
5. Pyoderma gangrenosum.
6. Graft versus host disease.
7. Toxic epidermal necrolysis.

Doses And Preparations :

- 5 or 7 mg/kg/dose i.v. alone or in combination with other agents
- REMICADE 100 mg injection

PREGNANCY CATEGORY – B :

It can be used in children > 6 years of age.

Side Effects :

Infusion reactions include pain or swelling at the injection site, flushing, urticaria, angioedema, breathlessness, fever with chills and headache. Premedication with antihistaminic and steroid injections is recommended before infusion.

Diarrhea, headache, upper respiratory tract infections, urinary tract infection, rash, may cause reactivation of tuberculosis or hepatitis B or fungal infections due to immunosuppression, demyelinating encephalitis / myelitis, autoimmune hepatitis.

Contraindications :

Known hypersensitivity, active serious infections, heart failure (NYHA grade 3 or 4), neurological disease like multiple sclerosis in patient or in 1st degree relative, malignancies, active or latent TB. Crohn's disease & ulcerative colitis.

Key Points :

- Infliximab may produce autoantibodies and autoimmune syndromes. Clinical SLE is rare.
- Subsequent infusions of infliximab may lead to the development of neutralizing antibodies in approximately 40% patients over one year, which may diminish its therapeutic effect when used alone in the absence of a concomitant immunosuppressive agent. These antibodies are responsible for infusion reactions.
- Infliximab therapy is /given at Week 0, Week 2, Week 6 and 2-3 monthly thereafter. Good response is achieved (PASI 75) in 73-82% patients.

ADALIMUMAB :

MECHANISM OF ACTION :

It is a fully human monoclonal antibody towards TNF-α produced by recombinant technology from chinese hamster kidney.

INDICATIONS :

1. Chronic plaque psoriasis.
2. Psoriatic arthritis.
3. Hidradenitis suppurativa.
4. Off label used for Nail psoriasis, Pyoderma gangrenosum, vasculitis and sarcoidosis.

Time for peak action : 5 hours.

Half life : 2 weeks.

SIDE EFFECTS :

Similar to aforementioned TNF-α inhibitors.

DOSAGE :

80 mg on day 0, 40 mg on day 8 followed by 40 mg every other week.

PREGNANCY CATEGORY – 'B' :

SECUKINUMAB :

It is a fully human monoclonal IgG_1 antibody against IL-17A molecule. IL-17A is a novel molecule produced by the TH17 cells involved in the pathogenesis of psoriasis and acts downstream on the keratinocytes to cause hyperproliferation. The newer models of psoriasis are skewing towards a predominance of TH_{17} response than TH_1 response in psoriasis.

INDICATIONS :

1. Chronic plaque psoriasis.
2. Arthritis.
3. Nail psoriasis.
4. Palmoplantar psoriasis.

DOSAGE :

150-300 mg subcutaneously, 0, 1, 2, 3, 4 weekly in induction phase followed by monthly indefinitely.

300 mg gives better clearance. Discontinuation of Secukinumab for 3 months warrants repetition of induction phase.

SIDE EFFECTS :

1. Injection site reaction (rare).
2. Anti drug antibodies is also less (< 1%) compared to other TNF-α blockers.
3. URTI's, Candidiasis, Herpes (no major infection).
4. Neutropenia (self limiting, resolves during the course of therapy).
5. Hypersensitivity, flare of IBD's.

PREGNANCY CATEGORY – not assigned as data is scarce

ETANERCEPT :

> MECHANISM OF ACTION :
>
> Fusion protein; inhibits cytokines TNF-α and TNF-β by blocking their receptors.

INDICATIONS :

1. Psoriasis and psoriatic arthritis, juvenile psoriasis.
2. Pustular psoriasis and its variants including acrodermatitis continua.

3. Rheumatoid arthritis.
4. Cicatricial pemphigoid (anecdotal)
5. Systemic scleroderma (experimental).
6. Behcet's disease (partially effective)

DOSES AND PREPARATIONS :

- ENBREL 25-50 mg s.c. twice weekly for minimum 12 weeks.
- Biosimilars : Etacept (Cipla) and Intacept (Intas).

Half time :

4.8 days; bioavailability - 58%.

PREGNANCY CATEGORY – B :

can be used in children > 4 years of age.

SIDE EFFECTS :

Injection site reactions, headache, nausea/vomiting, diarrhea upper respiratory tract infections, abdominal pain, rash.

KEY POINTS :

- Response to etanercept is slower as compared to infliximab in treatment of psoriasis.
- Etanercept is approved for use with methotrexate in the treatment of psoriatic arthritis. Methotrexate improves psoriasis/psoriatic arthritis and prevents the formation of blocking antibodies against etanercept thereby maintaining its efficacy.
- Chances of reactivation of TB is less than that with Infliximab or Adalimumab.
- It can be given in patients with coexistent Hepatitis C chronic infection and hepatitis B (along with antivirals).

APREMILAST :

MECHANISM OF ACTION :

Apremilast works at the intracellular level. It is a phosphodiesterase inhibitor which prevents degradation of cAMP. The increased levels of cAMP inturn downregulate the production of inflammatory cytokines like TNF-α, IL-23, INF-γ involved in the pathogenesis of psoriasis.

DOSAGE : 30 mg bd.

Recommended dose escalation is as follows :

Day	Morning dose	Evening dose
1	10 mg	—
2	10 mg	10 mg
3	10 mg	20 mg
4	20 mg	20 mg
5	20 mg	30 mg
6	30 mg	30 mg

However, lower dosages and slower escalation of doses are better tolerated.

Bioavailability : 73%

Half time : 6-9 hours

INDICATIONS :

- Psoriatic arthritis.
- Moderate to severe psoriasis.

Conditions that have been treated with apremilast with variable response include :

Atopic dermatitis, Lichen planus, alopecia areata, recurrent EM, vitiligo, Hidradenitis suppurativa, SAPHO syndrome, aphthous stomatitis, Behcet's disease, recalcitrant PG, inflammatory rosacea, chronic cutaneous sarcoidosis.

SIDE EFFECTS :

- Nausea, vomiting, diarrhea.
- Headache.
- URTI.
- Depression, suicidal thoughts.
- Weight loss and loss of appetite.

PREGNANCY CATEGORY – C :

CONTRAINDICATED IN LACTATION :

Avoided in children < 18 years due to inadequate data.

KEY POINTS :

- Dose reduction to 30 mg is required in case of severe renal impairment (creatinine clearance < 30 ml/min). No dose reduction for hepatic impairment.
- It is metabolized by CYP3A4 enzymes. Hence, concomitant administration with enzyme inducers like rifampicin, phenytoin, carbamazepine should be avoided.
- For patients with gastrointestinal symptoms, the 6 day titration can be extended to 2 weeks or longer.
- Maximum patients usually respond in the initial period. However, sustained efficacy after 6-8 months is yet to be established. It is recommended to stop apremilast if adequate response is not achieved in 16 weeks.
- Baseline CBC, LFT, RFT followed by quarterly repeat investigations are recommended despite no adverse effects on liver, kidney and bone marrow.

RITUXIMAB :

Chimeric monoclonal IgG1 antibody against CD20 antigen present on the pre-B cell and mature lymphocytes in the circulation.

DERMATOLOGICAL INDICATIONS :

1. Vesicobullous disorders like Pemphigus vulgaris, bullous pemphigoid, EBA, mucous membrane pemphigoid, paraneoplastic pemphigus.
2. Autoimmune CTD's like SLE, DM, vasculitis, cryoglobulinemia, GVHD as adjunctive treatment.
3. Cutaneous B cell Lymphoma.

Route : Intravenous.

Half life : 1.6-20 days.

Biological – Rituxan (Roche).

Biosimilar – Reditux RA (Dr. Reddys).
Mabtas (Intas).

METHOD OF ADMINISTRATION :

Premedication with Hydrocortisone 100 mg, Pheniramine maleate and paracetamol 500 mg 30 mins prior to starting infusion.

Start at 50 mg/hr, increase by 50 mg/hr if patient tolerates every 30 mins upto maximum 400 mg/hour.

CONTRAINDICATIONS :

1. Hypersensitivity to murine proteins.
2. Active infection.
3. HIV.
4. Heart failure.

PREGNANCY CATEGORY – 'C' : not recommended in children.

KEY POINTS :

- B cell depletion typically occurs after 2-3 weeks of infusion. Recovery begins at 6 months and continues till 12 months. Hence repeat infusions may be required at 12-18 months.
- Treatment protocols used for pemphigus :
    1. Modified lymphoma protocol- 375 mg/m^2 every week for 3 weeks followed by single dose after 3 months.
    2. Rheumatoid arthritis protocol- 1 g infusions at interval of 2 weeks.
    3. Combination therapy of rituximab with IVIG has been successful.
- Rituximab consistently reduces the dose and duration of systemic steroids and other immunosuppressive agents..

SIDE EFFECTS :

1. Infusion reaction :
    - ***Mild :*** nausea, fever, chills, rigors, tachycardia, dyspnea, rhinitis, pruritus- can be treated with injectable antihistamines and hydrocortisone and withholding the infusion.
    - ***Severe :*** Chest tightness, hypotension, cough, wheezing - stop the infusion and manage as anaphylaxis - s.c/i.m adrenaline (1:1000 dilution) every 5 mins i.v steroids.
2. Worsening of heart failure, Myocardial infarction, atrial fibrillation.
3. Worsening of active infections, reactivation of dormant infections like Hep B and TB if adequate screening has not been done.

4. Late onset neutropenia.
5. SJS and TEN (rare).
6. Progressive mutifocal leucoencephalopathy (rare).

OMALIZUMAB :

Recombinant humanized monoclonal antibody against IgE. It binds to the Fc portion of free circulating IgE and prevents in binding to FcER1. It also causes downregulation of FcER1 on basophils and mast cells.

Dermatological Indications :

- Chronic spontaneous urticaria > 12 years of age (third line for refractory patients).
- Atopic dermatitis.
- Bullous pemphigoid (anecdotal).
- Systemic mastocytosis (may not improve skin lesions).
- Hyperimmunoglobulin E syndrome.

Brands – Xolair (Novartis), Emzumab (Cipla).

Dose :

150-300 mg subcutaneously every 4 weeks irrespective of body weight. Doses in CS urticaria do not reliably correlate with serum IgE levels.

PREGNANCY CATEGORY – 'B' :

Side Effects :

- Headache, fatigue.
- Risk of anaphylaxis rash, urticaria.
- Thrombocytopenia.
- Injection site reactions.

KEY POINTS :

1. Duration of treatment is solely on the discretion of treating physicians. CS urticaria may become more manageable with other drugs.
2. Safety of treatment is documented upto 24 weeks use. Monthly 150 mg can be used as maintenance dose.
3. Higher doses are required for atopic dermatitis. Results have been variable.
4. It is used as adjunctive therapy for severe BP patients with raised IgE.

DUPILUMAB :

MECHANISM OF ACTION :

Human monoclonal antibody og IgG4 subclass, binds to IL-4 Ra subunit and inhibits IL-4 and IL-13 signalling.

INDICATIONS :

Recently approved for moderate to severe atopic dermatitis requiring repeated steroid courses.

DOSE :

600 mg subcutaneous followed by 300 mg every other week.

Bioavailability – 64%.

SIDE EFFECTS :

- Injection site reactions.
- Conjunctivitis, keratitis, dry eyes.
- Herpes simplex.
- Allergic reactions including urticaria.

CONTRAINDICATIONS :

Pregnancy, lactation, children (less than 6 years).

Avoid live vaccines.

JAK INHIBITORS (Janus kinase inhibitors) :

These are a new class of oral and topical agents used for disorders due to dysfunctional immune mechanisms. JAK are a family of tyrosine kinase receptors which bring about signal transduction through phosphorylation of intracellular proteins. Various cytokines, growth factors and hormones utilize this pathway.

DERMATOLOGICAL INDICATIONS :

Psoriasis and psoriatic arthritis.

Alopecia areata, Atopic dermatitis, vitiligo.

Few others like erythema multiforme, dermatomyositis, SLE, chronic actinic dermatitis, allergic contact dermatitis, GVHD, melanoma, cutaneous T cell lymphoma have shown variable response.

DRUGS :

- Tofacitinib (Tofajak, TFCT- NIB) - 5 mg bd
- Baricitinib (Barijak, Barinat) - 2-4 mg od
- Ruxolitinib (Novartis) - 5 mg bd

These agents are also being studied as topical formulations.

SIDE EFFECTS :

- Risk of infection - URTI, UTI, herpes simplex, VZV infections.
- Anemia, thrombocytopenia.
- Deranged lipid profile.
- Increased risk of malignancy.

PREGNANCY CATEGORY – 'C' :

CONTRAINDICATIONS :

- Hypersensitivity.
- Liver failure.
- Renal failure.

KEY POINTS :

- Tofacitinib 10 mg BD has shown similar efficacy to Adalimumab for PsA and similar to etanercept for psoriasis. However, the side effect profile at this dose is higher.
- Side effect profile is similar to biologicals but ease of oral administration and relative fewer side effects hold promise in future.
- For alopecia areata and vitiligo- they have shown to be effective over 3-4 months. However, majority patients relapsed after stoppage. Hence treatment may need to be continued for longer periods.

INTERFERONS :

Interferons (IFN) are a family of glycoproteins, which are synthesized naturally by leukocytes (IFN-α), fibroblasts (IFN-β), and immune cells (IFN-γ) against viral infections and other nonviral challenges that, in addition to having antiviral properties, also modulate various cellular functions. Interferon-α is mainly usedfor therapeutic purposes.

Interferons synthesized by recombinant techniques have therapeutic value in the treatment of viral infections of the skin and cutaneous malignancies. They are products of bacterial fermentation of particular strain of *E. coli* consisting genetically engineered plasmid containing a specific interferon gene from human leukocytes.

Mechanism Of Action :

Antiviral :

Induces enzyme 2′-5′ A synthetase; polymerizes ATP; activates cellular endonuclease; degrades both viral as well as cellular RNA.

Antiproliferative effect :

Inhibits mitosis of the cells and downregulates their growth factors.

Immunoregulatory effect :

1. Induces expression of class I and II MHC complexes antigens on immune cells.
2. Enhances number of natural killer (NK) cells.

Principal Indications Of Interferons (IFN-α_{2B}) In Dermatology :

Condylomata acuminata :

1 MU per lesion (maximum of five lesions in a single course). Intralesional injections should be three times weekly on alternate days for 3 weeks. An additional course may be administered at 12-16 weeks.

Technique for intralesional injection :

Insulin syringe or 25-30 G caliber needle directed toward the center of base of the wart and parallel to the plane of the wart which if done correctly will cause a small wheal and deliver the drug to the core of the lesion. Too deep (subcutaneous injection) and too superficial an injection needs to be avoided.

Malignant melanoma (adjuvant treatment) (Kirkwood regimen) :

Induction phase recommended dose :

- 20 MU/m^2 i.v. over 20 min for 5 consecutive days/week for 4 weeks.

- Solution formulations not recommended for i.v. use and shouldnot be used for the induction phase of malignant melanoma.

Maintenance phase recommended dose :

- 10 MU/m^2 s.c. injection three times/week for 48 weeks.

AIDS-related Kaposi's sarcoma :

30 MU/m^2/dose subcutaneously or intramuscularly three times a week for 16 weeks of treatment till maximum response. Dose reduction is frequently required thereafter.

Basal cell carcinoma : 1-3 mU intralesional 3 times a week for 3 weeks.

OTHER INDICATIONS :

Viral Infections :

- Common warts (Recalcitrant).
- Herpes zoster.
- Herpes simplex infections.

Cutaneous Malignancies :

- Keratoacanthoma.
- Actinic keratoses.
- Basal cell carcinoma.
- Squamous cell carcinoma.
- Cutaneous T-cell lymphoma.

Others :

- Hemangioma.
- Keloids.
- Atopic dermatitis.
- Behcet's disease.

- Systemic sclerosis.
- Chronic granulomatous disease of childhood.

Doses And Preparations Of Interferons IFN-ALPHA$_{2B}$:

IFN-alpha$_{2b}$ is supplied as :

1. Powder for injection/reconstitution :

TABLE 13.2 : **Doses and preparations of interferon alpha$_{2b}$**

Powder formulation

Viral strength million IU	ML diluent (sterile water)	Final concentrations after reconstitution million IU/ml	Route of administration
10	1	10	IM, SC, W, IL
18	1	18	IM, SC, IV
50	1	50	IM, SC, IV

Solutions formulations

Viral strength	Concentration	Route of administration
10 MIU single dose	10 million IU/1.0 ml	SC, IL
18 MIU multidose	3 million IU/0.5 ml	IM, SC
25 MIU multidose	5 million IU/0.5 ml	IM, SC, IL

2. Solution for injection in vials
3. Solution for injection in multidose pens

Side Effects :

1. Flu-like symptoms (can be avoided by the administration of paracetamol or other NSAIDs).
2. Hematological (neutropenia, thrombocytopenia).
3. Gastrointestinal disturbances.
4. Hepatotoxicity, nephrotoxicity.
5. Hypotension and arrhythmias.
6. Spastic paraplegia (may be related to preservatives).

TABLE 13.3 : **Immunostimulants in dermatology**

Agent	Mechanism of Action	Indications	Doses	Side Effects
Zinc sulfate (efficacy doubtful)	Enhances both B-cell and T-cell immunity increase in CD_8 cells Low serum zinc levels in some unresponsive patients.	Viral warts; Type II lepra reaction, Epiderma dysplasia verruciformis (EDV).	220 mg b.i.d./t.i.d. in addition to oral zinc, 10% cream applied bd for verruca.	Nausea; vomiting, epigastric distress may occur.
Cimetidine (efficacy doubtful)	IL-2 and IFN-γ expression	Viral warts Reversal of tolerance to DNCB or DPCP.	30-40 mg/kg/day for up to 4 months.	Mental confusion, loss of libido, gynecomastia, impotence, galactorrhea, elevation of liver enzymes and serum creatinine.
Levamisole (efficacy doubtful)	Increases delayed hypersensitivity (DHS) and CMI, increases E-rosette formation herpes, ENL.	Recurrent molluscum and verrucae; slowly spreading vitiligo and alopecia areata, recurrent.	150 mg/day on two consecutive days in a week.	Flu like symptoms, Pregnancy catagory C
BCG vaccination (live attenuated)	Induction of DHS and cell-mediated immunity	Lepromatous leprosy, cutaneous malignancies, melanoma, herpes genitalis, rheumatoid arthritis, verruca vulgaris, recalcitrant condyloma acuminata or warts.	0.05 ml intradermal, topical for genital warts	Injection reactions, BCG lymphadenitis, disseminated infection in Immunocompromised, inoculation lupus vulgaris Same as that of BCG

(Table 13.3 Continued)

INTERFERONS

INTERFERONS

(Table 13.3 Continued)

Agent	Mechanism of Action	Indications	Doses	Side Effects
Myco w vaccine IMMUVAC (heat-killed vaccine)	Enhances CMI, bacterial killing, and lesion clearance. Share antigens with Myco lepra and M. tuberculosis.	Adjunct to MDT in LL cases with high bacillary load and for leprosy prophylaxis. May have a role in management of cancer, HIV and TB.	0.5 ml/multidose vial. First dose : 0.1 ml intra dermal two injections each in right and left deltoid region. Subsequent doses: Similar dose at 3 months.	May increase frequency and severity of Type II lepra reactions.
MMR vaccine	Induction of cell mediated immunity against the wart antigen	Verruca vulgaris, palmoplantar and periungual warts, cutaneous malignancies.	0.1 ml/lesion injected every 2 weeks till complete resolution (max. 12 weeks)	Flu like symptoms, pain, edema. To be avoided in pregnant and lactating females, immunosuppressed patient, patients with hypersensitivity
PPD (purified protein derivative)	Same as above	Same as above	0.1 ml/lesion injected every 2 weeks till complete resolution.	Cheaper modality of treatments. Side effects rare through severe local reactions can occur.

7. Rhabdomyolysis (rare), autoimmune SLE, RA, Hypothyroidism.

PREGNANCY CATEGORY – C :

KEY POINTS :

- Longer duration of IFN therapy is required to achieve desired therapeutic effect (Table 13.3).
- Neutralizing antibodies formed in response to IFN therapy do not affect their efficacy and hence appear to have little clinical significance.
- Drug interactions concurrent use of IFNs with zidovudine may increase the risk of hematologic complications.
- Solution forms of interferons are not used for intravenous use as they contain preservatives like cresol, which can cause severe adverse reactions.

INTRAVENOUS IMMUNOGLOBULINS :

Intravenous immunoglobulins are heterogenous human gammaglobulins containing IgG with trace of IgA and IgM prepared by cold ethanol fractionalization of pooled human sera harvested from thousands of donors.

IVIG is an important safe, effective (but costly) therapeutic option as an immunomodulatory agent in the management of skin disorders where corticosteroids and immunosuppressive agents cannot be used.

MECHANISM OF ACTION :

Suppression of antibody production due to infusion of heavy doses of IVIG.

Suppression of idiotypic antibodies (idiotype-antiidiotype interactions regulate autoimmunity).

Saturation of Fc receptors on macrophages (Fc receptors play role in cytotoxic cell-mediated immunity and opsonization).

Neutralization of microbe or toxin.
Inhibition of cytokines like IL-I, IL-6, and TNF-α.
Superantigen neutralization.
Modulation of complement activation.
Acceleration of IgG catabolism.

TABLE 13.4 : **Indications and doses of intravenous immunoglobulins**

Indication	Doses Used
Autoimmune bullous disorders, *e.g.* pemphigus vulgaris	2 g/kg i.v. single dose monthly or 1 g/kg/day X 3 days every month, or 0.5 g/kg/day X 5 days every month.
Steven's Johnson syndrome and Toxic epidermal necrolysis	1 g/kg/day IV x 3 consecutive days.
Autoimmune connective tissue disorders, *e.g.* dermatomyositis	0.8-5.8 g/kg for 1-5 days.
Graft versus host disease (GVHD)	2 g/kg i.v. single dose monthly for 2-4 months.
Kawasaki disease	250-500 mg/kg weekly from day-8 to day-11 after BMT for prevention of GVHD.
Hypersensitive dermatoses, *e.g.* autoimmune urticaria	2 g/kg i.v. as single dose
Agammaglobulinemia/hypogammaglobulinemia : congenital or acquired	0.4 g/kg/day for 5 days
Scleromyxedema	> 0.25 g/kg every 3 weeks in childhood
Pyoderma gangrenosum	2 g/kg i.v. monthly for 3 months

BMT : Bone marrow transplantation

DOSES AND PREPARATIONS :

- GAMMA-I.V. 5% lyophilized powder to be dissolved in 5% dextrose, IMMUGLOB 2.5 g/100 ml, 5 g/200 ml vial.
- IVIG should be infused initially at the rate of 0.01-0.02 kg/min for 30 min; if well-tolerated, the infusion rate can

be increased to a maximum of 0.08 ml/kg/min. A separate peripheral venous line should be established without mixing with other fluids or medications. Since it is not compatible with normal saline, it has to be diluted with 5% dextrose in water.

PREGNANCY CATEGORY – C :

SIDE EFFECTS :

Side effects are rare, mild, and usually self-limited and may be related to the infusion rate. They can be prevented or minimized by slowing the infusion rates or by prior administration of intravenous corticosteroids and antihistamines.

Common side effects are :

- Headache, backache, nausea/vomiting, chills, fever, myalgia.
- Hypersensitivity reactions including anaphylaxis (due to IVIG or thimerosal, maltose, or sucrose in infusion solution).
- Acute renal failure (irreversible, IVIG containing sucrose more likely to lead to this complication).
- Fluid overload and electrolyte disturbances, MI, stroke.
- Hemolysis.
- Neutropenia.
- Cutaneous adverse effects : petechiae, pruritus, urticarial, lichenoid eruption, alopecia, pompholyx, vasculitis.

KEY POINTS :

- Peak serum concentrations of IVIG are achieved immediately following the intravenous injection and is dose related. 30% of the dose is eliminated by catabolism within 24 h. Serum half life is 3-5 weeks.
- All batches of IVIG should undergo testing for HIV,

syphilis, hepatitis B, and hepatitis C to minimize the risk of transmission. A small sample may be stored before infusion for 60 days when the donors are under observation for seroconversion.

- Anaphylaxis to IVIG is more common when IgA is deficient. IVIG are the immunoglobulins, which can interact with livevirus vaccine. Such vaccines should not be given 14 days before or 3 months after IVIG administration.
- IVIG has a theoretical risk of autoimmunity owing to infusion of antibodies.
- Sudden infusion of IVIG may suppress antibody production and rebound flare-up can occur after the discontinuation of therapy. Hence it should be used as a bridge to standard therapy.

x=x=x=x=x

14

Vitamins and Trace Elements

FAT-SOLUBLE VITAMINS :

Fat-soluble vitamins include vitamin A, D, E and K.

VITAMIN A (RETINOL) :

Vitamin A is a fat-soluble vitamin mainly required for night vision and maintenance of the integrity of the epithelia.

MECHANISM OF ACTION (PHYSIOLOGICAL) :

Normalizes keratinization (regulates cell growth, differentiation, and morphogenesis of keratinocytes).

Prevents tumorigenesis and carcinogenesis.

Maintain the integrity of epithelial membranes.

Antiinflammatory (stabilizes lysosomal membranes) action.

Stimulate humoral and cellular immunity.

Antioxidant effect (beta-carotene only).

INDICATIONS OF VITAMIN A IN DERMATOLOGY :

- Phrynoderma (vitamin A deficiency). (Table 14.1)

OF HIGH-DOSE VITAMIN A IN DERMATOLOGY :

1. Pityriasis rubra pilaris
2. Darier-White disease
3. Congenital ichthyosis
4. Keratosis pilaris.
5. Palmoplantar keratoderma.

VITAMIN A (RETINOL)

TABLE 14.1 : **Vitamins of relevance to dermatology**

	Therapeutic doses	RDA	Dietary sources (vegetarian)	Dietary sources (nonvegetarian)
Fat-soluble vitamins :				
Vitamin A (Retinol)	30,000 IU/day for neonates, 50,000 IU/day children and adults	5000 IU	Milk and milk products, spinach, amaranth, coriander, curry leaves, papaya, cabbage, tomato, mango	Egg yolk, liver, fish, polar bear, and cod liver oil
Vitamin D (Tocopherol)	800 IU/day	—	Butter and cheese	Liver, egg yolk, some fishes
Vitamin E (Tocopherol)	100-400 mg/day	0.8 mg/g of EFA	Cotton seed and sunflower seed oil, butter	Egg yolk
Vitamin K (Menadione)	5-10 mg i.m/day	1 μg/kg	Fresh green vegetables (spinach, cauliflower, cabbage), fruits	—
Water-soluble vitamins :				
Vitamin B_2 (Riboflavin)	10-30 mg/day in divided doses	1-2 mg	Milk and milk products, green leafy/vegetables	Liver, eggs, and kidney
Vitamin B_3 (Niacin)	1 g t.i.d for 3 days (maximum); 25 mg i.v. b.i.d./t.i.d.	10-20 mg	Legumes and groundnut	Liver, kidney meat, poultry, poultry, fish
Vitamin Bs (Pantothenic acid)	50 mg o.d/b.i.d.	10 mg	Peas, beans, whole grain cereals	Poultry, fish
Vitamin B_6 (Pyridoxine)	30-100 mg/day	1.5-2.5 mg	Milk, legumes, whole grain cereals, vegetables	Liver, meat, egg yolk, fish
Vitamin B_{12} (Cyanocobalamin)	1000 μg (1 mg) i.m./week	1 μg	Milk and fermented cheeses	Fish, seafood, egg yolk
Vitamin B_9 (Folic acid)	1-5 mg/day	50-100 μg	Green leafy vegetables, pulses	Liver, eggs
Vitamin H (Biotin)	5-10 mg/day	200-250 μg	Legumes, nuts, whole cereals, milk	Animal proteins
Vitamin C (Ascorbic acid)	300-1000 mg/day	200 mg	Amla, citrus fruits, germinating pulses	Traces in animal proteins

* RDA, recommended daily allowances.

6. Other disorders of keratinization, *e.g.*, pachyonychia, erythrokeratoderma.
7. Nodulocystic acne.
8. Pustular psoriasis.
9. Leukoplakia.

SIDE EFFECTS (HYPERVITAMINOSIS) :

Hypervitaminosis A may occur on consumption of high doses (more than 200,000 IU) for prolonged periods or on consumption of organ meat in large portions for prolonged periods. Initial symptoms are lassitude, lethargy, and headache. Later vomiting and hepatitis may occur. The skin becomes dry, erythematous, scaly, and cracked. Hair loss and mucosal bleeding may follow. Pseudotumor cerebri has also been reported.

KEY POINTS :

1. Vegetable sources of vitamin A contain retinal (two retinal molecules forming beta-carotene) while animal sources contain retinyl esters. Polar bear liver is the richest natural source of vitamin A.
2. Vitamin A is used for the treatment of night blindness as the dark pigment for night vision—rhodopsin—is synthesized from vitamin A.
3. Beta-carotene overdoses do not lead to hypervitaminosis A as beta-carotene is slowly converted to vitamin A so that there is no accumulation of toxic quantities of vitamin A in the body.
4. Hypervitaminosis A may clinically resemble vitamin A deficiency.

VITAMIN D (CHOLECALCIFEROL) :

Vitamin D is a fat-soluble vitamin predominantly required for mineralization of bones.

Mechanism Of Action (Physiological) :

Increases the absorption of calcium from the gastrointestinal tract and helps in mineralization of bones.

Indications :

- As a supplementation (800 units) during long-term systemic steroid therapy.
- Oral calcitriol (100,000-1,500,00 units daily) was used in the past for treatment of a variety of disorders including cutaneous tuberculosis, subcutaneous fungal infections, and psoriasis. However, this has now been given up due to its toxicity.

Side Effects :

- Excessive intake can cause hypervitaminosis D, which manifests as vomiting, muscle weakness, nephrolithiasis, and osteolysis.
- No cutaneous side effects are reported.

Key Points :

When used as a coprescription with systemic steroids, vitamin D is given with oral calcium 500 mg once or twice daily. Additionally in patients with osteopenia, osteoporosis or those at high risk for these, oral alendronate 35-70 mg/week may be given.

Vitamin D deficiency is reported to be associated with dry itchy skin that is prone to psoriasis, atopic dermatitis and hair loss. However, vitamin D supplementation may not be helpful in the treatment of these disorders.

VITAMIN E (TOCOPHEROL) :

Vitamin E or alpha-tocopherol is a fat-soluble vitamin with antioxidant properties.

MECHANISM OF ACTION (PHYSIOLOGICAL) :

Inhibits lipid peroxidation of membranes (antioxidant effect).

Protects stratum corneum against chemical and physical (UV rays) trauma, inhibits photoaging and cancer development.

Reduces prostaglandin synthesis (antiinflammatory effect).

Promotes phagocytosis, humoral, and cellular immunity (immunostimulant action).

Inhibits tyrosinase enzyme thus inhibiting melanogenesis.

INDICATIONS IN DERMATOLOGY :

Vitamin E is emperically or experimentally used in the following conditions with doubtful efficacy. No controlled studies are available.

DOSE :

Variable from 400-1200 IU/day

1. In keratinization disorders, vitamin E is used for its proposed synergistic action with vitamin A, *e.g.* pityriasis rubra pilaris, Darier's disease, Hailey Hailey disease.
2. Yellow nail syndrome.
3. Epidermolysis bullosa.
4. Morphea and Lichen sclerosus atrophicus.
5. Striae.
6. Pigmented purpuric dermatoses (topical).
7. It is reported to be useful topically for periorbital darkening; along with vitamin C and ferrulic acid as a photoprotective agent.

SIDE EFFECTS :

- Adverse side effects reported with high doses of vitamin

E are reduced platelet aggregation and bleeding tendencies.

KEY POINTS :

- Vitamin E deficiency is rare but can be encountered in premature infants, formula-fed infants, malabsorption syndromes, kwashiorkar, chronic alcoholics, pustular psoriasis, thalassemics, sickle cell anemia, and those on oral contraceptives.

VITAMIN K (MENADIONE) :

Vitamin K or phytonadione is a fat-soluble vitamin which plays a very important role in normal coagulation.

> MECHANISM OF ACTION (PHYSIOLOGICAL) :
>
> Vitamin K controls the synthesis of liver-dependent coagulation factors like factors II, VII, IX, and X and thus helps in coagulation.
>
> Vitamin K plays an indirect role in mineralization of bones.

INDICATIONS IN DERMATOLOGY :

1. Purpura, ecchymoses and hematoma secondary to vitamin K deficiency.
2. In topical formulations, it is useful in accelerating resolution of post procedure bruising in cosmetic procedures.
3. It is also useful in periorbital hyperpigmentation caused due to sluggish blood flow.

SIDE EFFECTS :

No cutaneous side effects noted with vitamin K.

Key Points :

- Vitamin K_1 is present in fresh vegetables while vitamin K_2 is synthesized by bacterial flora.
- Vitamin K deficiency is encountered in premature infants and infants whose mothers are on warfarin or phenytoin or broad-spectrum antibiotic therapy, cholestatic jaundice, malabsorption syndromes, and total parenteral nutrition.
- Vitamin K or menadione sulfate is the antidote of warfarin

WATER-SOLUBLE VITAMINS :

Water-soluble vitamins include vitamin B_2, B_3, B_6, B_{12}, folic acid, vitamin C, biotin, and pantothenic acid.

PREGNANCY CATEGORY : A, C (> RDA levels)

RIBOFLAVIN (VITAMIN B_2) :

Riboflavin or vitamin B_2 is a flavonoid.

Mechanism Of Action (Physiological) :

Vitamin B_2 converts pyridoxine to pyridoxal phosphate necessary for the activity of lysyl oxidase that initiates the crosslinking of collagen.

Affects metabolism of free fatty acids, tryptophan, and folic acid.

Indications In Dermatology :

- Mucocutaneous manifestations caused by riboflavin deficiency that include :
    1. Oro-oculo-genital syndrome
    2. Seborrheic dermatitis like rash
    3. Dyssebacea of nasolabial areas
- Lactic acidosis caused by antiretroviral drugs, *i.e.* protease inhibitors.

DOSES AND PREPARATIONS :

- 20-40 mg thrice daily, LIPOBOL 20 mg tablets.

SIDE EFFECTS :

None is reported.

KEY POINTS :

- Vitamin B_2 is called riboflavin because they are "yellow flavonoids" richly present in liver, ovary, and curd-yellowish in color.
- Riboflavin deficiency may be associated with zinc deficiency owing to common dietary source of both vitamins.

NIACIN (VITAMIN B_3) :

Niacin or nicotinic acid is a water-soluble B-complex vitamin and is also an hypolipidemic agent.

MECHANISM OF ACTION (PHYSIOLOGICAL AND PHARMACOLOGICAL) :

1. Tryptophan → Niacin → Nicotine-adenine-nucleotide (NAD, coenzyme l)

   ↓

   Nicotine-adenine-dinucleotide phosphate (NADP, coenzyme II)

   NADP is important for synthesis of fatty acid and collagen.
2. Nicotinamide inhibits eosinophilic chemotactic factor (ECF) to reduce eosinophilic chemotaxis thereby useful in bullous pemphigoid.
3. Nicotinic acid reduces blood triglyceride levels by increasing high-density lipoproteins.

INDICATIONS IN DERMATOLOGY :

1. Pellagra (niacin deficiency states).

2. Bullous pemphigoid.
3. Xanthomas (eruptive type due to hypertriglyceridemia).
4. Erythema elevatum diutinum (as one of the therapeutic options).
5. Acne (Topical niacin as anti-inflammatory and sebostatic).

Doses And Preparations :

- 1 g/day for 3 days in niacin deficiency.
- NIALIP (nicotinic acid) 375 mg tablet and 500 mg, (Antiinflammatory or hypolipimic dose - 1.5 g/day).
- Nicotinic acid 50 mg tablet twice daily for 2-4 weeks for pellagra
- Nicotinamide 100 mg capsules also provide Vit. B_3.

Side Effects :

- Hypotension and acid peptic disease, abnormal LFT, headache, syncope.
- Nicotinic acid causes pruritus, burning, and flushing of the skin.
- It is known to cause acanthosis nigricans when used as an hypolipimic agent has been replaced by Acipimox a new derivative of niacin free of its vascular side effects.

Key Points :

- Niacin deficiency is commonly encountered in chronic alcoholics, maize and sorghum eating populations, malabsorption syndromes, ulcerative colitis and Crohn's disease, post-bowel resection surgery, carcinoid syndrome, Hartnup disease, and patients on azathioprine or 6-mercaptopurine therapy.
- Nicotinic acid, a potent vasodilator, may potentiate hypotensive actions of ganglion blocking agents and other vasodilators.

PANTOTHENIC ACID (VITAMIN B_5) :

Pantothenic acid is mainly used in dermatology with unproven efficacy as adjuvant therapy for disorders of hairs.

Mechanism Of Action :

Pantothenic acid is a factor of coenzyme A required for the metabolism of carbohydrate, fat, and proteins. Recent work indicated its role in steroid biosynthesis.

Indications :

1. Burning feet syndrome (Gopalan's syndrome).
2. Graying of hairs (doubtful efficacy).
3. Disorders of hair shaft and telogen effluvium (doubtful efficacy).

Side Effects :

None is reported.

Key Points :

- Intake of pantothenic acid matches with excretion so that it is degraded in the body.
- Burning feet syndrome is characterized by severe burning, tingling, numbness of the feet that respond to pantothenic acid.

PYRIDOXINE (VITAMIN B_6) :

Pyridoxine or vitamin B_6 is a water-soluble B-complex vitamin with multiple physiological functions.

Mechanism Of Action (Physiological) :

Pyridoxine which is a component of coenzyme pyridoxal phosphate, helps in cross-linking of collagen.

Pyridoxine converts tryptophan to niacin.

INDICATIONS IN DERMATOLOGY :

1. During antituberculous therapy that contains isoniazid as a part of regimen.
2. Homocysteinuria.
3. Pyridoxine deficiency manifesting as seborrheic dermatitis like rash and/or pellagroid dermatitis.
4. Palmoplantar erythrodysthesia syndrome due to cytotoxic chemotherapy - 40 mg/day.

DOSES AND PREPARATIONS :

- 30-100 mg/day B-LONG 100 mg tablet.

SIDE EFFECTS :

Systemic : Sensory ataxia, hypoxemia.

Cutaneous : Subepidermal blisters, photosensitive dermatosis.

KEY POINTS :

- 60% of the circulating vitamin B_6 is pyridoxal phosphate.
- Pyridoxine deficiency is encountered in patients of malabsorption syndromes, chronic alcoholics, pregnant women, and patients on drugs like isoniazid, cycloserine and hydralazine (pyridoxine is antagonist of these drugs) oral contraceptives, and penicillamine.
- Pyridoxine deficiency leads to the "Chinese restaurant syndrome". It is a clinical syndrome characterized by headache, palpitations, tightness of the chest, tingling, and numbness. It is caused due to the accumulation of monosodium glutamate present in Chinese food metabolized by glutamic transaminases of which pyridoxine is a cofactor.
- Pyridoxine promotes peripheral decarboxylation of levodopa, reducing its efficacy.

BIOTIN :

Biotin is a water-soluble vitamin, which is mainly tried in dermatology for disorders of hairs and nails.

> **Mechanism Of Action :**
>
> Biotin is a coenzyme, which plays a major role in the metabolism of carbohydrates, fats, and proteins.
>
> Biotin activates folic acid.

Indications In Dermatology :

1. Biotin deficiency due to congenital (holocarboxylase synthetase deficiency and biotinidase deficiency) and acquired causes like excessive raw egg white intake, alcoholism, pregnancy, medications like isotretinoin, valproate, prolonged antibiotic usage.
2. Uncombable hair syndrome.
3. Supportive role for hair and nail disorders.

Doses And Preparations :

- BTN 5 mg tablet, ESSVIT 5 mg tablet.

ASCORBIC ACID (VITAMIN C) :

Ascorbic acid is a "versatile vitamin" with multiple biochemical and physiological functions. L- Ascorbic acid - active form.

> **Mechanism Of Action :**
>
> Cofactor of iron-containing enzymes like prolyl and lysyl hydroxylases that is involved in post-transational modification of collagen (widely present in blood vessels and capillaries, bone, and scar tissue).
>
> Ascorbic acid plays an important role in phenylalanine, tyrosine and carbohydrate metabolism. Useful as a depigmentary agent.

Scavenger of free radicals (antioxidant action).

Potentiate antioxidant action of vitamin E, Photoprotective agent.

Increases absorption of iron from gut.

Anti-inflammatory action.

Because of the multiple physiologic actions of ascorbic acid, it is called a "versatile vitamin".

Oral bioavailability - limited.

INDICATIONS IN DERMATOLOGY :

1. Scurvy with cutaneous manifestations like perifollicular petechiae, cork-screw hairs, and follicular keratosis.
2. Pigmented purpuric dermatosis and other hyperpigmentation disorders (efficacy not documented).
3. Wound healing (non-healing ulcers).

TOPICAL VIT C :

Vitamin C is hydrophilic and vitamin E is lipophilic.

Lipophilic forms of Vit. C :

Magnesium ascorbyl palmitate.

Ascorbyl 6 - palmitate.

Method of use : Regular 8 hourly application.

Half life is 4 days after achieving maximum concentration.

pH has to be maintained < 3.5.

Tyrosine, Zn, vitamin E, ferrulic acid increase the bioavailability of topical Vit C.

Uses : Collagen remodeling in atrophic acne scars.
Photoaging.
Depigmentary action.
Anti-inflammatory in Acne and rosacea.

Side Effects :

Urticaria and erythema multiforme after the use of topical Vit. C has been reported.

FOLIC ACID :

Folic acid naturally occurring and synthetic compound, is most commonly used in dermatology during methotrexate therapy for psoriasis.

Mechanism Of Action :

Synthesis of DNA and RNA.

Vitamin B_9 along with vitamins B_6 and B_{12} control blood levels of homocysteine (linked with heart disease and, possibly, depression and Alzheimer's disease).

Indications in Dermatology :

1. During methotrexate therapy for psoriasis (prevents mucosal and GI side effects).
2. As a supplementation in erythroderma (folate is lost in scales).
3. Diffuse pigmentation over palms and soles and depigmentation of hair.
4. Homocysteinuria.
5. Stomatitis, glossitis (folic acid deficiency).
6. Hyperhomocysteinemia.

Key Points :

- All vitamin B complex vitamins including folic acid get depleted during therapy with broad-spectrum antibiotics. Hence, vitamin B supplementation is routinely advocated during such therapy.
- Folic acid deficiency is the most common vitamin B deficiency. It is commonly seen in alcoholics, during pregnancy, irritable bowel syndrome, and celiac disease.

- Animal foods, with the exception of liver, are poor sources of folic acid. Folic acid-rich plant sources are not completely available in the diet.
- Folic acid should always be given with vitamin B_{12} supplementation (400-1000 μg daily) because folic acid can mask an underlying vitamin B_{12} deficiency, which may cause permanent damage to the nervous system.
- **Drug interactions :**
  1. Aspirin, ibuprofen and acetaminophen increases body requirement of folate.
  2. Cholestyramine, phenytoin, carbamazepine and OC pills reduce blood levels of folate.
  3. Antacids, cimetidine, ranitidine and metformin may inhibit the absorption of folic acid.
  4. Folate antagonists like methotrexate, sulfadoxine pyrimethamine may produce folate deficiency anemia.

VITAMIN B_{12} (CYANOCOBALAMIN) :

Vitamin B_{12} or cyanocobalamin is a water-soluble vitamin known for its neurotropic effects.

MECHANISM OF ACTION (PHYSIOLOGICAL) :

Vitamin B_{12} acts as a coenzyme for fat, protein and carbohydrate metabolism.

It is vital for cell growth, hematopoiesis, and nucleoprotein and myelin synthesis because of its effects on the metabolism of methionine, folic acid, and malonic acid.

INDICATIONS IN DERMATOLOGY :

1. Mucositis secondary to vitamin B_{12} deficiency anemia.
2. Addisonian pigmentation due to vitamin B_{12} deficiency anemia.

3. Canitis or premature graying of hairs.
4. As a neurotropic vitamin.
5. Vitiligo is associated with pernicious anemia another autoimmune disorder.

SIDE EFFECTS :

- Very rare, hypersensitivity, pruritus may occur.
- Vitamin B_{12} may unmask the signs of polycythemia vera.
- Acne, roasacea and allergic reactions.

PREGNANCY CATEGORY – C :

KEY POINTS :

- Dietary improvement, rather than supplementation, is indicated for the prophylaxis of vitamin B_{12} deficiency. Supplementation is preferred for treatment. Dose is 1000 microg daily for 5 days followed weekly for 8 weeks and then monthly for 3 months.
- Pigmentation in Vit B_{12} deficiency is usually over bony prominences and mucosa as against folic acid which is usually over skin creases.
- **Drug interactions :**
  1. Alcohol, aminosalicylates, colchicine (particularly in combination with aminoglycosides) may reduce absorption of vitamin B_{12} from the gut-enhancing requirements of vitamin B_{12}.
  2. Large and continuous doses of folic may reduce blood vitamin B_{12} concentration.
  3. Vitamin B_{12} can cause inactivation of certain antibiotics like streptomycin, tetracyclines, and erythromycin.

TRACE ELEMENTS :

(Refer to Table 14.2)

TABLE 14.2 : **Trace elements of clinical relevance in dermatology**

Micronutrients	Doses	RDA	Dietary sources
Zinc	2 mg/kg/day	15.5 mg	Shellfish, legumes, nutsi, whole grain, green leafy vegetable.
Iron	300 mg t.i.d.	10 mg	Green leafy vegetable, pulses, meat.
Selenium	100-150 mg/day in formulations	70 µg	Wheat, nuts, fish, kidney.
Copper	2 mg/day in formulations	2 mg	Normal Indian diet has sufficient copper.
Essential fatty acids	12 g/day for 6 weeks	0.5% of daily calories requirement	Groundnut oil, safflower oil, cottonseed oil, sunflower oil, and soya bean oil.

ZINC :

Zinc is essential for many physiological actions in the body and also has therapeutic actions in dermatological disorders.

Mechanism Of Action :

Antioxidant action :

i. Stabilization of cell membranes.

ii. Protects against free radicals.

Wound healing.

Immunomodulatory action.

Enhances T-cell mediated immunity.

Mild antiandrogenic action.

Indications In Dermatology :

1. Zinc deficiency congenital (acrodermatitis enteropathica) and acquired.
2. Chronic nonhealing ulcers.

DOSES AND PREPARATIONS :

- 2-3 mg/kg/day in deficiency states, anti-inflammatory dose - 5-10 mg/kg/day.
- ZINFATE (zinc sulfate) 220 mg tablet containing 50 mg elemental zinc.
- Zinc dosages are variable in different multivitamin formulations.

SIDE EFFECTS :

- No side effects with therapeutic dosages.
- Accidental exposure to high quantities of zinc may give rise to nausea, vomiting, diarrhea, abdominal pain, dizziness, acute renal failure, and muscular incoordination. Chronic toxicity includes anemia, neutropenia, and immunosuppression.

KEY POINTS :

Zinc deficiency states :

1. Congenital : acrodermatitis enteropathica is an autosomal recessive disorder of defective zinc absorption.
2. Zinc deficiency is commonly encountered in chronic alcoholics and liver disease, malabsorption syndromes, chronic renal failure, diabetes mellitus, malignancies, HIV infection, post-bowel resection surgery, and severe burns.
3. Deficiency can also occur in patients on antimetabolites, antianabolics, diuretics, sodium valproate, and OC pills.
4. Excess ingestion of iron, calcium, copper, and even tea or coffee can reduce absorption of zinc from the gastrointestinal tract.

Clinical features of acute zinc deficiency include vesiculobullous lesions on erythematous base in acral, periorificial, and perianal distribution. Chronic zinc deficiency manifests as subacute eczematous and psoriasiform dermatitis in similar distribution. Vesiculobullous lesions are thought to be due to apoptotic cell death. Other cutaneous features include alopecia, paronychia, delayed wound healing, and increased incidence of bacterial, fungal, and viral infections of skin.

- Serum value of less than 70 mg/dl and low alkaline phosphatase are some indicators of zinc deficiency.

IRON :

Iron is a micronutrient which is principally required for hemoglobin synthesis and has some indications in dermatology.

Indications Of Iron In Dermatology :

1. Many drugs and diseases cause anemia. Co-existing iron deficiency may compound the anemic state.
2. Telogen effluvium due to iron deficiency.
3. Supplementation for patients with erythroderma.
4. Koilonychia.
5. Plummer-Vinson syndrome.

Doses And Preparations :

(Refer to Table 14.3)

Side Effects :

Systemic :

Nausea, vomiting, upper abdominal pain, constipation, diarrhea, melena and black staining of the tongue.

Key Points :

- Iron deficiency is manifested by koilonychias, telogen effluvium, glossitis (bald tongue), pruritus, and angular stomatitis'.
- Microcytic hypochromic anemia, low serum ferritin, and micronormoblasts on bone marrow examination are indicators of iron deficiency (Table 14.3).

TABLE 14.3 : **Doses and preparations of iron**

Preparations	Doses	Remarks
Oral :		
Ferrous sulfate	2-3 mg/kg/day (300 mg t.i.d./day)	Available iron : 20%
Ferrous fumarate	2-3 mg/kg/day	Available iron : 33%
Ferrous gluconate	2-3 mg/kg/day (300 mg t.i.d./day)	Available iron : 12%
Parenteral		
Intramuscular iron dextran complex	50 mg/ml, 0.5 ml deep i.m. followed by incremental doses of not more than 2 ml/day for adults, 1 ml/day for children, and 0.5 ml/day for infants	Effects are seen after 1-2 weeks
Intravenous iron	Initial dose of 0.5 ml for 5 min followed by 2 ml/day till calculated dose is reached	Corrects iron deficiency rapidly, has risk of anaphylaxis

- Nausea and upper abdominal pain due to iron therapy are dose-dependent, while constipation and diarrhea are due to the changes in bacterial flora of lower GI tract.

COPPER :

Copper is an essential micronutrient, but has a limited therapeutic role in dermatology.

Mechanism Of Action :

It is a component of lysyl hydroxylase, an enzyme for posttranslational modification of collagen. It promotes angiogenesis, skin regeneration, stabilization of ECM proteins along with antibacterial and antifungal action.

Key Points :

- Copper helps in iron absorption.
- No cutaneous features of copper deficiency are reported.
- Menkes kinky hair or "steely hair syndrome" is an inborn error of metabolism with defective copper transport.

SELENIUM :

Selenium is an essential micronutrient and may play an important role in etiopathogenesis of many dermatological manifestations.

> **MECHANISM OF ACTION :**
>
> Selenium is an antioxidant, essential for the enzyme glutathione peroxidase.

DOSES :

- 100-150 mg/day.

KEY POINTS :

- Leukonychia, hypo-depigmentation of skin and hair, thinning and curling of hair (pseudoalbinism) are some of the reported cutaneous manifestations of selenium deficiency.
- Selenium deficiency occurs most commonly in protein energy malnutrition and in malabsorption syndromes.
- Selenium sulfide shampoo (1% and 2.5%) used in pityriasis versicolor, seborrheic dermatitis. Selenium toxicity (endemic selenosis) causes alopecia' anonychia, and xerosis of skin. Airborne exposure more common.

ESSENTIAL FATTY ACIDS (EFA) :

FUNCTION IN SKIN :

- EFA contributes to the formation of lamellar bodies by stratum granulosum, which form principal intercellular lipids stratum corneum.
- EFA, namely linoleic acid (w6), is a parent molecule of arachidonic acid which acts as a precursor of inflammatory mediators like prostaglandins, thromboxanes, and leukotrienes.

- Eicosapentaenoic acid (EFA) and DHA are w3 EFA which shift the inflammatory milleu towards anti-inflammatory.
- A ratio of 5:1 of w6:w3 EFA is optimum.

INDICATIONS :

1. EFA deficiency states.
2. Phrynoderma.
3. Psoriasis.
4. Atopic dermatitis.

Dietary sources :

Fish and fish oil, nuts and seeds (flax seeds, chia seeds, walnuts, plant oils).

DOSES :

- 12 g eicosapentaenoic acid daily for 6 weeks.

KEY POINTS :

- EFA deficiency manifests as generalized xerosis, eczematous dermatitis, erosions in intertriginous areas, and alopecia. Cutaneous features of EFA deficiency overlap with that of zinc deficiency.
- *5 g* of linoleic acid per day is required to prevent essential fatty acid deficiency.
- A ratio of more than 0.4 of eicosatrienoic acid to eicosatetraenoic acid is indicative of EFA deficiency.
- EFA deficiency is uncommon in India due to liberal use of edible oils in diet. However, chronic pancreatitic insufficiency (due to chronic alcoholism), bowel surgery and total Parenteral nutrition lacking lipid supplements can result in EFA deficiency.
- The role of EFAs in many dermatoses is speculative and higher doses may be required to achieve a therapeutic effect in the conditions for which they are supposed to be effective.

x=x=x=x=x

15

Antihistamines and Mast Cell Stabilizers

Antihistamines are widely used in dermatology for various allergic and pruritic dermatoses. (Table 15.1)

TABLE 15.2 : **Differences between 1st generation antihistamines 2nd generation antihistamines**

1st generation antihistamines	2nd generation antihistamines
Lipid soluble, cross blood brain barrier	Low lipid solubility and limited potential to cross BBB
Highly sedating	Low sedating
Has anti-cholinergic, anti-emetic effects	No anti-cholinergic, anti-emetic effects
Short acting, frequent dosing required	Long acting, No frequent dosing required
Early tachyphylaxis *e.g.* promethazine	No tachyphylaxis *e.g.* cetirizine

FIRST GENERATION ANTHIHISTAMINES :

MECHANISM OF ACTION :

Antihistamines act as inverse agonists at H_1 receptors.

INDICATIONS :

1. Allergic : skin disorders *e.g.* urticaria and angioedema, drug hypersensitivity.
2. Severe pruritus associated with skin lesions *e.g.* scabies lichen planus, atopic dermatitis, contact dermatitis, dermatitis herpetiformis.

FIRST GENERATION HI ANTHIHISTAMINES

TABLE 15.1 : **Classification of antihistamines**

	Doses	Peak plasma concentration (hrs)	Pregnancy Category	Half time
First generation antihistamines :				
Ethanolamines :				
Diphenhydramine	25-50 mg tid	0.6-2.8	B	2-9 hr
Clemastine	2 mg bid		B	
Alkylamines :				
Chlorpheniramine	4-8 mg bid	2.0-3.6	B	21-27 hrs
Pheniramine maleate	25-50 mg oral, i.m			
Piperidines :				
Cyproheptadine	4-8 mg bid	2-3	B	
Azatadine	1-2 mg tid		B	
Phenothiazines :				
Promethazine	12.5-25 mg tid	2-3	C	16-19 hrs
Piperazines :				
Hydroxyzine	12.5 mg-25 mg tid	1.7-2.5	C	20-25 hrs
Indene	1-2 mg tds oral,		B	
Dimethindene maleate	0.1% gel topical			

(Continued)

TABLE 15.1 : (Continued)

	Doses	Peak plasma concentration (hrs)	Pregnancy Category	Half time
Second generation antihistamines :				
Piperazines :				
Cetirizine	10 mg od/bid	0.5-1 5	B	6-8 hr
Levocetirizine	2.5-10 mg odd	1 hr	B	4 hrs
Piperidines :				
Loratadine	10 mg od	1-2.5	B	
Benzeneacetic acid-Fexofenadine	180 mg od	2-6	C	14 hrs
Desloratadine	5 mg od	3	C	21-24 hrs
Mizolastine	10 mg od	1.5	No adequate data	
Ebastine	10-20 mg od	2.6	No adequate data	8-12 hrs
Astemizole	10 mg od	Days	C	29 hrs
Monohydrochloride-Olapatadine	5-10 mg			7-9 hrs
Pyridine-Rupatadine	10-20 mg	5 hours		6 hrs
Bilastine	20 mg OD, upto QID	1-3 hours	C	14.5 hrs

3. Pruritus without skin lesions especially if interfering with sleep.

CONTRAINDICATIONS :

1. Drivers/Pilots (causes sedation).
2. Machine operators during work and those involved with moving machine parts (causes sedation).
3. Elderly individuals with benign prostatic hyperplasia (BPH) (precipitates urinary retention).
4. Glaucoma (precipitates glaucoma).

SIDE EFFECTS :

Central nervous system :

- Sedation (clemastine, diphenhydramine, promethazine) and weight gain. Sedation can last longer in the 2nd generation longer acting antihistammines.
- Paradoxical excitation and agitation.
- Increased appetite (Cyproheptadine).

Gastrointestinal :

- Nausea and vomiting.
- Constipation and pain in abdomen.
- Epigastric discomfort.

Anticholinergic effects (clemastine, diphenhydramine, promethazine, hydroxyzine) :

- Dryness of mucosae.
- Difficulty in micturition.
- Urinary retention (in elderly with benign prostatic hyperplasia).
- Impotence.
- Glaucoma.

Cutaneous (rare) :

- Urticaria, maculopapular rash (rare).
- Fixed drug eruption to cetirizine has been reported.
- Allergic contact dermatitis (with topical application).
- Photosensitivity.

KEY POINTS :

1. First generation antihistamines are sedative because they are lipophilic and easily cross blood brain barrier.
2. Alcohol, opioid analgesics like morphine and codeine, and benzodiazepines use is contraindicated in patients taking 1st generation antihistamines as it causes more CNS depression.
3. First generation antihistamines like diphenhydramine, chlorpheniramine, clemastine, promethazine and hydroxyzine inhibit CYP2D6 enzyme leading to increase in blood levels of other drugs.
4. Serum half life of 1st generation antihistamines is shorter in children and longer in elderly necessitating doses adjustments.
5. Cetirizine, levocetirizine, fexofenadine are generally considered safe in children. However, none of them are approved for use in children less than 2 years of age, (hydroxyzine- 6 months) while fexofenadine is now approved for use in children above 6 months for chronic urticaria.
6. Antihistamines are also available as topical preparations but they are less effective in reducing the pruritus of eczema.
7. There may be an increased chance of side effects such as dry mouth and constipation if sedating antihistamines are taken with other drugs like hyoscine (antispasmodic) or procyclidine (anti-cholinergic).

8. Should be used cautiously in cases of severe hepatic or renal injury and in the elderly as these patients have increased chances of sedation which can interfere with physician's assessment of their interval disease.
9. Efficacy of antihistamines varies from patient to patient. If an antihistamine fails to provide adequate relief, switch to a drug from a different chemical class.

SECOND GENERATION H_1 ANTIHISTAMINES :

Mechanism Of Action :

1. Inverse agonists of H_1 histamine receptors.
2. Affect cell trafficking in skin of eosinophils and neutrophils.
3. Alters expression of vascular adhesion molecules.

Indications :

1. Urticaria and angioedema.
2. Azelastine has mast cell stabilizing properties for which has been used in mastocytosis.
3. Cetirizine has antiinflammatory properties for which it has been tried in bullous pemphigoid, small vessel vasculitis and type II lepra reaction with limited success.

Side Effects :

Common side effects of 2nd generation AH-fatigue, dizziness, headache, dry mouth.

Other side effcts of 1st generation AH and their contraindications mentioned earlier also apply to 2nd generation AH albeit with lesser frequency.

Polymorphous ventricular tachycardia or torsades de pointes is seen with terfenadine, astemizole.

KEY POINTS :

1. Second generation antihistamines like terfinadine and astemizole (no longer in use) when used along with ketoconazole or itraconazole; -erythromycin or clarithromycin (not with azithromycin); lovastatin, protease inhibitors and flavonoids can cause polymorphous ventricular tachycardia.
2. Sedating potential of 2nd generation antihistamines is in the following order, cetirizine > levocetirizine > desloratidine > fexofenadine.
3. Potency of 2nd generation AH is in the following order Levocetirizine > Fexofenadine (short acting) > desloratidine (less potent, longer acting).
4. In cases of chronic spontaneous urticarias, if standard dosing with cetirizine, levocetirizine, desloratidine or fexofenadineor is ineffective, increasing the frequency of dosing (safe upto fourfold) is recommended.

H_2 ANTIHISTAMINES :

Include drugs like famotidine, ranitidine and cimetidine.

Drug	Doses	Pregnancy Category
Cimetidine	400 mg bid	B
Ranitidinc	150 mg bid	B
Famotidine	40 mg od	B

MECHANISM OF ACTION

Inhibit H_2 histamine receptors in cutaneous vasculature.

INDICATIONS IN DERMATOLOGY :

1. Refractory chronic idiopathic urticaria.
2. Physical urticarias.

3. As a co-prescription with oral steroids to prevent gastritis.
4. Mastocytosis.
5. Pruritus associated with polycythemia vera, myelofibrosis and carcinoid syndrome.
5. Immunomodulatory action in non genital warts and molluscum contagiosum is claimed to be of use.

SIDE EFFECTS :

Cimetidine (Not in use now) :

- Mental confusion.
- Loss of libido.
- Gynecomastia.
- Impotence.
- Galactorrhea in females due to raised prolactin levels.

Ranitidine :

- Increases blood alcohol levels.
- Reversible mental confusion.
- Susceptibility to arrhythmias.

KEY POINTS :

1. Cimetidine prolongs bleeding time and prothrombin time in patients on warfarin therapy.
2. Cimetidine increases blood levels of phenytoin, nifedipine diazepam and propranolol.
3. Cimetidine has immunomodulatory effects.
4. Ranitidine decreases diazepam absorption.

DOXEPIN :

Class - tricyclic antidepressant.

Mechanism Of Action :

Antihistaminic and anticholinergic action along with antidepressant effect. Amongst the TCA's, Doxepin has the highest affinity for H_1 receptors (800 times that of diphenhydramine).

Dose :

10 or 25 mg capsules, maximum 30 mg per day in divided doses or 25 mg at bedtime.

Indications :

Urticaria, atopic dermatitis, urticaria pigmentosa.

Side Effects :

Drowsiness, dry mouth, metallic taste, constipation, urinary retention, blurred vision, palpitation, tachycardia.

PREGNANCY CATEGORY – C, avoid in lactation.

MAST CELL STABILIZERS :

Mast cell stabilizers include drugs like ketotifen and disodium cromoglycate.

KETOTIFEN :

Mechanism of Action :

It is mast cell stabilizer. It is H_1 type antihistamine and calcium channel blocker, which prevents release of histamine from mast cells. Ketotifen inhibits the Ca^{++} pass through the mastocyte and basophil membrane.

Indications :

1. Chronic idiopathic urticaria.
2. Physical urticaria.

3. Mastocytosis.
4. Neurofibromatosis-associated pruritus.

DOSES :

- 1 mg bid, 50 micrograms/kg bid for infants and children upto 3 years of age.
- KETASMA 1 mg tab.

SIDE EFFECTS :

- Sedation
- Weight gain

KEY POINTS :

- It may take up to 10 weeks for complete effect of ketotifen to occur.

LEUKOTRIENE INHIBITORS :

DRUGS :

Leukotriene antagonists : Montelukast (available in India), Zafirlukast, Pranlukast.

Leukotriene synthesis inhibitors : Zileuton.

Levamisole has some inhibitory action against 5-LOX enzyme.

MECHANISM OF ACTION :

Leukotrienes are involved in the promotion and maintenance of histamine mediated allergic reactions. Their inhibition is of use in the following :

1. Allergic rhinitis and asthma (FDA approved).
2. Atopic dermatitis.
3. Refractory urticarias (along with H_1 AH) Drug of choice for aspirin and other NSAID induced urticaria -

angioedema. Other urticarias like cold urticaria, food and drug induced urticarias, delayed pressure urticaria, dermographism.

4. Systemic mastocytosis.

DOSE :

Avoided in children < 6 years

6-14 years : 5 mg Od

>14 years : 10 mg od

PREGNANCY CATEGORY – C :

SIDE EFFECTS :

URTI, nausea, abdominal pain and rarely psychiatric disturbances.

x=x=x=x=x

16
Miscellaneous Agents

Miscellaneous agents used included in this chapter are :

1. Psychotropic agents
2. Antiandrogens
3. Antiperspirants
4. Antiinflammatory agents

PSYCHOTROPIC AGENTS :

A number of dermatological diseases are believed to have strong psychiatric basis. Conversely, many dermatological disorders can have strong psychological impacts. Though counseling and behavioral therapy is required in almost all such cases, psychotropic agents may, at times, be required in some cases. Various psychotropic agents that are or can be used for psychodermatological conditions are given in Table 16.1.

ANTIANDROGENS :

Antiandrogens are the agents, that block androgen receptors (AR) or synthesis of androgens. (Table 16.2)

CAUSES OF ANDROGEN EXCESS can be due to :

1. *Adrenal :*
   - Congenital adrenal hyperplasia.
   - Cushing's syndrome (rare).
   - Adrenal tumors (rare).

2. *Ovarian :*

   Nontumorous :

   - Polycystic ovarian disease (commonest cause).

   Tumorous :

   - Androgen secreting tumors are renoblastoma.
   - Sertoli-Leydig cell tumors, hilus cell tumors, and lipoid cell tumors.

3. *Pituitary :*

   Hyperprolactinemia due to pituitary tumor.

4. *Iatrogenic :*

   Drugs causing hyperprolactinemia.

Hormonal evaluation panel should include :

- LH : FSH ratio.
- Serum DHEAS, Total and free testosterone, 17-hydroxy progesterone, androstenedione and prolactin levels.

USG (Abdomen and pelvis) to rule out polycystic ovarian disease.

INDICATIONS OF ANTIANDROGENS IN DERMATOLOGY :

- Recalcitrant Acne, seborrhea with history of premenstrual flare, deep seated nodules over lower face and neck.
- Hirsutism.
- Androgenetic alopecia.
- Hidradenitis suppurativa.
- For the treatment of the above in syndromes like PCOS, Cushings, HAIR-AN, SAHA, congenital adrenal hyperplasia, acromegaly.

KEY POINTS :

- Acne and seborrhea responds in 3-6 months, alopecia

ANTIANDROGENS

TABLE 16.1 : **Psychotropic drugs**

Drug (trade name)	Mechanism of Action	Doses	Side Effects	Key Points	Dermatological Indications
Anxiolytic :					
Clonazepam	Benzodiazepine, GABA agonist	0.25-0.5 mg at night	Sedation	Should be used for less than 4 weeks due to its addiction potential	Acute anxiety due to dermatological disorders
Buspirone	Exact action unknown; moderate affinity for 5-HT and D_2 receptors	5-10 mg t.i.d./ q.i.d.	Dizziness, nausea, headache, nervousness, light-headedness, and excitement	Nonsedating, no addiction potential 2-4 weeks required for action	Chronic anxiety due to psoriasis, HIV or severe pruritic dermatoses like atopic dermatitis
Antidepressants :					
Doxepine	Tricyclic antidepressant	25 mg HS	Sedation	Antipruritic, analgesic, and anticholinergic effect. Minimum 2 weeks required for effect, wide patient-to-patient variation in therapeutic effect	Severe pruritus with depression
Amitriptyline	Tricyclic antidepressant	75 mg o.d.	Drowsiness, dizziness, loss of coordination, and hypotension, QT prolongation	TCA and SSRTI inhibits liver microsomal enzymes, anticholinergics and MAO inhibitors when given with TCA may cause hyperpyrexia	Postherpetic neuralgia, complex regional pain syndromes
Fluoxetine	5-HT reuptake inhibitor	20 mg o.d.	Anxiety insomnia, nausea and diarrhea, orgasmic problems	No muscarinic/cholinergic effect, no sadation and no titration of doses required	Severe depression due to psoriasis, vitiligo, untreatable or pruritic skin conditions, dermatitis artefacta
Sertraline	5-HT reuptake inhibitor	25-200 mg o.d.	Nausea, diarrhea, orgasmic problems	Same as that of fluoxetine	Same as above

(Continued)

Table 16.1 : (Continued)

Drug (trade name)	Mechanism of Action	Doses	Side Effects	Key Points	Dermatological Indications
Citalopram	5-HT reuptake inhibitor	20 mg o.d. initially to 40 mg o.d. within a week	Nausea, diarrhea, orgasmic problems	Same as that of fluoxetine	Same as above
Venlafloxine	5-HT and NA reuptake inhibitor	75-225 mg b.i.d.	Insomnia, nervousness, nausea, sweating, dry mouth, constipation	—	Same as above
Bupropion	Weak psychostimulant by noradrenergic effect	100 mg b.i.d. f/b 100 mg t.i.d.	Agitation, dry mouth, insomnia, headache, nausea/vomiting	Primarily metabolized to hydroxybupropion by the CYP2B6 isoenzyme	Same as above
Antipsychotic drugs :					
Pimozide	Blocks central dopamine receptors	1 mg followed by 1 mg increment weekly	Extrapyramidal symptoms, pseudoparkinsonism	Benzotropine 1 mg or diphenhydramine 25 mg q.i.d. for side effects of pimozide	Delusions of parasitosis, dysmorphohobia
Risperidone	Dopaminergic and serotoninergic effect	1 mg b.i.d. followed by incremental weekly doses	Dizziness, anxiety, rhinitis, QT prolongation	5-6 mg/day 18 months	Same as above
Anti-OCD drugs :					
Fluoxetine	Described earlier	20 mg o.d.	Same as mentioned earlier	Same as mentioned earlier	Neurotic excoriations, trichotillomania
Sertraline	Described earlier	25-200 mg o.d.	Same as mentioned earlier	Same as mentioned earlier	Same as above
Citalopram	Described earlier	20 mg o.d. initially to 40 mg o.d. within a week	Same as mentioned earlier	Safe and newer drug for OCD	Same as above
Clomipramine	Tricyclic antidepressant	100 mg HS	Increases lipid levels	Same as other TCA	Acne excoriee

ANTIANDROGENS

ANTIANDROGENS

TABLE 16.2 : **Antiandrogens and androgen inhibitors in dermatology**

	Mechanism of action	Indications	Doses	Side Effects	Key Points
Antiandrogens :					
Spironolactone (aldactone)	Blocks androgen receptors and inhibits androgen biosynthesis	Androgenetic alopecia, recalcitrant acne due to androgen excess, hirsutism	50-200 mg/day	Hyperkalemia, gynecomastia, minor GI disturbances	Canrenone is the active aldosterone antagonist of spironolactone, serum K^+ levels and BP needed to during therapy for use in male
Flutamide	Inhibits binding of DHT to AR and androgen uptake	Hirsutism	250 mg tds	Hypersensitivity, gynecomastia, fluid retention, hepatotoxicity (rare)	70% effective in hirsutism. Mostly used in combination with ethyl estradiol 35 µg (Diane 35, 21 days pills), 80% improvement in seborrhea
Cyproterone acetate	Competitive inhibitor of DHT for binding to AR	Androgenetic alopecia, recalcitrant acne due to androgen excess, hirsutism	100-200 mg/day when used alone, 2-3 mg/day when used in combination	OCPs Occasional; weight gain, hepatotoxicity, tiredness, depression	Refer chapter "Antihistamines" for details

(Continued)

TABLE 16.2 : **(Continued)**

	Mechanism of action	Indications	Doses	Side Effects	Key Points
Oral contraceptive agents with 4th generation progesterone	Fourth generation progesterones like drospirone have antiandrogenic action	Same as above	Yaz (20 mg of ethinyl estradiol + 3 mg drospirone) Yasmin (30 mg EE + 3 mg drospirone)	Hepatotoxicity, Deep vein thrombosis	Should not be used in women > 35 years for fear of thromboembolic events
Androgen inhibitors :					
Finasteride	Inhibits enzyme type II 5-reductase which converts Testosterone + DHT	Androgenetic alopecia, hirsutism, hidradenitis suppurativa	1 mg/day in men and 5 mg/day in women	Hypersensitivity, reports of loss of libido, depression	Refer chapter "Systemic Antifungals" for details
Dutasteride	Non selective inhibitor of 5 alpha reductase	Androgenetic alopecia, some role in frontal fibrosing alopecia, hirsutism, acne vulgaris and HS	0.5-2.5 mg/day	Same as above	Pregnancy category X. Men on finasteride and dutasteride should not donate blood for 6 months after the last dose

takes 6-12 months, while hirsutism takes much longer hence combination with other forms of hair reduction like mechanical methods or lasers is necessary.

- Oral contraception is a must in women of child bearing age due to risk of feminization of male fetus.

SIDE EFFECTS :

- Hepatotoxicity is a major concern.
- Increased risk of DVT and pulmonary embolism with spironolactone and OC pills.
- Spironolactone causes electrolyte imbalance.
- Reversible effects of 5 alpha reductase inhibitors in men include loss of libido and erectile dysfunction (< 1.5% cases).
- Breast cancer and glandular hyperplasia in females with finasteride.

ANTIPERSPIRANTS :

Systemic antiperspirants for the treatment of eccrine hyperhidrosis are anticholinergic agents like glycopyrrolate and propantheline bromide. These drugs can be used for generalized hyperhidrosis, axillary, and palmoplantar hyperhidrosis.

GLYCOPYRROLATE AND PROPANTHELINE BROMIDE :

Glycopyrrolate and propantheline bromide are anticholinergic agents that are used for the treatment of hyperhidrosis.

MECHANISM OF ACTION :

Anticholinergic agent; blocks acetylcholine that acts as neurotransmitter in eccrine sweat glands.

DOSES AND PREPARATIONS :

- Glycopyrrolate 1-2 mg t.i.d. ROBINUL 1 mg tablet.

- Propantheline bromide 15 mg b.i.d./t.i.d. PRO-BANTHINE.
- Oxybutyrin 2.5-5 mg bd (Oxyspas).

Side Effects :

- Anticholinergic Side Effects : Dryness of mouth, blurring of vision, constipation, urinary retention, hyperthermia, glaucoma.
- Seizures, hypersensitivity.

Key Points :

- Interindividual variation of anticholinergic agents occurs due to poor and variable oral absorption.
- The use of anticholinergic agents is not advocated in children, pregnancy, and lactation unless considered to be absolutely necessary.
- Since anticholinergic agents can cause drowsiness and blurring of vision, they should not be used while driving or operating machines.
- In elderly patients with prostatic enlargement, anticholinergic agents can cause urinary retention.
- *Drug interactions :*
    1. Tricyclic antidepressants increase side effects of anticholinergic agents.
    2. Attenuates effects of atenolol and digoxin while decreases effect of phenothiazines.
    3. Glycopyrrolate and cyclopropane (anesthetic agent) have a higher risk of ventricular arrhythmias when given concurrently.

ANTIINFLAMMATORY AGENTS :

DAPSONE :

Dapsone, an antimetabolite drug, is an effective antiinflammatory drug used in the treatment of inflammatory disorders predominantly consisting of neutrophils.

MECHANISM OF ACTION :

Inhibition of PABA incorporation into folic acid.

Inhibits chemotaxis of neutrophils.

Inhibits release of histamine from mast cells.

INDICATIONS IN DERMATOLOGY :

1. *Dermatoses with predominant neutrophils :*
   - Dermatitis herpetiformis.
   - Linear IgA dermatosis.
   - Subcorneal pustular dermatosis.
   - Infantile acropustulosis.
   - Bullous SLE.
   - Pyoderma gangrenosum.
   - Sweet's syndrome.
   - Behcet's syndrome.

2. *Autoimmune bullous dermatoses :*
   - Bullous cicatricial etc.
   - Bullous SLE.
   - Chronic bullous disorder of childhood (CBDC).
   - Pemphigus vulgaris/foliaceous.

3. *Vasculitis :*
   - Leukocytoclastic vasculitis.
   - Urticarial vasculitis.
   - Erythema elevatum diutinum.

4. *Other dermatoses :*
   - Subacute cutaneous lupus erythematosus (SCLE).

- Relapsing polychondritis.
- Granuloma annulare.
- Reclusive spider bite.

DOSES :

- 50-200 mg/day as an anti-inflammatory agent.

SIDE EFFECTS :

Systemic :

Hematological :

- Hemolysis in G6PD deficient patients (common).
- Methemoglobinemia (not common).
- Agranulocytosis (rare).
- Thrombocytopenia (rare).
- Even when G6PD is normal dapsone (100 mg) reduces hemoglobin by 1-1.5 g%.

Neurological :

- 'Wooly' headache (light headedness) due to transient hemolysis hence bedtime dose is recommended.
- Psychosis.
- Peripheral neuropathy (distal axonal, motor, dose-related and reversible).

Renal :

- Nephrotic syndrome (uncommon).

Hepatic :

- Hepatitis (uncommon but common with 'dapsone syndrome').
- Cholestatic jaundice (uncommon).

Cutaneous :

- Maculopapular rash.
- Fixed drug eruption.
- Stevens Johnson syndrome.
- Toxic epidermal necrolysis (TEN).
- Dapsone hypersensitivity syndrome (dapsone syndrome).

DRUG INTERACTIONS :

1. Hematologic reactions may increase with folic acid antagonists, *e.g.* pyrimethamine (monitor for agranulocytosis during the second and third month of therapy).
2. Probenecid increases dapsone toxicity.
3. Dapsone levels may significantly decrease when administered concurrently with rifampicin.

KEY POINTS :

1. Dapsone is completely (more than 90%) absorbed taken orally. It is excreted freely in bile with enterohepatic recirculation so that it is mainly lost from the body through urine as the glucuronide.
2. Dapsone is preferably taken at night as it causes lightheadedness.
3. Dapsone had been given in pregnancy in the past without teratogenic side effects. In fact, it has the advantage of killing viable bacilli in the breast milk during lactations
4. Treatment of dapsone-induced methemoglobinemia is intravenous administration of methylene blue. Ascorbic acid is also recommended. Levels of methemoglobin below 20% do not produce signs and symptoms, while levels above 70% are usually fatal.
5. In G6PD deficient individuals, dapsone should be started at a low dose, 25 mg twice weekly, and gradually

increased to 50-100 mg daily over 34 weeks if no severe hemolysis.

6. Dapsone syndrome or sulfone hypersensitivity syndrome develops between 2 and 6 weeks after dapsone is started and is characterized by :
   - fever and constitutional symptoms.
   - lymphadenopathy.
   - hepatitis with elevated liver enzymes, hepatomegaly.
   - skin rash which may begin as a maculopapular rash and may progress to exfoliative dermatitis
   - eosinophilia and atypical lymphocytes in peripheral smear.
   - SJS/TEN like lesions (uncommon).

Management consists of immediate stoppage of the drug and, if required, oral steroids for 2-6 weeks. If allowed to progress without the omission of dapsone, the condition can be fatal. Hence, rechallenge with dapsone is not advocated.

CLOFAZIMINE :

Clofazimine is an iminophenazine dye which is used as an antileprosy agent as well as antiinflammatory agent.

Mechanism Of Action :

Acts probably with interfering with the template function of DNA.

Uses :

1. Pyoderma gangrenosum.
2. Recalcitrant type II lepra reaction.
3. Chronic cutaneous LE.
4. Sweet's syndrome.
5. Acne fulminans.

6. Orofacial granulomatosis.
7. Atypical mycobacterial infections.
8. Leishmaniasis.
9. Malakoplakia.
10. Rhinoscleroma.
11. Ashy dermatosis.
12. Lupus pernio.

DOSES AND PREPARATIONS :

Anti-inflammatory doses of clofazimine are higher than those used in leprosy.

- 100 mg b.i.d. or t.i.d.
- Half life is 10 days after 1 dose and 70 days after longterm use.
- HANSEPRAN 50, 100 mg capsule, LAMPRENE soft gelatin capsule to be taken with meals.

PREGNANCY CATEGORY – C :

Half time – 10 days after 1 dose, 70 days after longterm.

SIDE EFFECTS :

Systemic :

- When used in higher doses, the drug gets deposited in mesenteric lymph nodes and causes a syndrome of acute abdomen that may mimic appendicitis. Pain may be accompanied by vomiting, diarrhea, and GI hemorrhage.
- Eosinophilic enteritis.
- Renal failure.
- Splenic infarction.

Cutaneous :

- Brown pigmentation of the infiltrated skin,"mahogany red" followed by "charcoal black".

- Ichthyosis.
- Phototoxicity (rare).

KEY POINTS :

- 40-70% absorbed after oral administration. Accumulates especially in fat, in crystalline form.
- The severity of skin discoloration due to clofazimine depends upon the dose and degree of skin infiltration by leprosy. Due to discoloration, clofazimine may be avoided in fair-colored individuals. An alternative drug may be used in such patients.
- Pigmentation is blotchy and more pronounced in photo exposed areas. It requires 6-12 months for clearance after discontinuation of the drug. It can also be seen in the cornea and conjunctiva.
- Due to anticholinergic action, clofazimine can cause diminished sweating and tearing (leads to more dryness of skin and eyes).

COLCHICINE :

Alkaloid extract; predominantly used for the treatment of gout; colchicine has some dermatological indications as an antiinflammatory agent.

MECHANISM OF ACTION :

Bind to fibrillar protein tubulin and causes metaphase arrest. Inhibits neutrophilic chemotaxis at the site of the inflammation.

INDICATIONS :

1. Tophaceous gout with gouty arthritis.
2. Behcet's disease.
3. Aphthous stomatitis.
4. Dermatitis herpetiformis.

5. Sweet's syndrome.
6. Linear IgA bullous dermatosis, CBDC, EBA (as an alternative to dapsone).
7. Type 2 lepra reaction.
8. Palmoplantar pustulosis.
9. Leukocytoclastic vasculitis.
10. Urticarial vasculitis.
11. Dermatomyositis.
12. Scleroderma.
13. Relapsing polychondritis.
14. Pyoderma gangrenosum.
15. Psoriasis.
16. May prevent progression of primary cutaneous amyloidosis.

DOSES AND PREPARATIONS :

- 0.5-1.5 mg/day, GOUTNIL 0.5 mg tablet.

SIDE EFFECTS :

- Nausea, vomiting, watery or bloody diarrhea, abdominal cramps, and CNS depression.
- Chronic therapy : aplastic anemia, agranulocytosis, myopathy, hair loss. rhabdomyolysis, azoospermia.

PREGNANCY CATEGORY – C :

KEY POINT :

- Diarrhea marks the onset of the action of colchicine.

THALIDOMIDE :

Thalidomide, infamous for its teratogenic effects, has many dermatological uses and is found to be a very effective drug for the treatment of recalcitrant type II lepra reaction, if used judiciously.

MECHANISM OF ACTION :

Immunomodulatory and antiinflammatory : specific inhibition of TNF-alpha, IL-6, IL-12.

Inhibits angiogenesis.

Sedative.

USES :

1. Resistant erythema nodosum leprosum (ENL) in lepromatous leprosy.
2. AIDS-Stomatitis, Kaposi's sarcoma, Pruritic papular exanthem of HIV.
3. Prurigo nodularis.
4. Actinic prurigo.
5. Cutaneous LE.
6. Recalcitrant aphthous stomatitis.
7. Behcet's disease.
8. Pyoderma gangrenosum.
9. Erosive lichen planus.
10. Bullous pemphigoid, cicatricial pemphigoid.
11. Recurrent erythema multiforme.
12. Porphyria cutanea tarda.
13. Chronic GVHD.
14. Sarcoidosis.
15. Myeloproliferative disorders.

PREGNANCY CATEGORY – X :

DOSES :

- 100 mg 3-4 times daily for 2 weeks in ENL to be tapered over 1-3 months to a maintenance dose of 50-100 mg daily.
- HIV - related conditions : 100-300 mg/day for 2 weeks.

Side Effects :

- Teratogenicity, 100 mg of thalidomide results in a 100% incidence of birth defects.
- Nausea, vomiting, constipation, sedation.
- Peripheral neuropathy manifesting as paresthesia, pain, and motor weakness, irreversible in 50%.
- Leukopenia, thrombocytopenia.
- Hypothyroidism, hypoglycemia.
- Other side effects : mood changes, xerosis and xerostomia, brittle nails, peripheral edema, pruritus, menstrual irregularities, bradycardia, red palms, decreased libido.
- DVT and pulmonary embolism.

Key Points :

- Thalidomide is best avoided in women of childbearing age. However, if considered must then effective birth control must be in place for at least 1 month before and a negative pregnancy test be obtained before the beginning of therapy. The tablets may be started preferably on the 4th day of the menstrual cycle. The test will have to be repeated monthly. A baseline CBC with platelets should be obtained. Thalidomide is present in semen. Men on thalidomide should not have unprotected sex with women of child bearing potential.
- Thalidomide can also cause neuropathy, which is of both sensory and motor type and needs to be differentiated from neuropathy associated with leprosy in which it is commonly used. Signs of neuropathy are usually preceded by symptoms like tingling, pain, or paresthesia. When muscle weakness occurs, it commonly affects the proximal muscles of lower limbs. However, the sensory affection is more symmetric and distal.

LOW MOLECULAR WEIGHT DEXTRAN :

Dextran is a gum produced from cane or beet sugar dextran is a polymer of glucose from which is prepared low molecular weight (LMW) dextran, which is a mixture of dextrose polymers with an average molecular weight of 40,000 (Range 10,000-70,000).

MECHANISM OF ACTION :

1. It lowers viscosity of blood and improves flow by hemodilution.
2. Decrease platelet adhesion.
3. It decreases serum fibrinogen and clotting factors.
4. Decreases rouleux formation by RBCs.

INDICATIONS :

1. Deep vein thrombosis and thrombophlebitis.
2. Raynaud's phenomenon and impending gangrene as in systemic sclerosis.
3. Anti phospholipid antibody syndrome - impending digital gangrene.
4. Frost bite.
5. Cutaneous cholesterol emboli.
6. Livedoid vasculopathy, livedo reticularis with ulceration.

Half life – 24 hours.

DOSES AND PREPARATIONS :

- 10% dextran in 5% dextrose or in normal saline (NS) solution is infused intravenously. First inject 20 ml i.v. over 3 to 5 minutes to decrease the risk of anaphylaxis. Then infuse 20-30 ml per hour up to a maximum of to 3 liters per day. In Raynaud's phenomenon : infuse 500-1000 ml over 4-6 hours on day 1, 500 ml on day 2 and then on alternate days for 10 days.
- LOMODEX dextran inj if 0.90/0 NS solution, 540 mi.
- Storage is upto 10 years.

Side Effects :

Acute renal failure, bleeding tendency, anaphylaxis, nausea and vomiting, hypotension.

Key Points :

- Adequate hydration is to be maintained before LMW dextran therapy. Low specific gravity of urine indicates decreased renal excretion of LMWD, warrants stoppage of infusion.
- If the urine output is low or if the blood urea is 60 mg/ml or higher, therapy is not advisable.
- Dose should never exceed more than 10% of the blood volume.

STANOZOLOL :

Stanozolol is a synthetic anabolic steroid with highest anabolic : androgenic ratio.

Mechanism Of Action :

It promotes the synthesis of C_1 esterase inhibitor and has fibrinolytic activity.

Indications :

1. Hereditary angioedema (prophylaxis and treatment).
2. Livedoid vasculopathy.
3. Raynaud's phenomenon.
4. Lipodermatosclerosis.

PREGNANCY PRESCRIBING STATUS – X :

Side Effects :

Nausea, epigastric discomfort, liver dysfunction, headache, skin rash, fluid retention, weight gain, hirsutism in females.

DOSES :

- 2 mg thrice a day. Maintenance dose of 2 mg/day on alternate days or 2.5 mg thrice weekly.
- MENABOL 2 mg tablet.

KEY POINTS :

- Stanozolol increases the sensitivity to anticoagulants and may increase bleeding.

CALCIUM DOBESILATE :

Calcium dobesilate has been advocated in disorders of blood vessels although efficacy to be substantially proved.

MECHANISM OF ACTION :

Angio-protective effect by decreasing capillary permeability and blood viscosity.

Anti-platelet and fibrinolytic effect.

Increased endothelium dependent relaxation secondary to increased nitrous oxide synthesis.

Antioxidant effect.

INDICATIONS IN DERMATOLOGY :

Chronic venous insufficiency, pigmented purpuric dermatoses (shambergs disease) may improve partially.

DOSES AND PREPARATIONS :

- 500 mg twice daily.
- DOBESIL 500 mg cap.

SIDE EFFECTS :

Epigastric pain, drug induced fever, pruritus, skin rash etc.

x=x=x=x=x

Section 2

Topical Agents

17
Principles of Topical Therapy

Topical therapy is the mainstay of dermatological treatment. Understanding the principles of topical therapy is important for its judicious and effective use in dermatology.

Most topical agents, when applied to the skin, penetrate the skin barrier that is mainly composed of stratum corneum and intercellular lipids between corneocytes. Stratum corneum consists of anuclear, keratinized corneocytes containing keratin filaments, water, and natural moisturizing factor (NMF). NMF is made up of lactate, urea, and electrolytes. Intercellular lipids form a hydrophobic layer between corneocytes and are synthesized from lamellar bodies secreted by granular cells of stratum granulosum. Intercellular lipid is made up of ceramides, cholesterol and fatty acids.

PHARMACOKINETICS OF TOPICAL AGENTS :

Topical agent when applied to the surface of the skin, after the lag phase (when drugs remain in the stratum corneum without being detected in blood circulation), penetrates the skin barrier with increasing concentration in the epidermis and then enters papillary dermal vessels and hence blood circulation (rising phase). Since the amount of the applied drug is finite, the concentration of the drug in the stratum corneum and blood falls over a period of time (falling phase) leading to decreased efficacy.

FACTORS AFFECTING ABSORPTION OF TOPICAL AGENTS :

Potency :

Higher the concentration of the drug in topical formulation, better are the absorption and therapeutic effect.

Vehicle Used For Transcutaneous Delivery :

Ointments have better penetration than lotions, creams, gels, or pastes.

Site Of Application :

Absorption is better in the following sites in descending order:

Mucous membranes > scrotum > eyelids > face > trunk > arms and legs > hands and feet (dorsum) > palms and soles > nails.

Age Of Patient :

Absorption is more in neonates and children as compared to adults.

Occlusion And Occlusive Sites :

Occlusion or application over occlusive sites increases the hydration of the skin and increases the absorption by 10-100 times with most drugs.

Frequency Of Application :

Frequency of application does not significantly affect the absorption. Nevertheless, the effect of emollients is drastically increased by frequent applications.

Hydration Of Skin :

Hydration of skin prior to topical application enhances absorption.

BARRIER FUNCTION IN CERTAIN SKIN DISEASES :

Skin conditions with deranged barrier functions like atopic dermatitis, psoriasis, eczema, or abrasions have the likelihood of greater absorption.

OTHERS :

Rubbing or massaging after topical application, application at the site with more hair follicles, and use of micronized drugs (smaller particle size increases surface area) increase absorption of a topical agent.

TOPICAL FORMULATIONS :

Polano has simplified topical formulations in his book *Topical. Skin Therapeutics,* as follows :

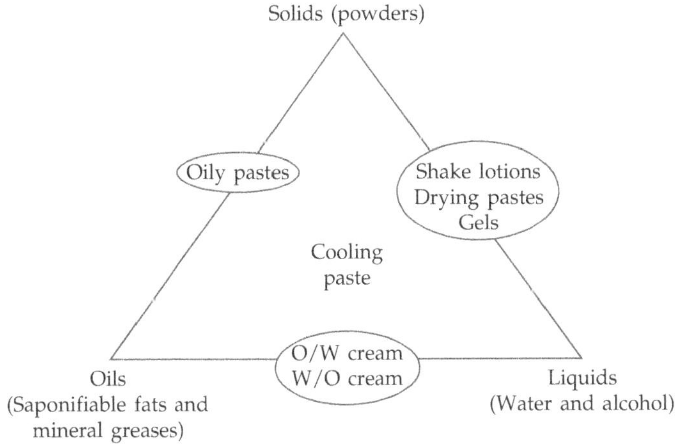

TOXICITY DUE TO TOPICAL AGENTS :

Local Effects :

- *Irritant :* irritation, burning, stinging, pruritus, pain, erythema, edema, vesicles, pustules, rarely bullae or burn, post inflammatory pigmentation is common.

- *Allergic :* allergic contact urticarial.
- *Others (neither irritant nor allergic) :* Comedogenicity, telangiectases, atrophy, contact purpura, etc.

Systemic Effects :

Systemic toxicity due to increased absorption of' the topical agents in systemic circulation. It may affect the central nervous system, the cardiovascular system, kidneys, and also include toxicity like teratogenicity, carcinogenicity, and drug interactions.

SOME CONCEPTUAL DEFINITIONS :

VEHICLE :

The substance that brings the active pharmaceutical agent or "specific drug" into skin contact is called a vehicle.

OINTMENT :

Any formulation which has an oily consistency or "greasy feel" is called an ointment, *e.g.* Whitfield's ointment.

SHAKE LOTION :

Lotions containing powders are referred to as shake lotions, *e.g.* calamine lotion.

SOLUTION :

Water- or alcohol-based lotions are referred to as solutions, tolnaftate solution.

TINCTURE :

When low concentration of active ingredients or principles of crude drugs are present in alcoholic liquid form, it is termed as a tincture, *e.g.* podophyllin tincture.

PAINT :

Paints are staining solutions, *e.g.* Castellani's paint.

EMULSION :

Suspensions of oily substances in water or vice versa in the presence of emulsifying agent. Emulsions have an outer continuous phase and an inner dispersed phase, *e.g.* cold creams (W/o type).

EMULSIFYING AGENT :

An agent that binds the dispersed phase with the continuous phase in an emulsion is called an emulsifying agent, *e.g.* sodium lauryl sulphate.

GELS :

Liquids with added gelling agents constitute gels, *e.g.* tazarotene in gel formulation. Many gels are temperature sensitive and on contact with skin spread easily like a liquid. Gels are aesthetic, cooling and cover large areas, may enhance penetration of active but are sometimes irritant.

MONOPHASIC VEHICLES :

TABLE 17.1 : **Monophasic vehicles**

Examples	
Powders :	
Inorganic	Zinc oxide, titanium dioxide, talc, bentonite, calamine (BP and USP)
Organic	Starch, zinc stearate
Liquids	Water, glycerol, glycerine, ethanol, propylene glycol, ether, chloroform, calcium hydroxide solution
Greases :	
Vegetable fat	Almond oil, arachis or peanut oil, castor oil, cottonseed oil, linseed oil, sesame oil, olive oil, theobroma oil
Animal fat	Cod-liver oil, wool fat or anhydrous lanolin, hydrous wool fat or lanolin, lard or pig fat, bees fat, emulsifying wax, cetostearyl alcohol, cetyl alcohol, cetyl ester wax
Mineral greases	Liquid paraffin, Macrogol 300, 1500-4000, soft paraffin (petrolatum)

INDICATIONS OF MONOPHASIC PREPARATIONS :

- Powders are used for hygienic and cosmetic purposes.
- Liquids are used for wet dressings, medicated bath and in tinctures, paints, lotions, gels, and solutions.
- Lotions are preferable over face, scalp, intertriginous areas, mucous membranes.
- Gels are preferred over mucous membranes and hairy areas.
- Greases are used predominantly as emollients for dry skin.

BIPHASIC VEHICLES :

A combination of two monophasic vehicles is present in biphasic vehicles. Examples of biphasic vehicles are shake lotions, drying pastes, greasy pastes, and creams.

TABLE 17.2 : **Biphasic vehicles**

Biphasic vehicles	Combination	Comments	Examples
Shake lotions	Powders + liquid	Powder is suspended in the liquid	Calamine lotion
Drying pastes	Powders + liquid	Proportion of powders and liquid is equal	Calamine paste
Greasy pastes	Powders + greases	Powders in greases in equal proportions	Lassar's paste
Liniments	Powders + greases	Powders in liquid greases	Calamine liniment
Creams	Liquids + greases	Mixtures of liquids and greases in the presence of emulsifring agents	—
O/W cream type	Liquids + greases	Oil (dispersed phase) in water (continuous phase)	Vanishing cream
W/O cream type	Liquids + greases	Water (dispersed phase) in oil (continuous phase)	Cold cream

ACTIONS OF BIPHASIC PREPARATIONS :

- Shake lotions (*e.g.* calamine lotion) is used as a bland and cooling lotion.
- Drying paste is used as a cooling paste.
- Vanishing creams are suited for oily skin.
- Cold creams are suited for dry skin.

TRIPHASIC VEHICLES :

Triphasic vehicles are a mixture of greases, liquids and powders. Examples of triphasic vehicles are cooling pastes and cream pastes.

TABLE 17.3 : **Triphasic vehicles**

Triphasic vehicles	Combination	Examples
Cooling pastes	Greases + liquids + powders	Unna's paste
Cream pastes	Greases + liquids + powders	Addition of zinc oxide to O/W or W/O creams

INDICATIONS OF TRIPHASIC PREPARATIONS :

Cooling pastes are extremely useful for their soothing properties on acutely inflamed skin.

SOME COMMON FORMULATIONS AND USES :

CALAMINE LOTION (USP) :

8% calamine, 8% zinc oxide, 2% glycerin, 25% bentonite. Add calcium hydroxide solution to make 100 ml of calamine lotion. Calamine lotion is a bland, soothing, and drying lotion mainly used in acute eczema, miliaria, vesicular lesions due to herpes Virus infections, urticaria, pityriasis rosea, etc.

ACNE LOTION :

3 g of precipitated sulfur, 3 g resorcinol, 3 g zinc oxide, 2 ml glycerine, and 10 ml methylated spirit. Acne lotion is used in

all grades of acne vulgaris and especially for the application over acne.

OILY CALAMINE LOTION (LINIMENT) :

Calamine lotion with peanut oil forms calamine liniment.

LASSER'S PASTE :

25% starch, 25% zinc oxide, and 2% salicylic acid in soft paraffin. (The idea of adding hard paraffin to Lasser's paste as a vehicle for anthralin for use in psoriasis to make stiff paste came later)

COAL TAR LOTION :

2% coal tar lotion in 90-95% alcohol (percentage of coal tar can be increased upto 10%. Coal tar lotion is used in psoriasis especially scalp psoriasis. It is also used occasionally for seborrheic dermatitis of the scalp. Goeckerman's regimen for psoriasis includes coal tar bath followed by UVB exposure.

BURROW'S SOLUTION :

6% aluminium subacetate solution, commonly used for open and closed wet dressings.

WHITFIELD'S OINTMENT :

12% benzoic acid and 6% salicylic acid; half strength Whitfield'S ointment is 6% benzoic acid and 3% salicylic acid. It is used for the treatment of superficial fungal infections of the skin.

CASTELLANI'S PAINT :

0.3% carbol fuchsin solution plus 4% phenol (antipruritic) and 10% resorcinol (antipruritic and keratolytic), 0.8% boric acid (antiseptic), in acetone (cleansing). It has local anesthetic, antifungal and antibacterial properties and hence was commonly used for superficial fungal infections of the skin mainly in intertriginous areas.

PODOPHYLLIN :

25% resinous extract of podophyllin in tincture benzoin. It is mainly used for genital warts.

WART LOTION :

16.7% salicylic acid and 16.7% lactic acid in flexible collodion base.

INGRAM'S DITHRANOL PASTE :

0.2-0.8% dithranol, 2% salicylic acid, 24% each of zinc oxide and starch, and 2.5% hard paraffin. Ingram regimen for psoriasis includes combination of coal tar bath, application of dithranolpaste, and UVB exposure.

DITHRANOL POMADE :

1% dithranol in 25% emulsifying wax, add liquid paraffin to make 100 ml.

10% GLUTARALDEHYDE SOLUTION :

10% glutaraldehyde solution is prepared by adding 50 ml of water to 10 ml of 25% glutaraldehyde solution. Solution is buffered by adding 1.65 g of sodium bicarbonate.

x=x=x=x=x

18

Topical Antibacterials

An ideal topical antibacterial : broad spectrum, quick and prolonged antibacterial effect, bactericidal, good penetration, minimal toxicity, low or null allergy, sparse activity against normal skin flora.

TABLE 18.1 : **Spectrum and indications of topical antibacterials in dermatology**

Organisms	Skin infections	Antibacterial used
Gram-positive organisms (mainly staphylococci and streptococci)	Bacterial folliculitis (including Bockhart's impetigo and chronic atrophic folliculitis), furunculosis, carbuncle, impetigo, ecthyma, erysipelas, cellulitis, intertrigo, acute paronychia	Mupirocin, fusidic acid, Retapamulin. Retapamulin
Gram-positive and Gram-negative organisms	Toe web infections, paronychia, secondarily infected eczemas, scabies, pediculosis, etc.	Neomycin B and C (framycetin), gentamicin, sisomycin, bacitracin, nadifloxacin, silver sulfadiazine
Gram-negative organisms mainly *Pseudomonas aeruginosa*	Gram-negative toe web infections, otitis externa, green nail, syndrome, Gram-negative folliculitis (also caused by *E. coli, Klebsiella, or Enterobacter)*	Polymyxin B; sisomycin
Corynebacterium species	Pitted keratolysis, erythrasma	Erythromycin and other macrolides
Propionibacterium acnes	Plays role in etiopathogenesis of acne vulgaris	Benzoyl peroxide, erythromycin, clindamycin, lincomycin, clarithromycin, nadifloxacin, azelaic acid
Anaerobes	Phagedena, cancrum oris, noma	Metronidazole (also antiparasitic and aerobic coverage), clindamycin

TABLE 18.2 : **Preparations, actions, and sensitization potential of topical antibacterials**

Antibacterial agent	Topical preparations	Sensitization potential
Aminoglycosides		
Gentamicin	0.1-0.3% cream	Yes
Neomycin	Neomycin B and 3% neomycin C	Yes, high (1-6%)
Framycetin	1% cream	Yes, high
Sisomycin (Ensamycin®)	0.1% cream	—
Macrolides		
Erythromycin	4% gel, cream, lotion	—
Clarithromycin	1% cream	—
Lincosamides		
Clindamycin	1% gel, 1% lotion, 1% solution	—
Lincomycin	2% gel	—
Fusidic acid	2% cream	Low
Mupirocin	2% cream	Low
Fluoroquinolones		
Nadifloxacin	1% cream	—
Sulfonamides		
Silver sulfadiazine	1% cream	Yes
Metronidazole	0.75% gel, 1% cream	—
Benzoyl peroxide	2.5%, 4%, 5%, gel, lotion	—
Azelaic acid	20% cream	—
Polymyxin B and Colistin	01. - 1% cream	— No
Bacitracin	20% in petrolatum	Yes
Retapamulin	1% cream/ointment	Not known

AMINOGLYCOSIDES :

Aminoglycosides that are available as topical preparations are neomycin, framycetin, gentamicin, and sisomycin.

MECHANISM OF ACTION :

Aminoglycosides inhibit bacterial protein synthesis by binding to 30-50S interface except for streptomycin that only binds to the 30S ribosomal subunit.

The cidal action of aminoglycosides is probably due to the secondary changes in the integrity of bacterial cell membrane.

INDICATIONS :

1. Localized cutaneous infections of skin caused by Gram negative bacteria (except pseudomonas and anaerobes) and staphylococci.
2. Mixed infections of skin caused by Gram-positive and Gram-negative bacteria. Resistance has been reported.

SIDE EFFECTS :

- Allergic contact dermatitis.

KEY POINTS :

- Certain aminoglycosides like sisomycin and framycetin has great efficacy for staphylococci thereby commonly used for staphylococcal skin infections. Sisomicin act synergistically with various beta lactam antibiotics against enterococci, staphylococci, enterobcateriaceae and non-fermentative gram negative bacilli. Sisomycin is effective against bacilli that are resistant to other aminoglycosides like gentamicin due to non-enzymatic mechanisms.
- Topical aminoglycosides are less commonly used now because of the risk of contact sensitization and development of resistance. Neomycin has systemic absorption.
- Allergic contact dermatitis is more common with neomycin as compared to framycetin. It is less common with gentamicin and sisomycin.

MACROLIDES :

Topical macrolides include erythromycin, azithromycin and clarithromycin.

> **MECHANISM OF ACTION :**
>
> Inhibits bacterial protein synthesis by binding to 50S ribosomal subunit.

INDICATIONS :

Localized cutaneous infections of skin caused by Gram-positive organisms.

KEY POINTS :

- Erythromycin resistance is fairly common and can be overcome by using a higher concentration of erythromycin or by combining it with benzoyl peroxide in the treatment of acne vulgaris.
- Mild erythema, scaling, burning, pruritus, irritation, oiliness, and dryness have been reported with erythromycin use.
- A few cases of pseudomembranous colitis have been reported even with topical clindamycin use.
- Clarithromycin is the most potent macrolide antibiotic for acne vulgaris.

SULFONAMIDES :

Topical sulfonamides include silver sulfadiazine and silver sulfacetamide.

> **MECHANISM OF ACTION :**
>
> Silver sulfadiazine competitively inhibits PABA of bacteria.

INDICATIONS :

Skin infections caused due to denuded skin in :

- Burns (including those caused by MRSA and Pseudomonas).
- Pemphigus vulgaris.
- Stevens Johnson syndrome.

KEY POINTS :

- Silver sulfadiazine is only effective in cutaneous infections with minimum bacterial load. This is because when bacterial load increases, increased concentration of PABA renders silver sulfadiazine ineffective. Silver sufadiazine competitively inhibits PABA of bacteria. Moreover, in many cases, it is used.
- Cross-reactions can occur in patients with sulfonamide allergy. Similarly, systemic contact dermatitis can occur in patients taking oral sulfonamides and having contact allergy to silver sulfadiazine.

MUPIROCIN :

Mupirocin is a naturally occurring antibiotic mainly effective against Gram-positive organisms.

MECHANISM OF ACTION :

It inhibits bacterial RNA, protein and cell wall synthesis by inhibiting enzyme isoleucyl tRNA synthetase of bacteria.

INDICATIONS :

Localized cutaneous infections of skin caused by Gram-positive bacteria especially staph aureus (bactericidal at 2%).

KEY POINTS :

- Systemically absorbed mupirocin (in small quantities) is

converted to monic acid and excreted in urine. Also due to the limited capacity of skin to metabolize, (below 3%) mupirocin, a majority of the drug is available on skin surface to exert antibacterial effect. However, it is ineffective against anaerobic organisms, minimally effective against corynebacteria, micrococci, and *propionbacteria* and less effective against streptococci.

- Mupirocin is highly effective at reducing the nasal carriage of S. aureus and MRSA and may lower the risk of related infections. To be applied twice daily at the nasal and anal openings, umbilicus for five days/month for 3-4 months, is advocated for recurrent furunculosis.
- Mupirocin does not cross-react with other topical antibacterials nor do bacteria develop resistance to it due to its unique structure and mechanism of action.
- Resistant strains have emerged though rare; Mupirocin resistant MRSA have been reported.

RETAPAMULIN :

Retapamulin is semi-synthetic occurring antibiotic derived from pleuromutilin produced by Pleurotusmutilins (now called Clitopilusscyphoides), an edible mushroom. It was approved by FDA in 2007 for topical treatment of impetigo.

Mechanism Of Action :

It inhibits bacterial protein synthesis at level of bacterial 50S ribosome.

Indications :

- Impetigo and infected wounds caused by S. pyogenes and Methicillin Sensitive Staphylococcus Aureus (MSSsA).
- Secondary infected dermatitis.

Preparation :

RETAREL 1% ointment – BD for 5 days. Dose : thin layer

(upto 100 cm^2 in adults and 2% BSA in paeds, > 9 months of age.

KEY POINTS :

1. It is active against bacteria resistant to methicillin, erythromycin, fusidic acid, mupirocin, azithromycin and levofloxacin.
2. Retapamulin is a bacteriostatic drug but said to be bactericidal at high concentration.
3. Retapamulin can be used in pregnancy with due to its Pregnancy prescribing category B.

SIDE EFFECTS :

- Most common – Pruritus at the site of application.
- Irritation, paresthesia, pain.

NADIFLOXACIN :

Nadifloxacin is a fluoroquinolone antibiotic employed for topical use in the treatment of skin infections.

MECHANISM OF ACTION :

Fluoroquinolones inhibit bacterial protein synthesis by interfering with bacterial DNA gyrase, which prevents uncoiling of DNA that is necessary for multiplication.

INDICATIONS :

Cutaneous infections caused by Gram-negative and Gram-positive organisms. A new related molecule, ozenoxacin has higher efficacy against Gram positive cocci.

KEY POINTS :

- Useful against infections caused by Gram-positive and Gram-negative organisms.
- No cross-sensitization has been noted with nadifloxacin.

METRONIDAZOLE :

Metronidazole is a synthetic 5-nitroimidazole antibacterial effective against anaerobic organisms.

MECHANISM OF ACTION :

Exact mechanism is unknown. It is supposed to cause rapid inhibition of DNA replication.

INDICATIONS :

1. Cutaneous infections caused by anerobic organisms.
2. Rosacea.
3. Acne vulgaris.
4. Hidradenitis suppurativa.

KEY POINTS :

- It is useful in rosacea for its antiinflammatory effect.
- Resistance to metronidazole is yet to be reported.

POLYMYXIN B :

Polymyxin B is a bactericidal, cationic polypeptide antibiotic effective against Gram-negative bacilli except *Proteus*.

MECHANISM OF ACTION :

Alters permeability of bacterial cytoplasmic membranes leading to leakage of ions and amino acids.

May neutralize endotoxins of bacteria.

INDICATIONS :

Cutaneous infections caused by Gram-negative organisms. Commonly used in combination with bacitracin, zinc and neomycin (Neosporin powder).

BACITRACIN :

Polypeptide antibiotic derived from cultures of *B. subtilise*. It is mainly effective against Gram-positive cocci and bacilli.

KEY POINTS :

- Because of high systemic toxicity, it is only used topically.
- Does not penetrate the intact skin, so less effective in furunculosis and folliculitis than open wounds.

MECHANISM OF ACTION :
Inhibits bacterial cell wall synthesis.

INDICATIONS :

Infections caused by Gram-positive organisms and a few Gram-negative organisms.

KEY POINTS :

- Allergic contact dermatitis may occur.
- Systemic absorption of bacitracin can lead to nephrotoxicity.

FUSIDIC ACID :

Fusidic acid is a steroidal antibiotic mainly effective against Gram-positive organisms.

MECHANISM OF ACTION :
Steroidal antibiotic; inhibits protein synthesis by inhibiting elongation of factor-G.
It interferes with transfer of amino acid from aminoacylsRNA to proteins on ribosomes.

INDICATIONS :

Skin infections caused by staphylococci, streptococci, and corynebacterium species and gram positive anaerobes.

Key Points :

- Fusidic acid has low sensitization potential and no cross-sensitization is reported.
- Fusidic acid cream contains fusidic acid, whereas fusidic acid ointment contains its salt-sodium fusidate.

Fusidic acid is virtually ineffective against Gram-negative organisms due to differences in cell wall permeability.

TOPICAL ANTIBACTERIALS USED FOR ACNE VULGARIS AND ROSACEA (TABLE 18.3) :

Indications In ACNE Vulgaris :

- Grade II and III acne vulgaris.
- Benzoyl peroxide and azelaic acid are also used in grade I acne vulgaris.

Key Points :

- Benzoyl peroxide is an excellent antiacne agent for Grade I and II acne vulgaris for the following reasons :
    1. Comedolytic effect apart from antibacterial action.
    2. Rapidly reduces bacterial count of *Propionibacterium acnes* through its bacteriostatic effect.
    3. No bacterial resistance and rarely contact allergy has been reported.
    4. It can be combined with other antimicrobials to prevent resistance. However, it has irritant potential and can cause dryness of skin and may not be tolerated by many.
- Erythromycin, apart from its antibacterial action, exerts anti-inflammatory effect increasing its efficacy.
- Clindamycin has a potential (albeit rare) of causing pseudo-membranous colitis even with topical application.

TABLE 18.3 : **Topical antiacne agents**

Antiacne agent	Mechanism of action	Topical preparation	PPS
Benzoyl peroxide	It inhibits *Propionibacterium acnes* and hydrolysis of triglycerides, Also it has comedolytic effect	2.5%, 4%, 5% gel, lotion	No data
Azelaic acid	Inhibits bacterial protein synthesis. Also it has comedolytic effect	20% cream	No data
Erythromycin	Inhibits bacterial protein synthesis by binding to 50S ribosomal subunit	4% gel, cream, lotion	B
Clindamycin	Inhibits bacterial protein synthesis by binding to 50S ribosomal subunit	1% gel, 1% lotion, 1% solution	B
Azithromycin	Inhibits bacterial protein synthesis by binding to 50S ribosomal subunit	2% gel	—
Lincomycin	Inhibits bacterial protein synthesis by binding to 50S ribosomal subunit	20/0 gel	B
Clarithromycin	Inhibits bacterial protein synthesis by binding to 50S ribosomal subunit	1% cream	C
Nadifloxacin	Inhibits bacterial protein synthesis by inhibiting DNA gyrase	1% cream	C
Metronidazole	Inhibits anaerobic bacteria. Supposedly causes rapid inhibition of DNA replication. Also has anti-inflammatory effect	0.75% gel, 1% cream	B

PPS : Pregnancy Prescribing Status

- Demelanizing action of azelaic acid adds to its utility in patients of acne vulgaris with post inflammatory hyperpigmentation secondary to acne lesions.
- Metronidazole is effective against aerobic and anaerobic bacteria, and the mite *Demodexfolliculorum* (some efficacy). It also has antiinflammatory action, thereby being useful in both acne vulgaris and rosacea, especially the latter.

x=x=x=x=x

19

Topical Antifungals

CLASSIFICATION OF TOPICAL ANTIFUNGALS :

MODERN ANTIFUNGALS :

1. *Antifungal antibiotics :*
   a. Polyenes : amphotericin B, nystatin.
   b. Others : hamycin, candicidin, natamycin.
2. *Azoles :*
   a. Imidazoles, *e.g.* ketoconazole, econazole, sertaconazole, miconazole, oxiconazole, luliconazole, eberconazole, fenticonazole.
   b. Triazole, *e.g.* fluconazole.
3. *Allylamine :* terbinafine, naftifine.
4. *Benzylamine :* butenafine.
5. *Morpholines :* amorolfine.
6. *Hydroxypyrodinones :* Ciclopirox olamine.
7. Tolnaftate.
8. Selenium sulfide.
9. Undecylenic acid.

TRADITIONAL ANTIFUNGAL REMEDIES :

1. Whitfield's ointment (3% salicylic acid + 6% benzoic acid).
2. Salicylic acid.
3. Castellanis paint.
4. Sulfur.

MECHANISM OF ACTION OF ANTIFUNGALS THAT INHIBIT ERGOSTEROL SYNTHESIS :

- Azoles prevent conversion of lanosterol to 4,14-dimethylzymosterol inhibiting ergosterol synthesis.
- Allylamines (terbinafine, naftifine), benzylamines (butenafine), and tolnaftate inhibit the enzyme squalene epoxidase required for ergosterol synthesis.
- Amorolfine inhibits 4-reductase and 7,8-isomerase enzymes involved in ergosterol synthesis.

MECHANISM OF ACTION OF ANTIFUNGALS THAT DO NOT INHIBIT :

Ergosterol Synthesis :

- Amphotericin, nystatin alter membrane permeability across fungal cell membranes.
- Ciclopirox olamine interferes with membrane transport of essential macromolecular precursors, cell membrane integrity, and cell respiratory processes.
- Selenium sulfide promotes shedding of fungi in stratum corneum via a reduction in cell-to-cell adhesion of epidermal cells and follicular epithelium.

INDICATIONS OF TOPICAL ANTIFUNGALS :

1. Localized superficial fungal infections of the skin :
   - Dermatophytosis.
   - Pityriasis versicolor (Table 19.1).
   - Candidiasis.
   - Tinea nigra.
2. Seborrheic dermatitis (*Pityrosporum ovale* is implicated in pathogenesis).

TABLE 19.1 : **Topical Antifungal agents**

Antifungal agent	Topical preparation	Frequency of application	Other formulations	PPS*
Amphotericin B	3% cream	—	Oral suspension 100 mg/ml (also i.v.)	B
Nystatin	100,000 USP units/g	Twice, thrush : 4-5 times	Powder, suspension, pastille	B
Hamycin	1% cream	Once a day	—	No data
Azoles				
Clotrimazole	1% cream	Twice, oral thrush : 4 times a day	1% solution/lotion/oral troches 100 mg, powder, spray, vaginal tablet 100 mg, 300 mg, 500 mg	B
Miconazole	2% cream, lotion	Twice daily, in P. versicolor once daily	Spray, powder , gel	B
Ketoconazole	1%, 2% cream, lotion	Once daily	1%, 2% shampoos, tablet 200 mg	B
Bifonazole	1% cream	Once daily	Shampoo	No data
Oxiconazole	1% cream	Once/twice daily	Lotion, cream	B
Econazole	1% cream	Once/twice daily	Gel, suppositories	B
Luliconazole	1% cream or lotion	Once/ twice daily	Spray, powder	No data
Fluconazole	2% gel	Frequency of application	2% lotion, 2% shampoo , powder	No data
Allylamine				
Terbinafine	1% cream	Twice daily	250 mg tablets, Gel, lotion, powder	B
Naftifine	1% cream	Once/twice daily		B

(Continued)

TRADITIONAL ANTIFUNGAL REMEDIES

TABLE 19.1 : (Continued)

Antifungal agent	Topical preparation	Frequency of application	Other formulations	PPS*
Benzlamine				
Butenaflne	1% cream	Once/twice daily	None	B
Morpholines				
Amorolfine	0.125-0.5% cream	Once daily	5% nail lacquer	No Data
Ciclopirox olamine	1% cream, lotion	Twice daily	8% nail lacquer	B
Others				
Tolnaftate	1%, 2% solution	Twice daily	Spray, cream, ointment	No Data
Selenium sulfide	1%, 2.5% shampoo based lotion	Twice weekly for first week and once weekly thereafter	—	C
Undecylenic acid (mixture of undecylenic acid and its salts zinc, calcium, or sodium)	10% powder	Twice a day	Lotion, spray, or solution	No data available
Oxaboroles – Tavaborole	5% nail solution	Once daily for 48 weeks	Solution	

*PPS : Pregnancy Prescribing Status

3. Confluent and reticulate papillomatosis of Gougerot and Carteaud (*P. ovale* is implicated in etiopathogenesis).
4. Pityrosporum folliculitis.

TABLE 19.2 : **Spectrum of topical antifungal agents**

Antifungal agent	Anticandidal action	Antipityrosporum effect	Antibacterial effect
Amphotericin B	Yes	No	Yes
Nystatin	Yes	No	Yes
Azoles			
Clotrimazole	Yes	Yes	Yes
Miconazole	Yes	Yes	Yes
Ketoconazole	Yes	Yes	Yes
Bifonazole	Yes	Yes	No
Oxiconazole	Yes	Yes	No
Econazole	Yes	Yes	Yes
Allylamine			
Terbinafine	No	No	No
Naftifine	No	No	No
Benzylamines			
Butenafine	No	No	No
Amorolfine	No	No	No
Ciclopirox olamine	Yes	No	No
Miscellaneous			
Tolnaftate	No	Yes	No
Selenium sulfide	No	Yes	No
Undecylenic acid	No	No	No

ADVERSE EFFECTS :

Topical antifungals are generally well-tolerated when applied locally with rare side effects of :

1. *Contact irritation.*
2. *Contact allergy.*
3. *Irritation or allergy to vehicle or preservatives* like propyiene glycol, sodium sulfite, etc.

Key Points :

- Topical antifungals have an advantage of high local concentration and minimal systemic absorption and thus less systemic side effects.
- Nystatin is insoluble in water and has no absorption from intact skin or mucosa, hence extremely effective in superficial mycoses of skin, oral mucosa, gut, and vagina.
- Terbinafine, naftifine, and butenafine are fungicidal agents with residual effect. Thus, cure rates were high and chances of recurrences of dermatophytosis are minimum with these agents as compared to azoles. However in the last 5 years.
- In vitro, ciclopirox olamine inhibits saprophytic fungi. Nail lacquer can penetrate nail plate, thereby useful in onychomycoses. Amorolfine 5% nail lacquer once a week is highly effective for onycomycoses.
- Selenium disulfide lotion has to be kept in contact with scalp for 5 min for the treatment of seborrheic dermatitis and 10 min for the treatment of pityriasis versicolor and confluent and reticulate papillomatosis of Gougerot and Carteaud. The shampoo preparation must be diluted with water to half strength for application on body for pityriasis versicolor, otherwise irrritant dermatitis may occur.
- *Antibacterial effect :* Azoles like clotrimazole, miconazole, econazole, and ketoconazole have antibacterial properties and hence can be used to treat erythrasma, mixed toe web infections, and impetiginized dermatophytosis.
- *Antiinflammatory effect :* Some of the topical antifungals (like bifonazole, ketoconazole, or ciclopirox) have anti-inflammatory action through their effects on prostaglandin.
- Medication is to be applied outside to inside starting 1-2 cm of peripheral normal skin. Choice of formulation affects compliance and absorption rates.

- Use of antifungal powders and soaps should be discouraged, as they are of little benefit and may promote antifungal resistance may regions of India have reported high frequency of terbinafine resistant strains thus turning the tide in favour of azoles.

TRADITIONAL ANTIFUNGAL REMEDIES :

TABLE 19.3 : **Traditional antifungal remedies**

Antifungal agent	Mechanism of action	Topical formulation
Whitfield's ointment	Unexplored mechanism of antifungal action for benzoic acid, whereas salicylic acid is keratolytic and promotes shedding of keratinocytes infected by the fungus	12% benzoic acid and 6% salicylic acid (full strength Whitfield's ointment); 6% benzoic acid and 3% salicylic acid (half strength Whitfield's ointment)
Castellani's paint	Fungicidal, bactericidal, anesthetic	0.3% carbol fuchsin solution + 4% phenol (antipruritic) + 10% resorcinol (antipruritic and keratolytic), 0.8% boric acid (antiseptic), acetone (cleansing)
Salicylic acid	Keratolytic and promotes shedding of keratinocytes infected by the fungus	6% and 3% ointment, lotion
Sulfur	Keratolytic and mild antifungal properties. Sulfur combines with cysteine in stratum corneum, to form hydrogen sulfide that causes keratolysis. Sulfur-treated epidermal cells release pentathionic acid, which is toxic to fungi	6% sulfur ointment

x=x=x=x=x

20
Topical Antivirals

Various topical agents are used for the treatment of viral infections of skin. Many of these agents may not be viricidal, but are still useful.

TABLE 20.1 : **Topical antivirals for cutaneous infections caused by HSV**

Antiviral agent	Topical preparation	Frequency of application	PPS*
Acyclovir	5% ointment	4 times a day	C
Penciclovir	1% cream	6 times a day	B
Cidofovir	1-3%, 5% gel	Once a day	C
Foscarnet	3% cream	8 times a day	C
Docosanol	OTC product	5 times a day	No data

***PPS** : Pregnancy

VIRICIDAL AGENTS EFFECTIVE AGAINST INFECTIONS CAUSED BY HERPES VIRUSES :

ACYCLOVIR :

ACYCLOVIR

MECHANISM OF ACTION :

Acyclovir —Viral thymidine kinase (TK)→ Acyclovir monophosphate (AMP).

Acyclovir monophosphate (AMP) —Cellular kinases→ Acyclovir triphosphate.

Acyclovir triphosphate inhibits 'Viral DNA polymerase inhibiting DNA synthesis.

ANTIVIRAL SPECTRUM :

HSV-1, HSV-2, and VZV.

INDICATIONS :

Primary and recurrent herpes simplex infections mainly herpes labialis and genital herpes.

KEY POINTS :

- Topical antivirals are not as effective as oral antivirals though they may reduce healing time and symptoms compared to placebo.
- In case of recurrent genital herpes, viral shedding is unaffected.
- Topical acyclovir is not recommended as sole therapy for treatment of herpes.

PENCICLOVIR :

MECHANISM OF ACTION :

Similar to that of acyclovir.

ANTIVIRAL SPECTRUM :

HSV-l, HSV-2, VZV, and HSV-4 (EBV).

KEY POINTS :

- Topical penciclovir can rarely cause side effects like irritation, hyperesthesia, or paresthesia.
- Penciclovir should not be used in patients with known hypersensitivity to the compound.
- Benefit : similar to acyclovir.

CIDOFOVIR :

Cidofovir, an antiviral agent, is a potent nucleoside analog.

MECHANISM OF ACTION :

Cidofovir reaches the cell in a monophosphorylated whereby it is activated by cellular kinases. Cidofovir targets viral DNA polymerase and prevents transcription.

ANTIVIRAL SPECTRUM :

HPV, HSV (including CMV), molluscum contagiosum virus (Mc virus) especially in HIV positive patients.

KEY POINTS :

- Systemic side effects like headache, nausea, and pharyngitis have been reported in patients on cidofovir therapy.

DRUGS EFFECTIVE AGAINST INFECTIONS CAUSED BY HUMANPAPILLOMA VIRUSES :

These include :

- Immunomodulatory agents.
- Keratolytics.
- Cytotoxic agents.
- Caustics (Table 20.2).

IMMUNOMODULATORY AGENTS :

IMIQUIMOD :

Imiquimod is a newer immunomodulatory agent.

MECHANISM OF ACTION :

Imiquimod is an inducer of interferonfl (IFN-y), which is a potent cytokine of cell-mediated immunity responsible for viral killing. Thus, imiquimod has immunomodulatory action.

TABLE 20.2 : **Topical agents used for cutaneous viral infections caused by HPV (shift table to hpv section)**

Agents	Topical preparation	Frequency of application	PPS*
Keratolytics :			
Salicylic acid	16-60% cream, lotion, plaster, collodion	Once a day	C
Lactic acid	16%		
Immunomodulatory agents :			
Imiquimod	5% cream	Thrice a week	B
Interferons	1 MU/lesion (not more than five injections in one sitting)	Alternate day thrice weekly	
DNCB/DPCP	0.1% in acetone	Weekly	C
Caustics :			
Trichloroacetic acid	50%	Once in a week	Teratogenic
Formaldehyde	3% formalin (37% formaldehyde gas in water) for 10 min	Every 2 Weeks	Not known
Glutaraldehyde	2% soaks	Daily	Not known
Cytotoxic antiviral agents :			
Bleomycin	Intralesional 0.1 ml aqueous solution (1 mg/ml) in normal saline	Every 2 weeks	D
5-fluorouracil	1%, 5% cream	Once/twice a week	X
Podophyllin	25% resin in tincture benzoin base, 0.5% podophyllotoxin	Once a week	C
Miscellaneous :			
Cantharidin	0.7-1% solution	Every 2-3 week	No data
Retinoic acid	0.05% cream	Daily at night	C

***PPS** : Pregnancy Prescribing Status

Antiviral Spectrum :

It is useful for infections with HPV, MC, and HSV viruses. It is FDA approved for external genital warts, actinic keratosis and superficial BCC.

KEY POINTS :

- Refer to chapter "Topical Immunomodulators" for details.
- Erythema, inflammation, tenderness, ulceration are reported as local side effects of imiquimod.
- Imiquimod therapy may take 6-12 weeks to show its full therapeutic effect.

CONTACT SENSITIZERS :

- Contact sensitizers used are DNCB, DPCP, and SADBE.
- Refer to chapter "Topical Immunomodulators" for details.

INTERFERONS :

Refer to chapter "Immunobiologicals" for further details.

AUTOVACCINE :

Biopsy of wart issue in normal saline is processed in the laboratory to obtain a solution of wart antigen (after autoclaving). This is then injected subcutaneously twice a week in increasing concentrations over 6 weeks. Refer to chapter "Immunobiologicals" for details.

KERATOLYTICS :

SALICYLIC ACID :

MECHANISM OF ACTION :

Keratolytic causes exfoliation of virally infected keratinocytes. Also exposes such cells to cellular immunity.

KEY POINT :

- Overuse of salicylic acid in children, high raw and inflamed areas can give rise to salicylate toxicity, salicylism, characterized by nausea, vomiting, stupor, tinnitus, and hyperventilation.

CYTOTOXIC AGENTS FOR WARTS :

BLEOMYCIN :

Bleomycin is a cytotoxic agent.

MECHANISM OF ACTION :

Bleomycin, a cytotoxic agent, binds directly to DNA in the mitotic and postmitotic phases of cell cycle to remove purine and pyrimidine bases.

KEY POINTS :

It is effective in the treatment of recalcitrant verrucae and keloids when used intralesionally.

- Bleomycin is available in lyophilized powder form in vials containing 15 IU. It is reconstituted with 5 ml distilled water making it 3 IU/ml. This can be stored at 4-8 C for 60 days. Before injecting it is further diluted with lignocaine in a ratio of 1:2 making the final concentration 1 IU/ml.
- *Method of use :* 0.1 ml of 1 U/ml bleomycin in a normal saline solution is intralesionally injected every 2-3 weeks till resolution occurs (usually 2 injections).
- Bleomycin injections can cause severe pain or ulceration or gangrene when used for the treatment of subungual or periungual warts.

TOPICAL 5-FLUOROURACIL :

Topical 5-fluorouracil is a cytotoxic agent. Available in 1% and 5% cream.

MECHANISM OF ACTION :

5-Fluorouracil, a cytotoxic agent, inhibits DNA synthesis.

KEY POINTS :

- Hyperpigmentation is an important side effect of 5-fluorouracil. It can also cause burning, irritation, erythema, and ulceration particularly when used for genital warts.
- When 5-fluorouracil is not tolerated due to its local side effects, it can be stopped for a few days until erythema and ulceration subside, and can be restarted with lower concentration and lesser frequency.
- May be significantly (about 20%) absorbed through damaged skin. It should be avoided in pregnancy.
- 5-Fluorouracil cream is also effective for the treatment of actinic keratoses, other precancerous dermatoses and even Bowen's disease. Sustained inflammation leading to burning, itching and even ulceration is not uncommon during therapy lasting several weeks.

PODOPHYLLIN :

Podophyllin is a plant resin.

MECHANISM OF ACTION :

Podophyllin, a cytotoxic agent, inhibits DNA synthesis in metaphase by binding to cell microtubules.

INDICATION :

Condyloma accumulata.

KEY POINTS :

- Podophyllin is obtained from resinous roots (may apple roots) of plant *Podophyllum peltatum* or *Podophyllum emodi* (in India).
- Podophyllotoxin is the active component of podophyllin, which is available as 1% cream or 0.5% lotion. It has an advantage of self-application, greater efficacy, and minimum side effects.

- For details of mode of application and side effects refer to the chapter "Topical Cytotoxics".
- Use of podophyllin for genital warts in pregnancy is contraindicated due to the risk of teratogenicity and CNS toxicity.

PREGNANCY CATEGORY – X :

MISCELLANEOUS AGENTS :

CANTHARIDIN :

Cantharidin (7%) is a vesiculating agent obtained from the blister beetle also called the "Spanish fly".

Mechanism Of Action :

Cantharidin, a vesiculating agent, produces acantholysis and sub-epidermal blister with subsequent removal of viral wart or molluscum contagiosum.

Key Points :

- Cantharidin needs to be occluded for 24 h after its application after which there is the formation of the blister.
- Cantharidin application is painless and hence can be used in children, but the blister formed after 24 h is painful.

Inadequate application of cantharidin may result in annular or ring-like wart with a flattening in the center. This is popularly known as the "doughnut wart" and may also be seen following other ablative therapies.

SINECATECHINS :

Standardized extract of green tea leaves containing polyphenols (catechins). The main ingredient is epigallocatechin galleate.

MECHANISM OF ACTION :

Antioxidant, pro-apoptotic, boosting of CMI.

INDICATIONS :

External genital and perianal warts.

Veregen 15% ointment applied twice to thrice daily to all lesions for maximum 4 months.

ADVERSE REACTION :

Local tissue erythema, swelling, pain.

x=x=x=x=x

21
Topical Antiparasitic Agents

Topical antiparasitic agents are used in scabies, pediculosis, cutaneous larva migrans, and leishmaniasis.

TABLE 21.1 : **Topical antiparasitic agents**

	Formulation
Antiscabetic agents :	
Permethrin	5% cream
Gamma-benzene hydrochloride	1% lotion
Benzyl benzoate	25% lotion
Crotamiton	10% cream, lotion
Precipitated sulfur	6% cream in petrolatum
Topical ivermectin	0.8% w/v cream in 15-25 ml of single dose
Malathion	0.5% lotion
Tetramethyl thiuram monosulfide	25% alcoholic lotion, 5% in antiscabetic soap
Pediculicidal agents :	
Gamma-benzene hexachloride	1% lotion
Permethrin	1% lotion
Malathion	0.5 lotion
Agents for cutaneous larva migrans :	
Thiabendazole	10% cream
Agents for cutaneous leishmaniasis :	
Paromomycin sulfate	15% cream

PERMETHRIN :

Permethrin, a synthetic pyrethroid derivative, is an effective antiscabetic agent.

MECHANISM OF ACTION :

Permethrin produces nerve paralysis and death in ectoparasites by causing delayed repolarization by disrupting Na^{+} current.

INDICATIONS :

Scabies and pediculosis.

FORMUNATIONS :

PERLICE/KERALICE 1% cream, PERMITE/HHMITE/NOSCAB 5% cream.

INSTRUCTIONS FOR USE PEDICULOSIS AND SCABIES :

FOR THE TREATMENT OF HEAD LICE (1% LOTION) INFESTATION :

1. Shampoo the hair and scalp using a regular shampoo.
2. Thoroughly rinse and dry the hair and the scalp using a towel.
3. Allow the hair to air dry for a few minutes.
4. Shake the permethrin lotion well before applying.
5. Thoroughly wet the hair and scalp with the permethrin lotion. Be sure to cover the areas behind the ears and also the back of the neck. Allow the lotion to remain in place for 10 min.
6. Then, rinse the hair and scalp thoroughly and dry with a clean towel.
7. When the hair is wet, you can comb the hair with fine-toothed comb to remove dead lice, any remaining nits (eggs) or nit shells.
8. Repeat application after 7-10 days.

THE TREATMENT OF SCABIES (5% CREAM) :

1. Thoroughly wash and dry the skin with clean towels.

2. Massage the cream into the skin from the neck to the soles of the feet, paying special attention to the web spaces, abdomen and flexures.
3. Scabies rarely infests the scalp of adults, but infants should be treated on the scalp, side of the head, and forehead.
4. Leave the permethrin cream on the skin for overnight (8-14 h).
5. Wash off by taking a bath in the morning.
6. Wash all clothes and bedding. Scabies mite cannot survive without human contact for more than 72 hours.
7. With widespread use of permethrin, stray cases of permethrin resistance arre reported. They respond to oral Nermectin and 5% topical tea tree oil.

SIDE EFFECTS :

- Burning, itching, numbness, rash, redness, stinging, tingling of the scalp. It is well tolerated compared to other antiscabitics.
- Hypersensitivity to permethrin.
- Cost is a very rare limiting factor.

PREGNANCY CATEGORY – B :

KEY POINTS :

- Systemic absorption of permethrin is minimal and less than 2%.
- Permethrin is an ovicidal agent thereby being effective as only single application. Two applications of permethrin are not better than one as shown by various controlled studies. However, current recommendations include 2 applications on consecutive days to be repeated after a gap of 7-10 days.
- Cure rates of single application of permethrin are high and range from 89% to 100% in various studies.

- Permethrin resistance in head louse is rare but looks increasingly possible. Various mutations in the KDR (knock down resistance) gene are described in some populations in Florii Indian studies are missing. Malathion is effective in such cases.

GAMMA-BENZENE HYDROCHLORIDE :

It is an ectoparasiticidal drug effective against *Sarcoptes scabies, Pediculus capitis,* and *Pediculus pubis.*

> **MECHANISM OF ACTION :**
>
> It inhibits inositol in scabies mite to produce CNS excitation and death of the parasite.

INDICATIONS :

Scabies and pediculosis.

PREGNANCY CATEGORY – 'C' :

DOSAGE AND INSTRUCTIONS :

Apply to cover all parts of the body from neck down to form a thin layer. If used in infants, prevent sucking or licking of lotion. Leave for 8-12 h (overnight and then wash off with a bath). Repeat application after 1 week.

ADVERSE EFFECTS :

CNS excitation, agitation, delirium, nervousness, giddiness, hematological abnormalities, tremors, convulsions, respiratory failure, coma, death (if systemic absorption takes place, may occur through the mucosa).

CONTRAINDICATIONS :

- Neonates and infants.
- Pregnant and lactating women.

- Norwegian scabies (higher systemic absorption may lead to toxicity).
- Hypersensitivity.
- Seizure disorders and other CNS disorder.
- Broken skin and wounds.

KEY POINTS :

- It is a cheaper alternative to permethrin.
- Should be stored in a cool, dry and dark place to maintain efficacy. It has shelf life of 2 years.
- Avoid contact with eyes and mucous membranes.
- Avoid over exposure and frequent reapplications as it may lead to toxicity.
- Avoid simultaneous application of oils and oily creams as they increase the systemic absorption of the drug.
- Diazepam or barbiturates can be used to control CNS excitation and convulsions due to systemic toxicity of gamma-benzene hydrochloride.

PRECIPITATED SULFUR :

Precipitated sulfur is an inexpensive and effective treatment for scabies.

MECHANISM OF ACTION :

Sulfur kills adult scabies mite.

INDICATIONS :

Scabies in infants < 2 months of age and pregnant or lactating women. However, permethrin 5% cream has rapidly replaced this drug in this indication.

FORMULATIONS AND APPLICATIONS :

Sulfur ointment with 6% precipitated sulfur in petroleum

(melphalan) to be applied to the entire body at night for three consecutive nights.

PREGNANCY PRESCRIBING STATUS – C :

Key Points :

- Sulfur is less acceptable to patients because of its odour and messy application. It can also cause irritation or dryness of the skin.
- Hypersensitivity to sulfur or sulfonamides is a contraindication for sulfur use.
- Cure rates of 65% and 97% were observed in one study after 8 and 14 days of sulfur application, respectively.

CROTAMITON :

Mechanism Of Action :

Not known.

Indications :

Scabies and as an antipruritic agent.

PREGNANCY CATEGORY – 'C' :

Formualations And Applications :

An application of thin layer of 10% cream or lotion from neck to toes; then gently massage into skin and leave on; a second application should be applied after 24 h; bathe 48 h after the last application. Better results are obtained with twice daily application for 5 consecutive days.

Side Effects :

Generally well tolerated. However, application may induce pruritus, redness, and swelling temporarily.

KEY POINTS :

- Multiple treatment failures were observed with crotamiton, when used in scabies. Cure rates with crotamiton are 40-50%.
- Crotamiton and hydrocortisone combination is an effective treatment for nodular scabies especially over the genitals.
- Do not apply to face, urethral meatus, eyes, mucous membranes, or swollen skin.

BENZYL BENZOATE :

MECHANISM OF ACTION :

It kills scabies mite by unexplored mechanism.

FORMULATIONS AND APPLICATIONS :

Overnight application of 25% emulsion lotion for three consecutive nights or three times application within 24 hours.

PREGNANCY CATEGORY – 'C' :

SIDE EFFECTS :

1. Pruritus, redness, and swelling and allergic contact dermatitis (derivative of balsam of Peru).
2. Seizures.

KEY POINTS :

- Resistance to benzoate is fairly common.
- Do not apply to raw areas or eyes.
- It is not ovicidal and hence repeated application is required.
- Useful in permethrin resistant cases.

TOPICAL IVERMECTIN :

Ivermectin is effective orally for scabies and can also be used topically as 1% cream including that for rosacea.

MECHANISM OF ACTION :

GABA agonistic action to block chloride channels and causes tonic paralysis.

TOPICAL FORMULATION :

0.8% w, v in a dose of 15-25 ml of single dose with second application after 5 days.

PREGNANCY CATEGORY – 'C' :

KEY POINTS :

- Avoid in children, pregnant women, and in old people.
- It is also used in rosacea 1% or 5% BD for 1-2 months.
- Refer to chapter "Oral Antiparasitic Agents" for details on ivermectin.

MALATHION :

MECHANISM OF ACTION :

Organophosphate compound causes cholinesterase inhibition in the parasite.

FORMULATIONS AND APPLICATIONS :

0.5% lotion OVIDE.

PREGNANCY CATEGORY – 'B' :

KEY POINTS :

- Potent ovicidal agent in pediculosis.

- It has an effective killing time of only 4-5 min, but has residual activity for up to 1 month after application. This occurs through a slow bonding of the malathion to the sulfur atoms in the hair shaft. As a result, its efficacy approaches 95% in pediculosis.
- It contains flammable solvent isopropyl alcohol. If it must be used, patients should be cautioned about the use of inflammable compounds.
- Approximately 8% of a topical dose is absorbed systemically.
- Not recommended nowadays as safer alternatives are available, except in permethrin resistant lice infestation.

THIABENDAZOLE :

MECHANISM OF ACTION :

It inhibits helminth-specific fumarate reductase.

INDICATIONS :

Cutaneous larva migrans due to *Ancylostoma braziliense.*

FORMULATIONS AND APPLICATIONS :

10% cream, 2-4 times a day for 2-7 days. Thiabendazole oral suspension (500 mg/5 ml) MINTEZOL can be used when thiabendazole topical suspension is prescribed.

METHOD OF APPLICATION OF TOPICAL THIABENDAZOLE IN CUTANEOUS LARVA MIGRANS :

Thiabendazole topical suspension should be applied directly to the slowly advancing end of the larval burrow or tunnel in the skin. Since the larvae may have advanced beyond the site of inflammation in the skin, topical thiabendazole should also be applied approximately 5-7.5 cm around the possible end of the burrow or tunnel.

PAROMOMYCIN SULFATE :

Mechanism Of Action :

Inhibits initiation and elongation during protein synthesis.

Indications :

Localized cutaneous leishmaniasis.

Topical Formulation :

15% cream till resolution occurs. Cure rate of 82% has been observed.

x=x=x=x=x

22
Topical and Intralesional Corticosteroids

Topical corticosteroids (TCS) are widely used in dermatology for varied Indications.

MECHANISM OF ACTION :

Corticosteroids exert their ***antiinflammatory*** effects through the following mechanisms :

1. Vasoconstriction.
2. Stabilization of lysosomal membranes.
3. Inhibition of prostaglandins and leukotriene synthesis by blocking phospholipases. (immediate)
4. Decreased chemotaxis of proinflammatory cells at the sites of inflammation.

Corticosteroids exert their ***immunosuppressive*** effects through the following mechanisms :

1. Induction of lymphocyte and eosinophil apoptosis.
2. Depletion of Langerhans cells in epidermis and dermis.
3. Decreased IL-2 production by T-cells.

Corticosteroids exert their ***antiproliferative*** effects through the following mechanisms :

1. Inhibition of mitosis of keratinocytes.
2. Inhibition of synthesis of dermal fibroblasts and subsequent collagen, elastin, and glycosaminoglycans.
3. Corticosteroids bind to cytosolic receptors and affect transcription and translation (delayed)

INDICATIONS :

1. *Eczematous dermatoses :*
   - Atopic dermatitis.
   - Allergic contact dermatitis and irritant contact dermatitis.
   - Phototoxic and photoallergic contact dermatitis.
   - Seborrheic dermatitis.
   - Lichen simplex chronicus.

2. *Autoimmune disorders :*
   - Localized bullous pemphigoid.
   - Pemphigus vulgaris.
   - Alopecia areata.
   - Localized vitiligo.

3. *Inflanunatory dermatoses :*
   - Aphthous ulcers.
   - Lichen planus.
   - Lichen sclerosus atrophicus.
   - Granuloma annulare.
   - Patch stage of mycosis fungoides.
   - Polymorphous light eruption.
   - Prurigo simplex.
   - Insect bite reaction.
   - Prurigo nodularis.
   - Plasma cell balanitis.
   - Nodular scabies.

4. *Miscellaneous :*
   - Melasma.
   - Postinflammatory pigmentation.
   - Hemangioma.

INDICATIONS OF SUPER POTENT STEROIDS :

Steroid responsive dermatoses not responding to potent or medium potent steroids :

- Prurigo nodularis.
- Lichen simplex chronicus.
- Pemphigus vulgaris.
- Bullous pemphigoid.
- Keloids and hypertrophic scar.
- Thick, lichenified dermatoses over palms and soles.
- Hypertrophic lichen planus.
- Vitiligo over palms and soles.
- Hemangiomas.
- Nodular scabies.
- Pyoderma gangrenosum.

INDICATIONS OF POTENT STEROIDS :

- Alopecia areata.
- Lichen planus.
- Subacute eczema.
- Vitiligo excluding palms and soles.
- Aphthous ulcers.
- Nodular scabies.

INDICATIONS OF MEDIUM POTENCY STEROIDS :

- Patch stage of mycosis fungoides.
- Seborrheic dermatitis.
- Acute eczema.
- Insect bite allergy.

INDICATIONS OF MILD STEROIDS :

- Dermatoses in infants and children, *e.g.* pityriasis alba, napkin dermatitis.

TABLE 22.1 : **Classification of topical steroids**

Steroid	Formulations
Class 1 – Super Potent	
Clobetasol propionate	0.05% cream, ointment, lotion
Halobetasol	0.05% cream, ointment
Betamethasone propionate	0.05% cream, ointment
Class 2 – Highly Potent	
Betamethasone valerate	0.1% cream
Betamethasone dipropionate	0.05% cream, ointment
Mometasone furoate ointment	0.1% ointment
Halcinonide	0.1% cream
Fluocinonide	0.05% cream, ointment
Desoximetasone	0.05% gel
Class 3 – Potent	
Triamcinolone acetonide	0.1% ointment
Fluocinonide	0.05 cream
Fluticasone propionate	0.005% ointment
Betamethasone dipropionate	0.05% cream
Class 4 – Moderately Potent	
Mometasone furoate	0.1% cream
Triamcinolone acetonide	0.1% cream
Fluocinolone acetonide	0.025% ointment
Hydrocortisone valerate	0.2% ointment
Methylprednisolone aceponate	0.1% cream
Class 5 – Mildly Potent	
Fluticasone propionate	0.05% cream
Betamethasone dipropionate	0.05% lotion
Triamcinolone acetonide	0.1% lotion
Hydrocortisone butyrate	0.1% cream
Hydrocortisone valerate	0.2% cream
Class 6 – Low Potency	
Desonide	0.05% cream
Fluocinolone acetonide	0.01% cream, lotion
Class 7 – Very Low Potency	
Hydrocortisone acetate	0.5 cream, 1% cream
Dexamethasone	0.1% cream

- Dermatoses over face and genitals.
- Perioral dermatitis.
- Melasma.
- Radiation dermatitis.
- Xerotic eczema. (Table 22.1, 22.2)

TABLE 22.2 : **Local side effects of topical steroids**

Local side effect	Remarks/predisposing factors
Skin atrophy	Thin skin of eyelids, genitals, children
Vascular purpura	Dependent areas, scurvy, collagen vascular disorders
Telangiectasia	Senile skin, infants and children
Hypopigmentation	Is commonly perilesional!
Striae	Obesity, pregnancy, potent steroids
Allergic contact dermatitis	Due to steroid molecule or more commonly due to vehicles
Hypertrichosis	Reversible
Folliculitis and other bacterial infection	Preexisting cutaneous infection, diabetes, neutropenic patients, immunodeficiency, steroids in ointment forms
Cutaneous candidiasis	Diabetes, patients on cytotoxic therapy, malignancies
Miliaria	TCS under occlusion, TCS over occluded sites like flexures
Perioral dermatitis	Fluorinated steroids and potent steroids over face, use of cosmetics
Steroid-induced rosacea	Fluorinated steroids and potent steroids over face
Acneiform eruptions	Monomorphic papules mostly on back, no comedones and inflammatory lesions
Poor wound healing	Diabetes
Addicted dermatoses (rebound phenomenon)	Potent TCS

PREGNANCY CATEGORY – C :

SYSTEMIC SIDE EFFECTS :

Super-potent and topical steroids can cause systemic absorption and give rise to side effects similar to systemic steroids or features similar to iatrogenic Cushing's syndrome. Refer to chapter "Systemic Steroids" for details.

KEY POINTS :

- *Steroid structure :* Hydrocortisone forms the core molecule and addition and alteration of hydroxy, ester, fluoro, chloro, acetonide, and ketone groups at specific positions lead to steroid molecules of varying potency and adverse effects.
- *Vehicle and bases used in the formulations influence absorption.*
  1. Ointment base increases absorption. Ointments are used for thick palmar or plantar skin and lichenified dermatoses.
  2. Creams are used for subacute dermatitis and over intertriginous areas.
  3. Lotions are used over face, scalp and in diffuse steroid responsive dermatoses. Solutions are used over scalp and other hairy areas and occluded areas.
  4. Gels are used over hairy areas and mucosa.
  5. "Orabase" is specially formulated for mucosal use.

SIDE EFFECTS :

Side effects of topical steroids are more common :

1. When superpotent steroids are used.
2. In infants, children and old patients.
3. When used over thin skin.
4. Over skin whose barrier function is breached.

- *Factors affecting action of topical steroids :*
  1. Potency.
  2. Vehicle used for transcutaneous delivery.
  3. Amount of application.
  4. Site of application.
  5. Age of patient.
  6. Occlusive sites.
  7. Duration of treatment.
  8. Frequency of application.
  9. Application under occlusion.
  10. Thickness of stratum corneum.
  11. Hydration of skin.
  12. Repeated use (tachyphylaxis).
  13. Barrier function of skin.
  14. Method of application.

FINGERTIP UNIT :

- In order to bring uniformity in application of amount of creams and ointments like steroid or sunscreens a rough measure of the amount of cream being applied was devised so that we can correlate it with safety and efficacy of topicals.
- One finger tip unit is the amount of cream expressed from a tube nozzle of 5 mm diameter taken over distal skin crease to the tip of the index finger of the adult patient. This amount to about 0.5 gms and is enough to cover a palm & fingers of that person.
- One FTU covers a palm with fingers while the whole upper limb needs four FTUs and the lower limb needs eight FTUs. The chest and abdomen need 7 FTUs to cover while the back & buttocks together need 7 FTUs. For most steroid creams the aim should be to apply a thin layer, the sunscreens need more amount.

INTRALESIONAL STEROIDS (ILS) :

INDICATIONS :

1. Keloids.
2. Alopecia areata.
3. Prurigo nodularis.
4. Lichen simplex chronicus.
5. Hypertrophic lichen planus.
6. Hemangiomas (periocular, nasal or subglottic hemangioma).
7. Pemphigus vulgaris (recalcitrant lesions).
8. Nodular scabies.
9. Localized recalcitrant psoriasis.
10. Plantar fasciitis (Reiter's disease).
11. Granulomatous cheilitis.
12. DLE, tumid LE.
13. Nodulocystic acne.
14. Pyoderma gangrenosum.

SIDE EFFECTS :

1. *Due to injections :*
    - Pain (even vasovagal or neurogenic shock can occur).

TABLE 22.3 : **Steroids used for intralesional injections, doses, and preparations**

Steroid	Doses	Preparations
Triamcinolone acetonide	10 mg IL, 40 mg every 4 weeks	KENACORT 10 mg/ml, 40 mg/ml IL injection
Hydrocortisone (depot preparation)	25 mg IL every 4 weeks	WYCORT 25 mg/ml vial IL injection
Methyl prednisolone acetate (depot preparation)	10 mg IL, every 4-8 weeks	DEPOMEDROl 10 mg/ml, 40 mg/ml IL injection

    - Swelling.
    - Infection and abscess.

2. *Due to steroids :*

Acute :

- Amaurosis fugax (Transient monocular blindness due to accidental intravascular injection).

Chronic :

- Purpura.
- Telangiectasia.
- Hypopigmentation (mostly along distribution of lymphatics).
- Atrophy-Epidermal (imflammatory necrotic nodule, ulceration leading to depression), dermal (thinning, hypopigmentation and telangiectasia) or subcutaneous, depressed skin.
- An interesting form of linear atrophy extending proximally from the site of injection is infrequently observed probably due to the absorption of the steroid into perilymphatic tissues. This takes several months to subside and may be disturbing to the patient.
- Striae-particularly when intralesional steroids are given over the breast area.

KEY POINTS :

- For antiinflammatory indications, dose of intralesional steroids is 5 mg/ml, while in keloids it is 40 mg/ml. it can be diluted with NS/lignocaine. Total dose injected is 1-2 ml/dose. Repeated every 4-6 weeks. Depth of injection depends upon indication.
- Intralesional delivery of steroids can be done with insulin syringe, with 25G needle or by fast, painless jet of steroid lotions into the skin by special instrument available for this purpose (Dermajet), the latter is especially helpful in children.

x=x=x=x=x

23
Topical Immunomodulators

TABLE 23.1 : **Nonsteroidal immunomodulatory agents**

Macrolactums
Tacrolimus
Pimecrolimus
Sirolimus
Contact sensitizers
Dinitrochlorobenzenes (DNCB)
Diphencyprone or diphenylcyclopropenone (DPCP)
Squaric acid dibutyl ester (SADBE)
Immunostimulators
Imiquimod
Miscellaneous agents
Calcipotriol
Anthralin
Topical zinc
Topical interferon
Intralesional interferon

Topical immunomodulators are agents that regulate and modify the local immune responses of the skin. They are now emerging as the safe therapeutic alternative for several immune-mediated dermatoses such as atopic dermatitis, contact allergic dermatitis, alopecia areata, psoriasis, vitiligo, connective tissue disorders such as morphea and lupus erythematosus, psoriasis and skin tumors.

Topical immunomodulators are molecules that can cause either upregulation (immunostimulation) or downregulation (immunosuppression) of the immune response. They are classified into steroidal and nonsteroidal immunomodulatory agents.

TACROLIMUS (FK 506) :

Mechanism Of Action :

Tacrolimus blocks calcineurin, inhibits transcription of interleukene (IL) 2, 4 and 5, downregulates IL-8 receptors on the keratinocytes.

Alters the expression of receptors on Langerhan's cells.

It causes activation of $TRPV_1$ channels followed by desensitization (causing initial burning sensation) causing reduction in pruritus.

Indications Of Tacrolimus (Except AD, All Are Off-Label Indications) :

1. Atopic dermatitis (AD), *Pimecrolimus 1% cream/ointment is also used.*
2. Vitiligo.
3. Psoriasis (flexural).
4. Alopecia areata.
5. Lichen planus : erosive mucosal LP.
6. Cutaneous lupus erythematosus and dermatomyositis.
7. Graft versus host disease.
8. Allergic contact dermatitis.
9. Rosacea.
10. Pyoderma gangrenosum : tacrolimus inhibits neutrophil Chemotaxis.

Preparations And Formulations :

- 0.1%, 0.03% ointment, applied twice daily. Lower concentrations are preferred in children and extensive AD where systemic absorption is likely.
- TACROZ, T-BIS ointment.

Liposomal Tacrolimus (LTAC) :

Liposomal drug delivery increases the penetration of tacrolimus into the skin and allows slow release if the active compound locally with diminished toxicity. Topical application of LTAC achieved nine times more concentration of the drug at the target site than systemic TAC.

Side Effects :

Burning, erythema, and skin infection. Flu-like symptoms and headache on excess systemic absorption. Tacrolimus ointment should not be applied over large body areas on inflamed or eroded skin.

Key Points :

- The name of the drug tacrolimus is a neologism, composed of tsukuba (*Streptomyces tsukubaensis* found initially in Mount Tsukuba), *macrolide* (TAC is macrolide), and *immunosuppression* (TAC causes Immunosuppression).
- It penetrates the skin barrier more effectively than cyclosporine, minimally absorbed and is not metabolized locally, thereby, more effective than topical cyclosporine. It is also longer acting and more efficacious than pimecrolimus.
- Topical TAC has shown to be effective in inverse psoriasis, but ineffective in chronic plaque psoriasis involving the trunk and extremities, proving its inability to penetrate the thick hyperkeratotic skin lesions.

Contraindications :

Pregnancy, lactation, Netherton syndrome, Organ transplant recipients.

PIMECROLIMUS :

Pimecrolimus, an ascomycin derivative, is a potent topical calcineurin inhibitor.

MECHANISM OF ACTION :

Potent calcineurin inhibitor, inhibits cytokine gene transcription, resulting in fewer activated T-cells.

INDICATIONS :

Indications are similar to that of tacrolimus. Pimecrolimus is approved in mild-moderate atopic dermatitis.

FORMULATIONS AND APPLICATIONS :

- Pimecrolimus 1% cream twice a day.
- ELIDEL, PSCON, PACROMA cream

SIDE EFFECTS :

- Burning, irritation can occur but is much less frequent than tacrolimus. Hence, safer for use on sensitive areas like lips, eyelids, genitalia etc.

PREGNANCY CATEGORY – C :

KEY POINT :

- Pimecrolimus has greater cutaneous penetration and less systemic absorption when applied to the skin. However it is less efficacious than tacrolimus.

SIROLIMUS / RAPAYCIN :

Sirolimus, is a potent VEGF inhibitor and also mTOR inhibitor. It is used in patients of angiomyolipoma, lymphangioleiomyomatosis and cutaneous angiofibromas to retard growth of vascular and fibrous tissues. It is most effective in early vascular angiofibromas in children when used as a 0.1% to 0.5% ointment in white soft paraffin base over 1-3 months as twice daily application.

CONTACT SENSITIZERS :

Contact sensitizers are immunomodulating agents. Various

contact sensitizers used in dermatology are dinitrochlorobenzene (DNCB diphenylcyclopropenone (DPCP), and squaric acid dibutyl ester (SADBE).

DINITROCHLOROBENZENE :

Indications And Mechanism Of Action :

1. *Alopecia areata :*

   It is based on the "antigenic competition" theory, which proposes that immune reaction to one antigen may inhibit the development of immune response to other antigens.

   - It alters CD_4 : CD_8 ratio of approximately 4:1 to 1:1 of peribulbar lymphocytic infiltrate. Suppressor T cells may then nonspecifically inhibit the immune reaction to an unidentified hair-associated antigen, which is assumed to be the main target in the pathogenesis of alopecia areata.
   - DNCB also reduces the abnormal expression of human leukocyte antigens (HLA)-A, -B, -C, and -DR in the epithelium of hair follicles.

2. *Warts :*

   The mechanism of action is not clear. It enhances the cell-mediated immune response, triggering virus-infected cell lysis and death. It is believed to induce long term immunity preventing recurrences.

3. *Skin malignancies, (BCC, melanoma, bowen's disease, and actinic keratoses) :*

   DNCB acts as a hapten and interacts with weak tumor antigens, which are not sufficiently immunogenic to evoke an effective immune response.

4. *HIV infection :*

   Immunostimulation and decreased viral load; especially useful in the treatment of prurigo nodularis in HIV.

ADVERSE EFFECTS :

- *Systemic :* Lymphadenopathy, fever with chills, flu-like symptoms, and impaired sleep.
- *Topical :* Severe contact Dermatitis with or without autosensitization eczema, contact leucoderma, hyperpigmentation, dyschromia en confetti, erythema multiforme, urticaria, and contact urticaria (rare).

KEY POINTS :

- It contains contaminants that are mutagenic and may be carcinogenic to animals. The Ames mutagenicity test is done to test the mutagenicity of DNCB. In Ames test, test substance or its extract and test organism (special strains of Salmonella sensitive to mutation) are mixed in a soft agar solution. Reverse mutations are then observed.
- When applied locally, more than 40% of the drug is absorbed systemically.
- DNCB, being mutagenic, female patients of child-bearing age should use reliable contraception during treatment period. It is however not recommended anymore.

DIPHENCYPRONE OR DIPHENYLCYCLOPROPENONE (DPCP) :

PREPARATION :

DPCP solution in acetone.

0.0001-2% in AA, 0.01-2% for warts.

METHOD OF USE :

- ALOPECIA AREATA : Patients are sensitized by applying 2% solution in acetone to a 2 X 2 cm area of the back/ arm with a cotton swab with or without occlusion. Often, an eczematous response is seen 5-7 days after the initial sensitization. If no eczematous response is obtained, a second or third application with the 2% solution is necessary. If no sensitization occurs after 12 weeks, it is avoided.

- Elicitation of allergic contact dermatitis can begin as early as 2 weeks after sensitization.
- DPCP is then applied weekly, using the lowest concentration (*e.g.* 0.00001%, 0.0001%, 0.001%, 0.01%, 0.05%, 0.10/0, 0.5%, or 2%) that maintains erythema, itching, and scaling for 2-3 days.
- To prevent photolysis, the patient's head should be covered with a scarf for at least 6 h, but preferably for 48 h after DPCP is washed off.
- Vellus hair usually appears within 12-16 weeks, which becomes thicker and darker with continued treatment over 4-17 months. Upon unilateral regrowth, the DPCP should be applied to the entire scalp.
- Treatment failure is considered if no regrowth occurs after 20 weeks. Treatment is stopped after 30 weeks of uninterrupted treatment after the first successful elicitation, since a good response later is unlikely.
- Eyebrows should be treated with extreme caution with a concentration one-10th of that used for the scalp. Eyelashes should not be treated.
- WARTS : suitable for periungual, palmoplantar warts; to be avoided on face and genitalia. Initial conc 0.01-0.1% after parring, covered with adhesive dressing for two days. Keratolytics should be used along with immunotherapy.

PREGNANCY CATEGORY – C, not recommended due to limited data

KEY POINTS :

- DPCP is not mutagenic, teratogenic, and has no organ toxicity.
- The inability to provoke an eczematous reaction despite initial successful sensitization (also known as tolerance)

develops in 10-12% cases after an interval of 7-18 months. This necessitates switching over to other contact sensitizers like squaric acid dibutyl ester (SADBE). SADBE is also nonmutagenic, but has a shorter shelf life.

- Relapse rate is around 66%. Remote reverse koebnerisation can also occur.

SQUARIC ACID DIBUTYL ESTER :

Method of application and indications of SADBE are similar that of DPCP and DNCB. An advantage is nonmutagenicity and a disadvantage is its shorter shelf life, and refrigeration is required. It is relatively expensive, unstable in acetone and requires special additives to maintain potency. Hence it is not first choice.

IMMUNOSTIMULATORS :

IMIQUIMOD :

> MECHANISM OF ACTION :
>
> It is an inducer of IFN-γ responsible for local antiviral, antitumor, and immunoregulatory activity.
>
> It also stimulates the natural killer and B cells and enhances migration of Langerhan's cells.

INDICATIONS :

1. *Viral infections of the skin :*
   - Genital warts.
   - Common warts.
   - Molluscum contagiosum.

2. *Malignant and premalignant conditions of skin :*
   - Basal cell carcinoma.
   - Actinic keratosis, Bowen's disease.

- Lentigo maligna.
- Extramammary Paget's disease.
- Bowenoid papulosis.
- Cutaneous T cell lymphoma.

3. *Keloids* (enhances keloidal collagenase activity, reduces keloidal fibroblast synthesis of collagen, reduces glycosaminoglycan synthesis).

PREGNANCY CATEGORY – C :

Adverse Effects :

Erythema, erosions, irritation, pain, ulceration. Fatigue, flu like symptoms.

Preparations And Applications :

IMIQUAD, 5% cream available in sachet to be applied at bed times washed after 6-10 hours with soap and water thrice a week.

Key Points :

- Resiquimod is a more potent analog of imiquimod, which was tried in recurrent genital herpes.
- 6-12 weeks are required to see clinical effects of imiquimode.
- The end point of imiquimod therapy is not yet defined.
- Combination with other modalities like cryo/cautery better than monotherapy.

MISCELLANEOUS TOPICAL IMMUNOMODULATORS :

TOPICAL CALCIPOTRIOL :

Refer to the chapter "Topical Vitamins" for details.

ANTHRALIN (DITHRANOL) : (refer miscellaneous topical agents for details)

MECHANISM OF ACTION :

Antimitotic effect and a nonspecific immunomodulatory action :

- Psoriasis.
- Alopecia areata.

SIDE EFFECTS :

- Irritant and allergic contact dermatitis.
- Staining of skin and clothes.
- Can precipitate bullous pemphigoid in psoriasis patients.

TOPICAL ZINC :

In combination with steroids or other medications in various dermatoses due to its immunomodulating and antiinflammatory properties.

- *Infections :* Warts, cutaneous leishmaniasis, herpes genitalis, dermatophytosis, pityriasis versicolor.
- *Inflammatory disorders :* Chronic plaque psoriasis, acne, HS, rosacea, eczema, AA, oral LP, vitiligo.
- *Malignant conditions :* Actinic keratosis, keloids, BCC.
- *Miscellaneous :* Bromhidrosis, ulcer healing, melasma.

TOPICAL INTERFERON (IFN) :

IU/g of IFN-alpha in hydrophilic ointment recurrent genital herpes simplex infection containing dimethyl sulfoxide leads to rapid cessation of viral shedding (experimental).

INTRALESIONAL INTERFERON :

Intralesional administration of IFN-alpha2b (5 MU/dose) and

recombinant IFNβ-1a (1 MU) thrice a week has been effectively used in cases of lentigo maligna, cutaneous leishmaniasis, genital warts, verruca plana, actinic keratoses, squamous and basal cell carcinoma, keloids and hypertrophic scars, recalcitrant plaques of DLE, and hemangiomas.

Refer to the chapter "Immunobiologicals" for details about interferons.

INTRALESIONAL AND TOPICAL BACILLUS CALMETTE-GUERIN :

A pooled analysis of the efficacy of intralesional Bacillus Calmette-Guérin (BCG) immunotherapy in malignant melanoma showed complete response in 19% cases, partial response in 26% and extended survival in 13% of patients with Stage III melanoma (metastatic disease). It is useful in the immunotherapy of recalcitrant genital (topically) and common warts (intralesional).

x=x=x=x=x

24
Topical Retinoids

Topical retinoids have been widely used for dermatological indications for many years. Topical retinoids are similar to vitamin A (retinol) in terms of their activity (functional analog) and retinoids are natural or synthetic derivatives of retinol (structural analogs). Retinol and retinal are first generation retinoids that have lower efficacy but higher safety and are a common ingradient of cosmetic antiageing creams.

MECHANISM OF ACTION :

Topical retinoids bind to nuclear retinoic acid receptors.

Transcription of regulatory genes of epidermopoiesis and keratinization by direct or indirect activation.

Normalize the pattern of keratinization.

Regulate epidermal proliferation and differentiation.

TABLE 24.1 : **Classification of topical retinoids**

Classification	Retinoid	Formulation
First-generation topical retinoids	Tretinoin (all-trans retinoic acid)	0.025%, 0.01% gel, 0.025%, 0.05%, 0.01% cream
	9-cis. retinoic acid (Alitretinoin)	0.1% gel
	Isotretinoin (3-cis)	0.5% gel
Second-generation topical retinoids	No second generation is available	No second generation is available
Third-generation topical retinoids	Adapalene and tazarotene	Adapalene 0.1-% gel, tazarotene 0.05% gel, and 0.1% cream
	Bexarotene	1.0% gel

RECEPTOR SPECIFICITY OF COMMONLY USED TOPICAL RETINOIDS :

Tretinoin : No retinoic acid receptor sensitivity.

Adapalene : RAR-β and RAR-γ/ (strong aflinity) > RAR-α (poor affinity).

Tazarotene : RAR-β >RAR-γ >RAR-α.

TRETINOIN :

All-trans retinoic acid is available as a cream 0.025%, 0.05% (RetinoA, Tretin).

INDICATIONS :

1. Acne vulgaris.
2. Melasma (hypopigmenting agent) and post inflammatory hyperpigmentation.
3. Antiaging and antiphotoaging : fine wrinkles and dyspigmentation, actinic elastosis, solar comedones, telangiectasia.
4. For priming of skin prior to peels (keratolytic).
5. Actinic keratoses (keratolytic, protection against tumorigenesis), arsenical keratoses, radiation keratoses.
6. Viral warts (keratolytic) especially flat warts.
7. Lichen amyloidosus (keratolytic, hypopigmenting agent).
8. Molluscum contagiosum (causes irritation, stimulates immunity).
9. Keratinization disorders : Keratosis pilaris, Darier's disease, ichthyoses, porokeratosis, PRP, etc.

ADAPALENE :

INDICATION :

Same as tretinoin.

TAZAROTENE :

Indications :

1. Psoriasis (stable plaque type) : 0.1% cream.
2. Acne vulgaris 0.05% gel.
3. Other indications of tretinoin especially for keratolysis and keratinization disorders.

Side Effects of Topical Retinoids :

Side effects of topical retinoids are similar except that their severity differs from preparation to preparation. In the order of decreasing severity commonly used topical retinoids can be arranged as tazarotene > adapalene.

- Local irritation in the form of erythema, desquamation, and dryness (retinoid dermatitis).
- Burning of the skin tanning, itching.
- Temporary worsening of acne.
- Exacerbation of psoriasis (tazarotene) due to irritation.
- Photosensitivity erythema, edema, peeling.

Contraindications of Topical Retinoids :

1. Koebnerizing psoriasis (koebnerization noted with tazarotene) or unstable psoriasis.
2. Tretinoin : eczematous skin, sunburn, permanent wave solutions, electrolysis, hair depilatories waxes.
3. Pregnancy. All topical retinoids are contraindicated during pregnancy.
4. Concurrent administration of photosensitizing drugs like thiazides, tetracyclines, fluoroquinolones, phenothiazines, and sulfonamides.
5. Concurrent application of topical sulfur, resorcinol, salicylic acid, alcohol, astringents, abrasives, and irritant cosmetic products or face washes may potentiate topical retinoid side effects.

KEY POINTS :

- Topical retinoids can also be used in all types of acne including inflammatory acne (Grade II), if used judiciously.
- The skin condition following topical retinoid application in the form of erythema, desquamation, dryness, pruritus, burning and postinflammatory channges occurring within the first month of therapy, is called retinoid dermatitis. This is due to irritation potential of topical retinoids.
- The chance of developing retinoid dermatitis can be minimized by :
  a. Application of the retinoid in the night.
  b. Application of smaller quantities (use pea-sized or even lesser amount for the entire face avoiding eyelids and lips).
  c. Do not apply immediately after bath.
  d. If available, use a lesser concentration in the beginning.
  e. Use alternate day or less frequently in the initiation phase.
  f. Lotions are more irritating than gels and gels are more irritating than creams.
  g. In cases of psoriasis, the retinoid application may be alternated or combined with a steroid application.
  h. Use with caution in persons with atopic background or dry skin.
  i. Using topical retinoids in the newly available micromized forms.
- Ketoconazole inhibits enzyme retinoic acid 4-hydroxylase responsible for retinoid degradation in the skin. Hence, the concurrent use of azoles and topical retinoids increases local side effects of topical retinoids.

- Photosensitivity commonly attributed to retinoids application is not as common or troublesome in the pigmented skin. However retinoids, particularly tretinoin, are preferably applied at evening or at night.
- Adapalene and tazarotene are photostable compounds and therefore can be applied twice daily.
- Topical retinoids have a protective role in the prevention of malignant and pre-malignant conditions due to ultraviolet light'.

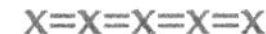

25

Sunscreens

Sunscreens are agents which form a protective "screen" from the harmful effects of ultraviolet radiation of the "sun", either completely or partially. They protect from sunburns and cumulative solar damage to the skin resulting in photoaging or heliosis. Sunscreens are also essential for the protection of the skin in photoinduced or photoaggravated dermatoses. Sun protection from sunscreens is not absolute. There are other components of sun-protection program which include :

- Staying indoors during periods of peak ultraviolet B exposure (11 am to 2 pm).
- Avoiding indirect ultraviolet exposure from lamps and tube lights.
- Minimizing the exposure to infrared radiation, *i.e.* heat.
- Use of umbrellas.
- Wearing wide brimmed hats or caps.
- Wearing protective clothing, *e.g.* 'palloos' worn by women in India.

INDICATIONS OF SUNSCREENS IN DERMATOLOGY :

- Prevention of sunburn.
- Prevention of aging.
- Prevention of tanning.
- Aging and skin Cancer.
- Polymorphic light eruption.
- Solar urticaria/actinic prurigo, sunburn.
- Cutaneous and systemic lupus erythematosus.

- Dermatomyositis.
- Phototoxic and photoallergic reactions.
- Melasma treatment and prevention of new lesions
- Vitiligo with photo-koebnerization and after PUVA therapy.
- Xeroderma pigmentosum, Bloom's syndrome, Photosensitive genodermatoses.
- Organ transplant recipients.
- Co-prescription to topical or oral retinoids to prevent photosensitivity or tanning. (Table 25.1)
- Actinic lichen planus and other photoaggravated conditions.
- To prevent solar aging.

Sunscreening agents are arbitrarily classified into UV-absorbing and UVblocking sunscreens. UV-absorbing sunscreens are known as chemical sunscreens or chemical absorbers, while UV-blocking sunscreens are known as physical, opaque, reflectors, or nonchemical blockers.

MECHANISM OF ACTION OF SUNSCREENS :

Chemical sunscreens absorb high-energy UV to move to higher energy state. This energy is dissipated by resonance delocalization and conversion to lower energy long-wave radiation, which is then re-emitted as heat. Certain amount of UV still enters the epidermis.

Physical sunscreens reflect and scatter ultraviolet radiation and visible radiation.

SUN PROTECTION FACTOR (SPF) OF A SUNSCREEN :

The protection provided by a sunscreen is measured by its SPF.

$$\text{SPF} = \frac{\textit{Minimal erythema dose of UVB light with sunscreen applied}}{\textit{Minimal erythema dose of UVB light without sunscreen}}$$

TABLE 25.1 : **Sunscreens**

	Protection from UV-B	Protection from UV-A	Remarks
Chemical sunscreens :			
Avobenzone	No	Yes	Exclusive UVA protection.
Oxybenzone (benzophenones)	No	Yes	Both avobenzone and oxybenzone are not photostable degrades in 30 minutes of sun exposure and may irritate the skin and need frequent reapplication.
Cinnamates (ethyihexyl p-methoxy cinnamate and octyl methoxy cinnamate)	Yes	No	Insoluble in water, rare sensitization.
PABA	Yes	No	Frequent sensitization, poor substantivity, stains clothes yellow, photoallergic contact dermatitis.
Octyl dimethyl PABA	Yes	No	Soluble and rare sensitization.
Salicylates (homosalate and octyl salicylate)	Yes	No	Insoluble in water, safe but weak sunscreen.
Tinosorb M & S	Yes	Yes	Highly effective, organic oil based sunscreens that blend well with other organic and inorganic compounds water resistant.
Physical sunscreens :			
Titanium dioxide	Yes	Yes	Safe, potent and no sensitization, less acceptable to patients. Micronized T102 or nanoparticles of titanium dioxide or even zinc oxide are available which is less opaque, greasy, and hence cosmetically acceptable.
Zinc oxide	Yes	Yes	Same as above

Sunscreen-protected skin is defined as the skin to which 2 mg/cm^2 of sunscreen is applied. SPF is determined after calculating the doses that produce minimum erythema (MED, dose that produces minimum perceptible erythema) for sun protected skin (by sunscreens) and sun-nonprotected skin.

In practice, much lesser amounts of the sunscreen are applied by people, hence the extent and duration of protection gets reduced.

According to this definition, theoretically, a person who burns after 15 min of sun exposure can extend the period of time until a burn begins after 3 h 45 min with an SPF 15 sunscreen. (15 min X 15). In theory, an SPF 15 sunscreen may absorb more than 92% of incident UVB radiation. An SPF 30 sunscreen may absorb 96.7%, and an SPF 40, 97.50/0 of incident U VB radiation SPF is the measure of protection from UVB and short UVA (320-340 nm) and does not refer to protection from long UVA(340-400 nm) light.

UVA protecting action of sunscreens is difficult to determine as erythema or tanning as an endpoint of induced damage is difficult to estimate. Various in vivo and in vitro methods have been proposed, but none of them has proved to be useful for assessing protection from UVA light.

UVA PROTECTION FACTOR :

$$\frac{\textit{Minimal response dose of UVA light to produce erythema with sunscreen applied}}{\textit{Minimal response dose of UVA light to produce erythema without sunscreen}}$$

The UVA protection factor does not relate to full UVA protection and relates more to protection from short UVA or UVA II, which is also suggested by SPF. Another method called "persistent pigment darkening" considers tanning as the endpoint of UV effect and thus perhaps may be a good measure of full UVA protection in dark-skinned individuals.

High SPF (>30 SPF) *sunscreens* are necessary in individuals with hypersensitivity to sunlight as in light eruptions or photoallergic dermatitis or those with a high risk of intense sun exposure or when sun exposure is expected to be extensive, or when substantivity of sunscreens is poor and when one expects time-dependent diminution of the SPF effect, independent of substantivity.

SUBSTANTIVITY OF SUNSCREEN (Waterproof/Water-Resistant) :

- The ability of the sunscreen to adhere to the skin is known as substantivity. Sunscreens with good SPF values should also require good substantivity for excellent sun protection.
- "Water-resistant" sunscreens allow maximum 40 min of water exposure to maintain substantivity (2 X 20 mins).
- "Waterproof" sunscreens allow maximum 80 min of water exposure to maintain substantivity. (4X20 mins). Durability and water resistance are vehicle dependent.

SUNSCREENS AND THEIR PROPER USE :

- Sunscreens should be applied 30 min prior to UV exposure except for pure physical sunscreens.
- Repeated applications of sunscreens are necessary to provide adequate protection.
- Sunscreens are also to be applied in rainy season or winters even when there is lesser apparent sun exposure.
- Sunscreens should be applied adequately all over the face and photoexposed areas. (2 mg/cm^2)
- Sunscreens are no guarantee that 100% protection from ultra-violet light is acquired. In other words, sunscreens do not allow complete freedom from ultraviolet exposure. They are just a part of a sun-protection program.
- Avoiding sunburn allows individuals to spend greater amount of time in the sun without burning albeit with

greater cumulative UVA exposure, which contributes to Ca and aging.

- Produce aesthetics play a large role in patient compliance.

SIDE EFFECTS OF SUNSCREENS :

- Irritant contact dermatitis.
- Allergic contact reactions.
- Contact urticaria.
- Photocontact reactions.
- Acneiform eruptions.

CONTRAINDICATIONS :

Known sensitivity, infants < 6 months of age.

KEY POINTS :

Sunscreen and Tanning :

As no transparent sunscreen absolutely blocks UV, some tanning or limited tanning will occur. This limited tanning will have a synergistic UV protective effect since sunscreens essentially enhance natural resistance to UV damage that is intrinsically present in the skin. In other words, people using strong sunscreens continuously get less total ultraviolet exposure, less total DNA damage than they would with natural tanning.

Sunscreens and Ageing :

In animal studies, it was found that continuous sunscreen use decreases the abnormal elastotic layer (solar elastoses) characteristic of the actinically induced damage.

Sunscreens And Immune Effects Of UV :

DNA damage leading to pyrimidine dimer formation is one of the factors responsible for adverse immune consequences of ultraviolet exposure. Since sunscreens prevent pyrimidine dimer formation, they can also prevent the principal adverse immunologic consequences of ultraviolet exposure including epidermal Langerhan's cell depletion, loss of contact hypersensitivity, and enhanced susceptibility to transplanted tumor cells.

Ectoin is a natural, water binding organic molecule, that protects against UVA damage including tanning, freckling, photoaging and even depletion of Langerhans cells.

Sunscreens And Vitamin D Deficiency In India :

When sunscreens are used extensively and multiple times in a day (every 2 hours) as advocated, in susceptible individuals, there are chances of vitamin D deficiency as skin is the principal site in formation of active vitamin D on exposure to UVB radiation in the sunlight. As high SPF sunscreens blocks UVB radiation, chances of vitamin D synthesis have been documented by many colleagues in Western countries where sun exposure is typically low throughout the year. However, occurrence of vitamin D deficiency in India has not been proven due to lack of data.

Sunscreen Use And Skin Cancer Risk :

Sunscreens prevent DNA damage and, in particular, pyrimidine dimer formation. Sunscreens may prevent ultraviolet-related cancers but confirmed data are definitely lacking. But prevention of skin malignancies by the use of sunscreens is particularly important in high-risk individuals like military personnel, outdoor sports persons, trekkers and high exposure situations like high altitude winter months, and windburn as well as conditions with a high risk of skin cancers such as xeroderma pigmentosum.

Naturally derived chemicals like polyphenols (green tea, fresh fruits, vegetables) and beta carotene (fruits and vegetables) have mild to moderate broad spectrum UV protective properties. Their oral consumption and topical formulations have been shown to have the property of preventing and even repairing photodamage and preventing ageing and skin cancer.

Sunscreens against visible light and Infrared radiation :

They are still in the experimental stage. The non micronized optically opaque zinc oxide, titanium oxide and ferric oxide are able to block visible light. Antioxidants like grape seed extract, flavonoids, procyanidins, phenolic acids etc and extracts of scutellaria baicalensis and polygonium aviculare have some IR blocking effect. Tinted sunscreens are a complex mixture of iron oxides and pigmentary titanium dioxide in nanoparticle form. Their different formulations produce different tints which allows them to be used tinted cosmetics as well.

x=x=x=x=x

26
Hypopigmenting Agents

Hypopigmenting agents are chemicals that reduce epidermal pigmentation but don't have any significant effect on dermal pigmentation. Most of them have temporary effect on melanin production or transfer or reduce epidermal melanin through peeling of upper epidermal layers. Notable exception is monobenzyl ether of hydroquinone which can cause irreversible depigmentation of skin.

TABLE 26.1 : **Hypopigmenting Agents**

Agent	Formulation	PPS
Hydroquinone	2-4% cream	C
Glycolic acid	6% cream, 12% lotion	No data
Retinoic acid	0.0540/0	C
Azelaic acid	20% cream	No data
Kojic acid	0.75-1% cream	No data
Magnesium ascorbyl phosphate	10%	No data

HYDROQUINONE :

Hydroquinone is a hydroxyphenolic compound, which is frequently used for hypermelanization.

Mechanism Of Action :

It inhibits enzyme tyrosinase, which is the rate-limiting enzyme in melanin synthesis.

Inhibits the formation and melanization of melanosomes.

Is toxic to melanocytes.

INDICATIONS :

It is useful for causes of epidermal hyperpigmentation like :

1. Melasma (epidermal or mixed).
2. Postinflammatory pigmentation due to :
   - Acne vulgaris.
   - Dermatitis.
3. Periorbital hypermelanosis (dark circles around eyes).
4. Freckles and lentigines.

SIDE EFFECTS :

- Burning, pruritus, irritation.
- Allergic contact dermatitis.
- Confetti like depigmentation (Fitzpatrick macules).
- Exogenous ochronosis (grey-black macules and papules).

KEY POINTS :

- 2% hydroquinone is a component of Kligman's regimen for melasma, which also contains 1% hydrocortisone and 0.05% tretinoin.
- Exposure to sunlight or UV light causes repigmentation in patients on hydroquinone, which may be prevented by broad-spectrum sunscreen agents.
- Exogenous ochronosis is an uncommon and late side effect of hydroquinone observed with higher concentrations. It can be diagnosed with skin biopsy showing yellow-brown colored collagen bundles described as banana bodies.
- Hydroquinone is an oxidizing agent, turning the color of formulations from white to brown. Such products should be discarded.

AZELAIC ACID :

Which is mainly used for vulgaris and hyperpigmentation of skin.

MECHANISM OF ACTION :

It inhibits thie enzyme tyrosinase of melanin synthesis.

Cytotoxicoxic to melanocytes, reduces free radical formation. It has no depigmentary effect on normally pigmented skin attributed to its selective effect on abnormal melanocytes

Comedolytic and antibacterial.

Recently, it is found to be a potent inhibitor of enzyme 5-alpha reductase that is responsible for androgenetic alopecia.

INDICATIONS :

- Inflammatory and noninflammatory acne vulgaris.
- Melasma.
- Postinflammatory hyperpigmentation.
- Combination with tretinoin, glycolic acid earlier produced pronounced skin lightening.

SIDE EFFECTS :

Burning, irritation, allergic contact dermatitis.

PREGNANCY CATEGORY – B :

RETINOIC ACID :

MECHANISM OF ACTION :

Pigment dilution effect which is due to increased epidermal turnover with decreased contact time between melanocytes and keratinocytes.

INDICATIONS :

1. Pigmented acne scars.

2. Melasma.
3. Postinflammatory hyperpigmentation due to macular amyloidosis.
4. Freckles and lentigines.
5. Fine Wrinkles (antiaging action).

SIDE EFFECTS :

Burning, irritation, erythema, and peeling.

KEY POINTS :

- The original Kligman's formula for treatment of melasma had a combination of 0.1% retinoic acid with hydroquinone 2% and hydrocortisone 1%. Due to its irritant potential concentration of retinoic acid was reduced to 0.05%.
- Retinoic acid should be applied at night to avoid photosensitivity occurring due to thinning of stratum corneum and reduced melanin synthesis.
- Tretinoin is photodegradable. Sunscreens should be regularly applied during tretinoin use for hyperpigmentation lest it may result in worsening.
- Should not be applied near eyes, nose, and open wounds.
- Application needs to be continued for about 1-2 months to show visible effects.

PREGNACY CATEGORY – C :

GLYCOLIC ACID :

Glycolic acid is an alpha-hydroxy acid or fruit acid that is found in sugarcane, sugar beets, or unripe grapes. Available as 6% and 12% creams for hyperpigmentation disorders (GLYCO).

MECHANISM OF ACTION :
Hyperproliferation or peeling effect due to glycolic acid leads to the premature loss of melanin during desquamation useful for epidermal hyperpigmentation.

INDICATIONS :
1. Pigmented superficial acne scars.
2. Facial hypermelanosis.
3. Postinflammatory hyperpigmentation.
4. Periorbital hypermelanosis (potential for irritation).
5. Fine Wrinkles.

SIDE EFFECTS :
Burning and irritation.

KEY POINTS :
- Glycolic acid causes exfoliation by interfering with the ionic bonding between keratinocytes.
- Glycolic acid is popularly used as a safe peeling agent during chemical peels.

KOJIC ACID :

Kojic acid, widely used in Japan as a food preservative, is not an alpha-hydroxy acid. It has the same mechanism of action as that of hydroquinone. It was isolated from "Koji" or malted rice in Japan at the beginning of 1900 and hence the name. However, it is currently not in use in Japan due to concern regarding its potential for cancer promotion.

MECHANISM OF ACTION :
- It inhibits tyrosinase enzyme of melanin synthesis possibly by the chelation of copper ions.
- Potent antioxidant.
- Antimicrobial properties.

INDICATIONS :
- Melasma.
- Antiaging cream.
- Postinflammatory hyperpigmentation.

SIDE EFFECTS :
- Burning.
- Allergic contact dermatitis.

KEY POINTS :
- Kojic acid is an extremely unstable ingredient in cosmetic formulations. Upon exposure to air or sunlight, it loses its efficacy. Many cosmetic companies use kojic dipalmitate as an alternative because it is far more stable in formulations. Recommended concentration of Kojic acid in lightening creams is 1-2%.

MONOBENZYL ETHER OF HYDROQUINONE :

This is a derivative of hydroquinone.

MECHANISM OF ACTION :
It causes demelanization by being toxic to melanocytes leading to their death and hence inducing permanent depigmentation.

Concentration : 20%, 40% cream.
Brand : Benzoquin, Benoquin.

INDICATIONS :
The only indication is generalized vitiligo with sparing of only a few islands of normal skin. In such cases, cosmetic appearance can be enhanced by inducing permanent depigmentation of the spared normal skin so as to get uniformly depigmented skin. Effect is gradual over 6-12 months.

CONTRAINDICATIONS :

It should not be used for other causes of hyperpigmentation as thehypo- or de-pigmentation induced by it may be permanent.

SIDE EFFECTS :

Depigmentation of treated skin.

KEY POINTS :

While choosing vitiligo patients for permanent depigmentation with monobenzyl ether of hydroquinone, it is important to ensure that their vitiligo is stable and they understand that the effects of the treatment will be irreversible, even if their vitiligo may improve with time. For this reason, it is essential to avoid patients who are unsure or who are mentally unstable.

Apart from above mentioned demelanizing agents in this chapter, there are various other plant derived agents or phytochemicals that are claimed to have demelanizing properties. However, they have no documented evidence of their efficacy as monotherapy in the treatment of pigmentation. These include tetrahydrocurcumin, licorice 0.1% extract etc. Some of them are mentioned here.

TETRAHYDRO CURCUMIN :

Tetrahydrocurcumin is derived from rhizomes of the plant Curcuma longa hydrogenated to form tetrahydro curcumin.

MECHANISM OF ACTION :

- Inhibits tyrosinase thereby slowing down melanin formation.
- Scavenges and prevents formation of free radicals.
- Promotes production of transforming growth factor beta (TGF α), collagen and regeneration of epidermal cells.

USES :

- Hypopigmenting agent as a part of many lightening creams.
- Antioxidant.
- Repair of wounds.

x=x=x=x=x

27

Moisturizers and Keratolytic Agents

Moisturizers are substances known to moisturize or hydrate the skin. Moisturizers are generally classified into occlusives, emollients and humectants with considerable overlap.

Occlusives : Vegetable or animal fats, mineral greases, fatty acids (linoleic acid, stearic acid), fatty alcohols (cetyl alcohol, lanolin alcohol), propylene glycol, wax esters, vegetable waxes, phospholipids, and cholesterol.

Emollients : Dimethicone, Cyclomethicone, propylene glycol, isopropyl myristate, ceramides.

Humectants : Glycerin, lactic acid, sodium lactate, urea, propylene glycol, sorbitol, gelatin, pyrrolidone carboxylic acid, and hyaluronic acid.

Hydrophilic matrices : Colloidal oatmeal bath and hyaluronic acid.

OCCLUSIVES :

Occlusives are greasy substances, which hydrate stratum corneum by forming a greasy layer over the skin surface, thereby preventing transepidermal water loss and retaining moisture in the skin. They are the greasy bases, which include true fats and waxes of vegetable or animal origin and mineral greases obtained from mineral sources.

CLASSIFICATION OF TRUE FATS AND WAXES :

1. True fats and waxes of vegetable origin.

2. True fats and waxes of animal origin.
3. Synthetic waxes.
4. Mineral greases.

TABLE 27.1 : **True fats and waxes of vegetable origin**

Material	Consistency	Remarks
Almond oil	Liquid	Mild, cicar, expensive, and tends to become rancid
Arachis or peanut oil	Liquid	Triglycerides of oleic and linoleic acid
Castor oil	Liquid	Obtained from *Ricinus communis* seeds
Cottonseed oil	Liquid	Obtained from *Gossypium* seeds
Linseed oil	Liquid	Previously used for burns, rich source of vitamin E
Olive oil	Liquid	Obtained from pressing olives
Sesame oil	Liquid	Obtained from sesame. Can cause sensitization
Hydrogenated vegetable oils	Unctuous fat	Vegetable oils hydrogenated to change phase
Theobroma oil	Solid	Obtained from roasted coca beans. Triglycerides of palmitic, stearic, and oleic acids
Vegetable waxes	Semisolid	Carnauba, candelilla

TABLE 27.2 : **True fats and waxes of animal origin**

Material	Consistency	Remarks
Cod-liver oil	Liquid	Obtained from cod-liver
Wool fat or anhydrous lanolin	Unctuous	Stiff sticky fat from sheep which when mixed with other greases can be applied to skin
Hydrous wool fat or lanolin	Unctuous	Wool fat to which 30% water is added (BP)
Lard or pig fat	Unctuous	Purified abdominal fat of pig
Bees wax	Solid	White and yellow wax from honeycomb of Bees

TABLE 27.3 : **Synthetic waxes**

Material	Consistency	Remarks
Emulsifying wax	Solid	1:9 mixture of sodium lauryl sulfate and cetostearyl alcohol
Cetostearyl alcohol	Solid	Constituent of emulsifying wax
Cetyl alcohol	Solid	Synthetic, emollient with melting point 48-50%
Cetyl ester wax	Solid	Synthetic, hydrophilic ointment with melting point 56-60%

TABLE 27.4 : **Mineral greases**

Mineral greases	Consistency	Remarks
Liquid paraffin	Liquid	Mixture of liquid hydrocarbons, also called mineral oil
Macrogol 300	Liquid	Polyethylene glycols with chain length of 300, hydrophilic and can be easily washed off
Soft paraffin (petrolatum) yellow or white	Soft or semisolid	White or yellow semisolid mass of crude mineral oils. Decolorization is done to remove irritants from yellow soft paraffin
Macrogol 1500-4000	Soft or semisolid	Polyethylene glycols with chain length of 1500-4000
Solid paraffin	Solid	Hard paraffin added to soft paraffin to make it solid
Macrogol 4000	Solid	Polyethylene glycols with chain Length 4000

EMOLLIENTS :

They are long chain saturated fatty acids and phospholipids which spread between the keratinocytes and hydrate the stratum corneum and also have an occlusive effect. They have a favourable effect on skin barrier function, repairing damaged skin. They are classified as :

- *Dry emollients :* Isopropyl palmitate, isosteryl alcohol.

- *Fatty emollients :* Propylene glycol, jojoba oil, castor oil, glyceryl stearate.
- *Astringent emollients :* Dimethicone, cyclomethicone, isopropyl myristate.
- *Protective emollients :* Isopropyl isostearate.

INDICATIONS :

1. Atopic dermatitis.
2. Psoriasis.
3. Xerotic eczema and xerosis.
4. Congenital and acquired ichthyosis.
5. Pityriasis rubra pilaris.
6. Pityriasis rosea.
7. Patch stage of mycosis fungoides.
8. Erythroderma.
9. Erythrokeratoderma variabilis.
10. Progressive symmetric erythrokeratoderma.
11. As a hydrophobic base for patch test materials.
12. As a vehicle for topical steroids to increase absorption.
13. As a diluent for topical steroids and other fat soluble actives.

SIDE EFFECTS :

- Occlusion miliaria.
- Occlusion folliculitis and furunculosis.
- Acneiform eruptions.
- Contact sensitivity (rare).
- Greasy skin.

KEY POINTS :

- Liberal use of occlusives and emollients is essential in patients of defective barrier function (increased transepidermal water loss, TEWL) like atopic dermatitis or psoriasis.

- Occlusives retain moisture and do not create it! Hence emollients are best applied immediately after bath or after hydrating skin.
- Oil-in-water formulations are suitable for an oily or acne-prone skin, while type of emollients are best suited for normal or dry skin.

HUMECTANTS :

Humectants are the substances which hydrate stratum corneum by absorbing water from the external environment or from deeper layers of the skin.

- Glycerin.
- Urea.
- Lactic acid and sodium lactate, Ammonium lactate.
- Pyrrolidone carboxylic acid.
- Honey.

Key Points :

- Humectant should not be applied in a dry weather with low humidity. In such conditions, it can absorb moisture from skin itself to promote more dryness.
- The natural moisturizing factors (NMF) consist of a mixture of pyrrolidone carboxylic acid, amino acids, lactate, urea, uric acid, citrate and a family of phosphates, peptides and chlorides. The moisturizing property of individual components and their penetration into stratum corneum is not adequately demonstrated.

KERATOLYTIC AGENTS :

Keratolytic agents are used for treatment of hyperkeratosis of skin.

TABLE 27.5 : **Keratolytic agents**

Keratolytic agent	Keratolytic concentration
Salicylic acid	3-6%, higher concentration, for nails, warts (Upto 60%)
Glycolic acid	6-12%, higher concentration 20-50% in peels
Urea	10-40%, higher concentration- 40% only for nails
Lactic acid	6-12%, higher concentration 16.7% in wart lotion
Sulphur	2-10%
Topical retinoids	Tretinoin 0.1%, Adapalene 0.1%, Tazarotene 0.05-0.1%
Propylene glycol	Mild keratolytic

KEY POINTS :

- Plastic occlusive dressing enhances the therapeutic effect of keratolytic agents.
- Topical steroids should be stable in the presence of acids like salicylic acid or lactic acid to exert their therapeutic effect. Fluocinolone is particularly stable in the presence of acids.
- Preparations of higher concentrations of keratolytic agents are not universally available.

SALICYLIC ACID :

Salicylic acid is a beta-hydroxy acid. It is the main keratolytic agent used in dermatology. At concentrations < 3% it acts as a keratoplastic agent.

MECHANISM OF ACTION :

Salicylic acid supposedly :

1. Reduces adhesion between corneocytes.
2. Dissolves intercellular cement substances between corneocytes.

INDICATIONS :

1. Disorders associated with hyperkeratosis like :
   - Congenital and acquired palmoplantar keratoderma.

- Ichthyoses, Darier's disease, porokeratosis and other keratinization disorders.
- Corn, calluses, warts, and various types of keratoses.

2. Papulosquamous disorders :
   - Psoriasis (particularly of the scalp, volar skin and bony prominences).
   - Seborrheic dermatitis (particularly of the scalp).
3. Dermatophyte infection (tinea pedis manuum).
4. As a peeling or exfoliating agent :
   - Acne vulgaris.
   - Rejuvenation of skin (see chemical peels).

PREPARATIONS AND FORMULATIONS :

SALICYLIX 6% and 12% ointment, SALACTIN 16.7% lotion, CORNCAP 40% salicylic acid in plaster base. Also availabe in bulk as powder. As a part of Whitfield ointment (6% salicylic acid and 12% benzoic acid) WHITOLYN DS ointment (half strength Whitfield oint is more commonly used in treatment of tinea corporis, cruvis, manuum or pedis as it is less irritant to the skin).

KEY POINTS :

1. Salicylic acid is a beta-hydroxy acid, which is lipid soluble and mixes with epidermal lipids and lipids of the sebaceous glands. Hence, it acts more superficially in superficial lipid rich layers of epidermis.
2. Salicylic acid should not be applied on raw areas, fissures, or wounds as it causes more irritations and more systemic absorption.
3. Salicylic acid should not be overused in children (not more than 30 g of 6% salicylic acid ointment in a day) due to the risk of salicylism, which include features like fever, confusion, delirium, psychosis, stupor, coma, tinnitus, metabolic acidosis, nausea, and vomiting.

PREGNANCY CATEGORY – C :

LACTIC ACID :

Lactic acid is an alpha-hydroxy acid, which is used as a humectant and a keratolytic agent.

MECHANISM OF ACTION :

It causes the breakdown of intercellular cement substances.

Lactic acid is also a humectant, which absorbs moisture from the environment into the skin.

INDICATIONS :

Same as those for emollients :

- Disorders associated with hyperkeratosis and dryness.
- Keratosis pilaris.

UREA :

Urea is a keratolytic or exfoliating agent as well as a humectant, and the effects of urea depend upon its concentration. Available as a cream or Lotion.

MECHANISM OF ACTION :

Disperses keratin in stratum corneum.

INDICATIONS :

As a humectant, the indications are those of an emollient. In higher concentrations it is useful for treating :

- Xerosis and ichthyosis (10-20%).
- Palmoplantar keratoderma (10-25%).
- Keratosis pilaris (10-25%).
- Phrynoderma (10-25%).

- Chemical avulsion of nails (40% under occlusion for 24-48 hours).
- Callosities (40%).

KEY POINTS :

Irritation is a common unwanted effect of urea that is concentration dependent. Patients with sensitive skin or atopic dermatitis may not tolerate it.

COMBINED PREPARATION OF UREA, PROPYLENE GLYCOL AND LACTIC ACID :

MOISTUREX urea 10%, lactic acid 10%, propylene glycol 100/0, liquid paraffin 10% (w/w). Many other combinations are now available.

TOPICAL RETINOIDS :

Topical retinoids have exfoliating or peeling effect on the skin.

MECHANISM OF ACTION :

Reduces cell-to-cell adhesion between corneocyte of follicular epithelium.

Promotes mitosis of basal keratinocytes and epidermal proliferation.

INDICATIONS :

- Acne vulgaris.
- Psoriasis.
- Congenital ichthyosis.

See chapter on topical retinoids.

PREPARATIONS :

0.01-0.1% tretinoin gel or cream, tazarotene gel or cream (0.05-0.1%).

Key Points :

Refer to the chapter "Topical Retinoids" for details.

PRECIPITATED SULFUR OINTMENT :

Sulfur ointment has been used since ancient times for various dermatological conditions for its emollient, keratolytic and antimicrobial properties.

Mechanism Of Action :

The exact mechanism of keratolytic action is not known.

Indications :

1. Scabies.
2. Seborrheic dermatitis and dandruff.
3. Fungal infections of the skin (it has antifungal properties).
4. Acne vulgaris (used in combination in calamine lotion).
5. Stable Psoriasis and chronic eczema.

Formulations And Applications :

Sulfur ointment with 6% precipitated sulfur in petroleum.

Key Points :

- Sulfur is less acceptable to patients because of its odor and messy application. It can also cause dryness and irritation of the skin.
- Hypersensitivity to sulfur is a contraindication for sulfur use.

x=x=x=x=x

28

Miscellaneous Topical Agents

TOPICAL VITAMINS :

Various vitamins and their derivatives used as topical agents in dermatology are as follows :

- Vitamin A and its derivatives like tretinoin, adapalene, and tazarotene.
- Vitamin B_3 (nicotinamide).
- Vitamin B_{12}.
- Vitamin C.
- Vitamin D derivatives (calcipotriol, calcitriol, tacalcitol).
- Vitamin E.
- Vitamin K.

Topical vitamins, though used popularly, have not been proved to be beneficial for skin conditions as compared to systemic vitamins. Many topical vitamins are not stable and have inadequate cutaneous penetration or absorption across the skin barrier to exert clinical effects.

TOPICAL VITAMIN A DERIVATIVES (RETINOIDS) :

Please see the chapter on "Topical Retinoids".

TOPICAL VITAMIN B_3 (NIACINAMIDE) :

INDICATIONS :

Many of the indications are experimental and not substantially proved. Used commonly in combination with clindamycin.

1. Acne vulgaris (papular and pustular acne).

2. Rosacea.
3. As a lightening agent for post-acne hyperpigmentation.
4. Antiaging medications (retains moisture in epidermis).

Side effects include local irritation.

TOPICAL PANTOTHENIC ACID :

Mechanism Of Action :

Antioxidant effect of pantothenic acid is due to its stimulation of increased cellular levels of coenzyme A.

Coenzyme A may facilitate the removal of lipid peroxides by increasing the mobilization of fatty acids.

Promote repair of plasma membranes by activating phospholipid synthesis.

Indications :

A topical form of the provitamin, dexpanthenol (pantothenol) is used for the treatment of minor skin disorders, including for the promotion of wound healing.

Contraindication : hypersensitivity.

TOPICAL VITAMIN B_{12} :

Mechanism Of Action :

It is an effective scavenger of nitric oxide (NO).

Indications :

Atopic dermatitis has increased levels of inflammatory cytokines mediated through inducible nitric oxide synthetase (NOS), which in turn, increases NO. NO can stimulate vasodilation, erythema, and edema and has a role in T-lymphocyte function, cell proliferation, and differentiation.

TOPICAL VITAMIN K (PHYTONADIONE) :

Mechanism Of Action :

Unknown efficacy unproved.

Indications :

1. Actinic purpura.
2. Postoperative purpura.
3. Telangiectasias.
4. Progressive pigmented purpura and traumatic purpura.

Key Points :

- 2% cream contains propylene glycol and paraben in the vehicle and has to be applied twice daily for 2 weeks.
- Systemic absorption can cause alteration of prothrombin time.

TOPICAL VITAMIN D_2 DERIVATIVES (CALCIPOTRIOL, CALCITRIOL) :

Mechanism Of Action :

Vitamin D_3 – 1;25 dihydroxyvitamin D_3 acts through vitamin D receptors to regulate cell growth, differentiation, and Immune function. Inhibit keratinocytes and modulate epidermal differentiation. Inhibits production of cytokines IL2, IL6 by T-cells. Blocks transcription of IFN-γ and GM-CSF mRNA. Inhibits cytotoxic and natural killer T-cell activity.

Indications :

Apart from psoriasis other indications are anecdotal

1. *Psoriasis :* plaque, nail, scalp, childhood psoriasis (calcipotriene).

2. *Morphea :* improvement in dyspigmentation, induration, erythema, and telangiectasia.
3. Vitiligos in combination with UVB exposure.
4. Lichen sclerosus et atrophicus.
5. *Disorders of keratinization :* congenital ichthyosis, hereditary palmoplantar keratoderma, keratosis pilaris, and Darier's disease.
6. *Acanthosis nigricans :* apply twice daily for 3 months.
7. Confluent and reticulated papillomatosis of Gougerot and Carteaud.
8. Grover's disease.
9. Inflammatory linear verrucous epidermal nevus (ILVEN).
10. Prurigo nodularis.
11. Verruca.

FORMULATIONS AND APPLICATIONS :

- *Calcipotriene (Calciportiol)* : 0.005% cream, (PASITREX ointment 0.01%), 0.005% lotion for scalp use (ALPSOR lotion).
- *Tacalcitol :* 0.004%, 0.002% ointment.
- Calcitriol oint 0.0003% (SORVATE).

SIDE EFFECTS :

- Hypercalcemia.
- Irritation.
- Photosensitivity (uncommon).
- Allergic contact dermatitis (rare).

KEY POINTS :

- Ultraviolet A light causes degradation of calcipotriol reducing its efficacy.

Topical vitamin D_2 derivatives can be combined with salicylic acid to increase tissue levels for short term use.

MINOXIDIL :

Topical minoxidil is a vasodilator which is commonly used to stimulate hair growth.

Mechanism Of Action :

Topical minoxidil increases microcirculation at the root of hair follicle thereby stimulating hair growth. Direct stimulation of follicle is also proposed.

It supposedly maintains hair in anagen phase for prolonged periods.

Indications :

1. Androgenetic alopecia (male and female pattern baldness).
2. Alopecia areata.
3. Chronic telogen effluvium.
4. Telogen effluvium, drug induced hair loss, hair loss in thyroid disorders are optional indications.

Doses And Preparations :

- Minoxidil lotion (2% or 5%), 1 ml to be applied twice daily over dry scalp, preferably after hair wash.
- MINTOP, PILOMIN 2% lotion, REGAIN, Mx 5% lotion. TUGAIN 5% gel and 5% foam.

Side Effects :

- Stickiness or dryness, irritation, itching (as most available lotions are alcohol based), scaling of scalp.
- Headaches are common.
- Allergic contact dermatitis may occur. Try switching to gel.

- Excess hair growth (hypertrichosis) over adjoining or distant areas especially sideburns and forehead is an alarming side effect. Avoid using more than 5% lotion.
- Hypotension (if excessive systemic absorption occurs).

KEY POINTS :

- There may be initial apparent loss of hair after minoxidil application as existing hair in telogen may be lost. The increased hair loss may resemble talogen effluvium.
- No effect other than reduction in rate of hair loss may be seen during the first months of therapy. Minimum of 6 months is required for hair regrowth to be seen after continuous minoxidil application. Greater the concentration of minoxidil earlier is the hair regrowth. However, more than 5% lotion is associated with greater chance of side effect.
- Stoppage of minoxidil application revert hair to the pretreatment state. Hence minoxidil has to be applied for a minimum period of 3 years or lifelong to sustain hair regrowth.

BRIMONIDINE :

Brimonidine tartrate 0.33% gel is a locally effective sympathomimetic agent that has become available recently for the treatment of rosacea. It works by causing vasoconstriction of the small vessels in the skin on application. Its effect starts after half an hour, peaks around 3 hours and may sustain for the rest of the day. Burning, pruritus, dermatitis are the common side effects though occasionally photosensitivity, blurring of vision or headache may occur.

EFLORNITHINE :

Eflornithine, also known as difluoromethylornithine or DFMO is the only topical agent available for the treatment of excessive hair growth.

Mechanism Of Action :

Eflornithine is an irreversible inhibitor of ornithine decarboxylase, the enzyme which prolongs anagen phase of the hair.

Indications :

As an adjunct to laser treatment for :

1. Hirsutism as an adjunct to laser treatment.
2. Hypertrichosis.

Doses And Preparations :

- Eflornithine 13.9% cream up to 24 weeks of treatment.
- ELYN, EFLORA 13.9% cream for twice daily application.

Side Effects :

Burning, stinging or tingling may occur occasionally.

PREGNANCY CATEGORY – C :

Key Points :

- Percutaneous absorption of eflornithine is minimal and most of the drug which is absorbed is excreted unchanged in the urine without metabolism.
- Eflornithine 13.9% cream can slow hair growth and may reduce the frequency of the need for hair removal by other means.
- Hair removing lasers can be used simultaneously. However, coarse hair respond better to laser therapy. Apart from this, eflornithine can be used for treating vellus hair that are unresponsive to laser therapy.

PLACENTAL EXTRACT :

Topical placental extract is obtained from the human placenta.

MECHANISM OF ACTION :

Placental extract stimulate the growth of melanocytes.

It promotes. DNA synthesis.

Biostimulant, and it also contains trace elements like Zn, Cu and tyrosine (a precursor of melanin).

INDICATIONS :

1. Vitiligo.
2. Wound healing.

DOSES AND PREPARATIONS :

- Aqueous gel or lotion for thrice daily application.
- PLACENTRIX gel, lotion consist of DNA 10-15 mcg/ml, RNA 5-10 mcg/ml, Tyrosine 0.25 to 0.35 mcg/ml.

SIDE EFFECTS :

None are reported.

KEY POINTS :

- Alcoholic placental extract (Melagenina® and Melagenina®) lotion has been found to be more effective in stimulating melanocyte growth as compared to aqueous preparations although efficacy of both the preparations remain to be substantially proved.

BASIC FIBROBLAST GROWTH FACTOR (b FGF) :

Basic fibroblast growth factor is a decapeptide that has been tried in the treatment of vitiligo.

MECHANISM OF ACTION :

Basic FGF is a selective growth factor for melanocytes.

INDICATIONS :

1. Vitiligo.

DOSES AND PREPARATIONS :

- Deca-peptide lotion for once daily application (roll on) for 6-8 weeks.
- MELGAIN, MELBILD lotion (1 mg/ml).

SIDE EFFECTS :

None are reported.

KEY POINTS :

- Basic FGF is recommended to be used at bed time followed by sun exposure for 10-15 minutes on the next day.
- Basic FGF is recommended to be used for minimum 6-8 weeks to show response.

ANTHRALIN (DITHRANOL) :

Anthralin is used traditionally for the treatment of psoriasis.

MECHANISM OF ACTION :

It inhibits DNA synthesis exerting anti-mitotic effect.

INDICATIONS :

1. Chronic plaque psoriasis.
2. Localized alopecia areata (as a contact irritant).

DOSES AND PREPARATIONS :

- 0.025-1.15% cream once daily application.
- PSORANOL, 1.15% ointment.
- DERO-ACT Microemulsion cream, Dithranol 0.5%, Salicylic acid 1.15%, Coal tar 0.58%.

- DEROBIN OINTMENT Dithranol 1.15%, Salicylic acid 1.15%, coal tar 5.3%, WSP.

Side Effects :

- Skin irritation is the most common side effect of topical anthralin. It is contraindicated in unstable or pustular or erythrodermic psoriasis.
- It also stains skin, hair or fabrics and bath tiles.

PREGNANCY CATEGORY – C :

Key Points :

- Irritation potential of anthralin is directly proportional to its concentration.
- Short contact anthralin therapy is commonly used to prevent irritation. It consists of application of anthralin by applicator for a short period of 20-30 minutes to avoid an irritation. Surrounding area is smeared with white soft paraffin prior to the application of anthralin. After 20-30 minutes, anthralin is washed with the help of cotton swab soaked in liquid paraffin or other oil.
- Resolution of the psoriatic lesions is suggested by "mahogany brown" discoloration of the psoriatic plaques.
- **Ingram's dithranol paste** 0.2-0.8% dithranol, 2% salicylic acid, 24% each of zinc oxide and starch and 2.5% hard paraffin. Ingram regimen for psoriasis consists of application of dithranol paste followed by coal tar bath on the next day. This is followed by dithranol paste application and UVB exposure. This form of treatment required hospitalization, therefore not popular.
- Extensive application of anthralin may result in significant systemic absorption and rarely may lead to nephrotoxicity.
- Liposomal anthralin and microemulsion preparation have an advantage of greater efficacy and lesser irritation.

COAL TAR :

Coal tar is used traditionally for the treatment of psoriasis.

Mechanism Of Action :

Exact mechanism of action not known affects granular layer of the skin by causing liberation of lysosomes.

Combined with UVB, it inhibits epidermal DNA synthesis.

Indications :

1. Chronic plaque psoriasis.
2. Subacute eczema.
3. Seborrheic dermatitis.
4. Atopic dermatitis.

Doses And Preparations :

- EXOREX coal tar lotion.
- FONGITAR liquid 1% coal tar plus 1% zinc pyrithione, IONEX-T lotion 5% coal tar lotion.
- SALYTAR-WS Ointment, coal tar 6% plus 3% salicylic acid.

Side Effects :

Phototoxicity, irritation, precipitation of pustular psoriasis. Avoid in unstable psoriasis coal tar does have potential for carcinogenicity and is to be avoided in pregnancy.

Key Points :

- Addition of sulfuric acid and ammonia to shale oil produces ichthammol (Ammonium ichthysulfonate).
- Goekerman regimen for psoriasis include coal tar bath followed by UVB exposure.
- Photosensitizing action of coal tar is due to anthracene.

TOPICAL TESTOSTERONE :

Testosterone is extensively metabolized when administered orally. Hence it is used topically or intramuscularly to exert therapeutic effects. Efficacy of topical testosterone not completely proved.

Indications In Dermatovenereology :

1. Erectile dysfunction—5 g gel once daily till symptoms improve.
2. Gynecomastia—5 g gel daily for 3 months on the breast area.
3. Lichen sclerosus atrophicus—25 g gel twice daily application for 6-8 months over lesions and adjacent areas.

Formulations :

ANDRACTIM 80 g gel.

Side Effects :

Virilization, priapism, increased libido, acne, precocious puberty.

PREGNANCY PRESCRIBING STATUS – X :

Contraindications :

Carcinoma of prostate, carcinoma breast (males), hepatic and renal dysfunction.

Key Points :

- In case of side effects from topical testosterone, 1% progesterone cream is advocated.
- Should not be used in females due to the risk of virilization.
- Concurrent use of corticosteroids and testosterone increases edema formation, and hence should be used cautiously in patients of cardiac or renal failure.

- Androgens may decrease serum glucose levels and insulin requirements in patients of diabetes mellitus.

TOPICAL ANTIPRURITIC AGENTS :

Topical Antihistamines	Remarks
Diphenhydramine	Inconsistent results
Doxepin 5%	Drowsiness is a side effect
Topical Neuromodulators :	
Lidocaine 5%	Used as a eutectic mixture
Pramoxine 1%	Very useful in uremic pruritus Also known as pramocaine, it is a relatively safe antipruritic agent that is sometimes added to soothing calamine lotion for treatment of many inflammatory pruritic dermatoses.
Polidocanol 3%	Combined with humectants in AD, psoriasis
Capsaicin	Transient burning sensation, useful for post-herpetic neuralgia.
Menthol 1-3%	Produces a cold sensation, ameliorates itch

x=x=x=x=x

29
Cosmeceuticals

Kligman introduced the term "Cosmeceuticai" to describe agents that are intended to enhance or preserve the cosmetic appearance of the skin. A cosmeceutical is a cosmetic product whose active ingredient is meant to have a beneficial physiological effect resulting from an enhanced pharmacologic action when compared with an inert cosmetic. Thus, cosmeceutical achieves a borderline position between pharmaceutical and cosmetic product. This term has invited a lot of debate among dermatologists, cosmetologists, pharmacologists, and FDA authorities.

These products are widely used by patients and hence it is important for dermatologists to be informed. Cosmetics and cosmeceuticals, in contrast to drugs, are not regulated by agencies such as the US Food and Drug Administration (FDA). It is not mandatory for cosmeceutical companies to provide safety and efficacy data to validate claims for their products. The contents of this chapter are mostly derived from various available sources of information on the subject and a sincere attempt has been made to bring forward the information of clinical importance to practitioners and Postgraduate students about the ever-expanding list of cosmeceuticals. However, this chapter should be looked at as only a compilation of such available, albeit unauthenticated, information about these Products and not as an endorsement of their efficacy or safety.

COSMECEUTICALS **include :**

- Moisturizers.

- Topical retinoids.

TABLE 29.1 : **Classification of newer cosmeceuticals**

Classification	Agents
Epidermal exfoliants	Amino acids filaggrin-based antioxidant (AFAs)
Dermal repair agents	Retinoids/retinol Growth factor preparations Engineered peptides
Antioxidants	Licorice, soy, isoflavone genistein, alpha-lipoic acid, green tea Dehydroepiandrosterone (DHEA), ubiquinone, silymarin

- Epidermal exfoliants including alpha- and beta-hydroxy acids, amino fruit acids.
- Bleaching or lightening agents.
- Antioxidants.
- Topical sunscreens.
- Dermal repair agents.

Many of the drugs that belong to these categories have already been covered in the preceding chapters. This chapter deals with the cosmeceuticals that have not been covered elsewhere (Table 29.1).

EPIDERMAL EXFOLIANTS :

AMINO ACID FILAGGRIN-BASED ANTIOXIDANTS (AFAs) :

MECHANISM OF ACTION :

Acidic amino acids, which constitute the protein filaggrinact as antioxidant, exfoliating agents and are a part of natural moisturizirig factor required for retaining moisture.

INDICATIONS :

AFA peels are used for :

1. Sun-damaged skin and for pigmentation.
2. Superficial acne scars.
3. Fine wrinkles.
4. Rejuvenation.

KEY POINTS :

- As compared to alpha-hydroxy acids, AFA has more acidic pH with more keratolytic effect and better skin penetration.
- Similar to glycolic acids, AFAs are derived from sugarcane.
- It does not cause photosensitivity, as the degradation product of AFA is urocanic acid which acts as a UV filter.

DERMAL REPAIR AGENTS :

Agents which cause dermal repair are retinoids/retinol, growth factor preparations, and engineered peptides. Some of these like retinol and growth factors may also act on the epidermis.

RETINOL :

Retinol is a precursor of retinoic acid.

MECHANISM OF ACTION :

1. Regulates epidermal proliferation and differentiation.
2. Stimulates fibroblasts and collagen synthesis.

INDICATIONS :

1. Solar aging.
2. Early and superficial actinic keratoses.

PREPARATIONS :

ROC Retinol Actif Pur and Neutrogena Healthy skin® retinol).

Alustra® (Medicis) combination of 4% hydroxyquinone and 0.3% retinol.

KEY POINTS :

- Retinol has greater penetration and lesser irritation potential.
- Retinol is 20 times lesser potent than retinoic acid.

GROWTH FACTOR PREPARATIONS :

Topical epidermal growth factors are useful for the repair of the skin and wound healing.

MECHANISM OF ACTION :

1. Increases mitotic rate of the epidermis, hastening growth and regeneration of the skin.
2. Can stimulate fibroblasts and transforming growth factor-beta (TGF).

PREPARATIONS :

The TNS Recovery Complex System by SkinMedica® (Carlsbad, CA, USA).

TNS Recovery Complex System with NouriCel-MD®.

INDICATIONS :

Fine wrinkles and photodamaged skin.

KINERASE :

Kinerase contains kinetin, which is a member of cytokinin family.

Mechanism Of Action :

1. Antioxidant.
2. Effects resemble that of topical retinoids.

Preparations :

0.01%, 0.05%, 0.10% cream or lotion.

Indications :

Fine wrinkles and photodamaged skin.

ENGINEERED PEPTIDES :

Peptides are molecules made up of amino acids. The use of biological active peptides is a matter of current interest in the field of dermatology for the prevention or treatment of aging.

Mechanism Of Action :

Peptides supposedly have hormonal, immunological, and metabolic properties.

COPPER PEPTIDES :

Copper peptides are copper salts added with GHK tripeptide (glycyl-L-histidyl-L-lysine complex) and mechanism of action is as follows :

Mechanism Of Action :

1. Stimulate collagen synthesis by transcription of collagen, elastin, proteoglycans, and glycosaminoglycans.
2. Attracts macrophages and mast cell for tissue repair.
3. Antiinflammatory effect.
4. Regulate hair follicle cycle.

PREPARATIONS :

The Neova® line of antiaging products (Procyte) provides GHK Copper Peptide Complex™ in cosmetically elegant formulations for daily skin care. Neutrogena Visibly Firm Night Cream and Eye Cream®.

INDICATIONS :

Copper peptide is used as a :

- Wound healer.
- Moisturizer.
- Antiager.
- Alopecia.

PENTAPEPTIDES :

Pentapeptides are combinations of peptides.

PAL-KTTKS :

Peptide containing lysine, threonine, threonine, lysine, and serine (KTTKS) is a breakdown product of procollagen-I that is combined with palmitic acid. Hence it is termed as pal-KTTKS.

MECHANISM OF ACTION :

1. Increases collagen synthesis and glycosaminoglycans.
2. Down regulation of collagenase.

INDICATIONS :

Fine wrinkles and antiaging.

PREPARATIONS :

Strivectin-SD® (Klein-Becker USA) and Oil of Olay's Regenerist®.

KEY POINTS :

Pal-KTTKS is used in combination with other agents like

panthenol, vitamin E, allantoin to exert humectant, antioxidant, and immunomodulatory properties.

ARGIRELINE :

Argireline is a synthetic peptide.

MECHANISM OF ACTION :
It exerts botulinum toxin-like effect of inhibiting acetylcholine release at neuromuscular junction to cause muscle relaxation.

PREPARATIONS :

Avotox® 5%, DDF's Wrinkle Relax (EIDS® Cosmetics Inc.), and Inhibit® (20%) by Natura Bissé, Reclaim (Principal Secret), Serutox® (Valeant).

ANTIOXIDANTS :

Oxidative stress and free oxygen radicals are responsible for aging, photoaging, and carcinogenesis. Antioxidants are therefore used to prevent or treat tissue damage caused by oxidative stress. Vitamin E and C are well regarded as antioxidants. Apart from these agents, others are extensively studied for their antioxidant properties. Many of them are phytochemicals or so called "Botaniceuticals" and are explored for their antioxidant and other properties.

TOPICAL VITAMIN E (ALPHA-TOCOPHEROL) :

MECHANISM OF ACTION :
Lipid-soluble antioxidant for the protection of cell membranes. It is a free radical scavenger.

INDICATIONS :

- Reduction in wrinkling and roughness associated with photoaging.
- As a component of sunscreen.
- Wound healing.
- Lichen sclerosus atrophicus.

TOPICAL VITAMIN C (ASCORBIC ACID) :

Humans lack L-gulono-γ-lactone oxidase and hence vitamin C is indispensable. Epidermis has more vitamin C than dermis and the level increases from stratum corneum to basal layer. It is the only antioxidant which acts on enzymatic (catalase, glutathione peroxidase and superoxide dismutase) and non-enzymatic (vitamin E, glutathione, carotenoids) antioxidant mechanisms.

MECHANISM OF ACTION :

Inhibits melanogenesis (inhibits tyrosinase), stimulates collagenogenesis and stabilizes collagen, antioxidant, protects against UV damage and ozone exposure, has anti-inflammatory properties.

INDICATIONS :

1. In treatinent of fine lines and wrinkles (antiaging).
2. Wound healing (as it aids in stabilizing collagen).
3. To decrease severity of sunburns.
4. To decrease pigmentation.

KEY POINTS :

- The correct formulation of topical vitamin C is difficult to make and costly process.
- Vitamin C is most commonly found in L-ascorbic acid

form, which is highly unstable when exposed to O_2, making it ineffective.

- Many currently available topical vitamin C preparations do not penetrate the skin sufficiently to exert a therapeutic response.

LIMITATIONS TO PERCUTANEOUS ABSORPTION :

1. Vitamin C is water soluble and rapidly oxidizes on exposure to air.
2. pH of preparation should be below 3.5 for stability and penetration.
3. As the pKa value is low (4.2), unionized form alone penetrates skin. L-ascorbic acid form is consistently absorbed through epidermis.
4. Phosphate derivatives, ascorbyl glucoside and lipophilic (palmitate) preparation confer better stability and permeability but the conversion to L-ascorbic acid (active form) is unpredictable.
5. Maximal percutaneous absorption was observed with 20% concentration of vitamin C.
6. If the plasma levels of vitamin C is saturated then, vitamin C is not absorbed topically; hence, systemic preparation are supposed to be more efficacious than topical.

Steps to improvise stability and penetration of vitamin C :

1. Vitamin C is packed in airless or amber colored container.
2. More stable preparations viz., 3-O ethyl ascorbic acid (more lipophilic, reduces ionization).
3. Better penetration viz., ascorbic acid loaded dissolving microneedle patches, liposomal ascorbic acid, pretreatment with CO_2 laser (5W) or Erb:YAG (3.8-5.0J/cm^2), microdermabrasion, microneedling.

4. Addition of co-molecules to enhance vitamin C function : Vitamin E, ferulic acid, AHA.

Formulations available :

Creams, serum, silicone sheets impregnated with vitamin C.

Strength of formulations : 1%-30%.

TABLE 29.2 : **Newer antioxidants**

Antioxidants	Remarks	Mechanism of Action
Licorice	Botanical name of licorice is *Glycyrrhiza glabra*, glabridin is hydrophobic fraction while glycyrrhizin and glycyrrhetinic acid are hydrophilic fraction	Glabridin inhibits melanogenesis and superoxide anion formation while liquirtin (flavonoids) acts as antioxidant
Soy	Soy is a botaniceutical	Inhibits transfer of melanosome to keratinocytes, acts as moisturizer
Isoflavone genistein	Soy is rich in flavonoids like isoflavone genistein	Flavanoid, antioxidant, anticancer, and photoprotective agent
Alpha-lipoic acid	Biological and universal antioxidant has excellent skin penetration	Chelates metals, scavenges O2 radicals, repair oxidative damage, inhibits cross-linking of proteins
Green tea	Obtained by steaming and drying of the fresh leaves of the tea plant Camellia sinensis	Catechin, has antioxidant, photoprotective, antiinflammatory and anticancer properties
Dehydro-epiandrosterone	DHEA is derived from Disscorea plants	Antioxidant, photoprotective, immunomodulatory and anticancer properties
Ubiquinone	Naturally occurring antioxidant in skin	Combats free radicals
Silymarin	Bioflavonoid; extract of milk thistle plant	Antioxidant and tumor-protective agent

KEY POINTS :

Licorice :

BAN A TAN cream® (Arbutin 0.5%, Licorice extract 0.1%, Cosmoperine 0.1%), Fairever cream®.

- Licorice extract is available in certain cosmetic formulations as 0.1% while topical liquirtin is 2% flavonoidal extract.

SOY :

Aveeno skin brightening daily moisturizer® (Johnson & Johnson) Soy Soft daily moisturizing lotion® (Soy Soft Inc.), Neutrogena Fine Fairness.

- Though soy proteins like soybean (trypsin inhibitor (ST I) and Bowman-Birk inhibitor (I'BI) inhibit illelanin production, soy also exerts sonne estrogen-type effects and hence can worsen melasma, which is thought to be mediated by estrogens.
- Soy proteins, lecithin, and phytosterols are believed to improve barrier function.

ISOFLAVONE GENISTEIN :

Dietary supplement "Nutrilite®" contains isoflavone genistein.

- It has excellent bioavailability as compared to other antioxidants.

ALPHA-LIPOIC ACID :

- Dihydrolipoic acid (DHLA) is an active component of alphalipoic acid.
- It is soluble in both water and lipids and hence called a universal antioxidant.
- Available as 1-7% in cosmetic preparations, alpha-lipoic acid is less irritating than tretinoin and hydroxy acids; also used for superficial peeling especially around the eyes. However, it can cause skin inflammation.

GREEN TEA :

- Green tea oil is a popular antioxidant ingredient of moisturizers, cleansers, shower gels, toothpastes, depilatories, shampoos, and perfumes.

COSMECEUTICALS FOR ACNE :

Seboregulatory effect : Niacinamide, L-Carnitine, Bakurchiol, epigallolcatechin-3 gallate, Phyco-saccharide.

Anti-P. acnes effect : Niacinamide, 1, 2-decanediol, Bakuchiol, Tea tree oil, Lactobacillus plantarum.

Anti-inflammatory effect : Licochalcone A, Bakuchiol, Soy isoflavones (Genistin, Daidzin), Nicotinamide, Enoxolone, Zinc, Ginkgo biloba, Probiotics (Lactobacillus fermented Chamaecyparis obtuse, Lactobacillus Plantarum), Epidermal growth factor, Vitamin CG.

Antioxidant effect : Epigallocatechin-3-gallate, Fullerene.

Keratinization regulator effect : Gluconolactone.

COSMECEUTICALS FOR HYPERPIGMENTATION :

Tyrosinase inhibitor : Thiamidol, Kojic acid (chelates copper required by tyrosinase), Arbutin, Resorcinol, Licorice extract (liquiritin, isoliquertin), Rutin, Quercetin, Caffeic acid, Ferulic acid, Epigallocatechin, Rosmarinic acid, Gallic acid, Epicatechin.

Antioxidant effect : Vitamin C, Kojic acid, Ferulic acid, Soybean extract.

Melanosome transfer inhibition : Soybean extract.

Cosmeceutical products for hyperpigmentation also have various plant based (A. montana, A. dracunculus, Artocarpus spp., C. sappan, C. tinctorius, J. chinensis, K. pandurate, M. fragrans, P. nodiflora, R. rosea, R. verniciflua, S. indicum, S. indicum, and T. avellanedae), marine algae based (I. foliacea) and fungus based (A. alternata var. monosporus, Monascus spp.) molecules which have significant melanosuppressive effect.

COSMECEUTICALS FOR ANTIAGING :

DNA damage modifiers : Polypodium leucotomos (7.5 mg oral, topical), ascorbic acid, ferulic acid, vitamin E. niacinamide, green tea (epigallocatechin – oral, topical).

Mitochondrial DNA damage modifiers : Coenzyme Q. 10 (oral, topical), curcumin.

Anti-inflammatory agents : Argan oil, Chamomile, Feverfew, caffeine, green tea, licorice extract, aloe, linoleic acid (argan oil and safflower oil have high concentration), niacinamide, polypodium leucotomos.

Retinoids (retinol, tretinoin, adaplene, tazarotene penetrate better into dermis than retinyl palmitate. retinyl linoleate), alpha hydroxyacids, peptides (GHK-cu, palmitoyl pentapeptide *i.e.,* Pal-KTTKS) and ascorbic acid stimulate neocollagenogenesis. Heparan sulfate binds to growth factor, protects and facilitates its transport to target site thereby acts as antiaging molecule. LRG + stem cells of hair follicles and defensin, a peptide which stimulates these stem cells are used for antiaging purpose.

x=x=x=x=x

30

Commonly Used Chemical Agents in Dermatological Practice

POTASSIUM HYDROXIDE (KOH) :

It is an ionic salt, which is commercially available as crystals that are soluble in water. To obtain 1000 concentration, 10 gm of KOH crystals are dissolved in 10 ml glycerin and 80 ml of distilled water.

MECHANISM OF ACTION :
Potassium hydroxide dissolves keratin.

DIAGNOSTIC USES :

- For demonstration of fungal elements in skin scrapings of pityriasis versicolor ('spaghetti and meat ball appearance'), cutaneous candidiasis (budding yeast, pseudohyphae) and dermatophyte infections (refractile branching hyphae and arthrospores). Similarly KOH mount can also be used for demonstration of fungal elements in nail clippings.
- To demonstrate organisms in crush smear of grains in cases of eumycotic mycetoma.
- Imprint smear in suspected subcutaneous and deep fungal infections via, cryptococcosis (capsulated yeast), chromoblastomycosis (muriform/sclerotic/fumagoid bodies), blastomycosis (round, refractile spores broad based buds).

- For demonstration of *Sarcopti scabiei* (mite) in scabies.
- For demonstration of *Demodex folliculorum* (mite) in cheesy material expressed from follicular papules or pustules in rosacea and demodicidosis.
- Whiff test-Drops of potassium hydroxide are added on the slide smeared with a sample of vaginal discharge. Fishy smell suggests the diagnosis of bacterial vaginosis.

MODIFICATIONS OF KOH USED FOR DIAGNOSTIC PURPOSES :

1. Parker's ink when added to KOH stains hyphae blue and hence makes it more visible.
2. Eosin 1% when added to KOH stains keratinocytes and hyphae stand out unstained.

THERAPEUTIC USES :

In concentration of 5-1000, KOH is used for the treatment of molluscum contagiosum, particularly in children. KOH solution is applied once/twice daily over the lesions. It induces inflammation that supposedly helps in faster resolution. Notable improvement is expected in 2-3 months of application. Over-application and higher concentration of KOH may lead to irritation.

SILVER NITRATE :

Silver nitrate is available as transparent, hygroscopic crystals in amber colored bottles and pencil sticks (95% w/w) wrapped in brown colored paper.

To obtain 0.25% concentration, 5 ml of stock solution (50%) is added to 1000 ml distilled water.

MECHANISM OF ACTION :

1. Caustic.
2. Bacterial inactivation due to interaction of Ag^+ with thiol groups.

METHOD OF APPLICATION :

- Surrounding areas of healthy skin should be protected with a wet pad or petroleum jelly prior to use.
- The tip of a silver nitrate stick is moistened with suitably clean water and applied to the area to be treated for up to 2 minutes. End point is frosting due to denaturation of proteins.

USES :

1. As a caustic (pencil sticks, 0.1-0.5% solution) :
    - Pyogenic granuloma, hyperplastic granulation tissue.
    - Cysts—Bartholin cyst, pilonidal cyst, mucous cyst.
    - Others—viral warts, molluscum contagiosum, herpes genitalis, aphthous stomatitis, and tattoo removal.
2. Antibacterial—0.5% solution is used (active against *S. aureus*, hemolytic streptococci and generally against *P. aeruginosa* and *E. coli*) for dressing non-healing ulcers.
3. Prophylactic :
    - Prophylaxis with 1% silver nitrate eye drops against chlamydial (Credé's technique) and gonococcal infection of the eye neonates.
    - Decrease radiation/chemotherapy associated mucositis, stimulates cells to divide before radiotherapy and hence reduces radiation induced damage.

SIDE EFFECTS :

1. Irritant—burning, pain, erythema, blistering, oozing.
2. Argyria is an accumulation of silver metal or compounds in the connective tissues resulting in a local or general grayish or blackish-blue appearance after repeated use of

silver nitrate in large quantities. The pigmentation is accentuated over sun exposed areas and mucosae.

3. Methemoglobinemia (rare, occurs after extensive topical application of nitrate).

KEY POINTS :

- Unopened stock solution of silver nitrate has a shelf life of 5 years. Silver nitrate needs to be protected from moisture and light to preserve efficacy.
- *Silver nitrate poisoning :* Symptoms are pain in the mouth, increased salivation (sialorrhea), diarrhea, nausea, vomiting, coma or convulsions. For treatment, stomach wash is given with 1% sodium chloride solution followed by purgative administration such as 30 g of sodium sulfate in 250 ml of water, to be allowed to remain in the stomach. Demulcents such as egg-white, milk or liquid paraffin may be administered. Pethidine or morphine is given to allay stress. Monitoring for renal function and maintenance of fluid balance is required.
- The disadvantage of silver nitrate is its limited solubility, because of which it cannot be used to treat established infection.
- Silver nitrate stains skin brown-black. It also stains overlying dressing materials brown or black. Skin stains can be removed by sodium hyposulfite.
- Caustics are not suitable for use near the eyes or other sensitive areas.

PHENOL (CARBOLIC ACID) :

Phenol is aromatic hydrocarbon derived from coal tar or manufactured from monochlorobenzene.

MECHANISM OF ACTION :

It causes denaturation of proteins.

USES :

1. ***Chemical cauterization (88% phenol) :***
   - Infectious lesions warts, molluscum contagiosum. seborrheic keratosis, adenoma.
   - Benign neoplasms sebaceum, trichoepithelioma etc.
   - Vascular lesions pyogenic granuloma. steatocystoma, mucocele.
   - Cysts.
2. Spot peeling (88% phenol) of hyperpigmented patches *e.g.* melasma, post inflammatory epidermal hyperpigmentation, freckles, lentigines.
3. Acne scar revision (88% phenol).
4. Alopecia areata (88%) as an irritant.
5. Lichen simplex chronicus, prurigo nodularis and lichen amyloidosis (88% phenol).
6. Ear lobe repair (88% phenol).
7. Vitiligo (88% phenol is used to produce therapeutic wound healing).
8. Facial rejuvenation (50% phenol).

SPECIAL FEATURES OF PHENOL :

1. Phenol 88% causes protein (epidermal keratin) denaturation, which prevents further deep penetration of phenol and protects deep reticular dermis. On diluting phenol, it causes keratolysis rather than keratin coagulation and hence phenol penetrates into deep reticular dermis. Thus, cutaneous penetration of phenol is inversely proportional to its concentration.
2. Phenol toxicity is related to the total surface area to which phenol is applied rather than its concentration. Hence it is essential to divide the entire face into smaller areas and a gap of 15 minutes should be given while peeling consecutive areas.

3. Phenol toxicity can be alleviated or prevented by advising the patient to have plenty of oral fluids pre- and post-peel. Alternatively, the patient can be infused 1 pint of Ringer lactate before procedure and 2 pints during and after peel.
4. Phenol has anesthetic properties.
5. Observe patients for 30 mins after procedure as arrhythmias can occur in immediate post-procedure period too.

PHENOL TOXICITY :

Phenol is a Protoplasmic poison and causes progressive renal failure, cardiac arrhythmia, central nervous depression, respiratory embarrassment and hepatotoxicity.

ACETIC ACID/VINEGAR :

For compresses, 0.25% solution of acetic acid is prepared from distilled white vinegar (5% acetic acid solution) by diluting it with distilled water in 1 :1 ratio. The resultant pH is 3.

MECHANISM OF ACTION :

It inhibits growth of *Pseudomonas spp.* due to its acidic pH.

Astringent-precipitates proteins.

USES :

1. Infections caused by *Pseudomonas spp. e.g.* wound infection, hot tub folliculitis, green nail syndrome and pseudomonal intertrigo (as an astringent which dries and heals the maceration).
2. Vinegar is used to dissolve cement for removing nits in pediculosis.
3. Candidal onychomycosis.

4. Used to elute the dye for patch testing in cases of clothing dermatitis.
5. Used to wash clothes to destroy jelly fish nematocytes in cases of recurrent swimmer's itch.
6. Used as a soothing agent in cases of sunburn or after photo-dynamic therapy induced blistering. Tepid vinegar bath is advised immediately after sun exposure.

BURROW'S SOLUTION (ALUMINIUM SUBACETATE SOLUTION) :

It is 1:10-1:40 dilution of 5% solution; one tablet of the compound added in a pint of water yields 1:40 concentration. It should be prepared fresh and used immediately.

Method of use : Commonly used as compresses or soaks.

USES :

1. To decrease edema and exudates in acute eczema, pompholyx.
2. Gram negative toe web space infection.
3. Used as an astringent for treating maceration in cases with vesiculobullous type of athlete's foot due to *T. mentagrophytes.*
4. Used as a soothing agent in poison ivy bite.

CONDY'S LOTION POTASSIUM PERMANGANATE) :

Condy's lotion is potassium permanganate.

MECHANISM OF ACTION :

Disinfectant due to its oxidizing effect.

Astringent – precipitates proteins.

Fungicidal action.

Deodorizer.

Method of use :

Commonly used as open wet compresses or soaks.

USES :

1. Cold compresses of potassium permanganate (1:4000 to 1:16,000 strength) are commonly used in exudative skin lesions like acute eczema. Used as open wet compresses, it is cooling, soothing, drying and relieves itching. Open wet compresses soften and loosen crusts and remove them, thereby reducing the bacterial load. Through evaporation of water, they cause cooling and vasoconstriction, thereby reducing oozing.
2. Mouth wash (1:10,000 strength) in cases with erosions (pemphigus vulgaris), ulcers (aphthous ulcers), and oral candidiasis.
3. Medicated bath – 8 g of crystals is dissolved in 200 lts of water to give a concentration of 1:25,000.
4. Sietz bath for treatment of perianal or scrotal/vulval painful exudative/ulcerative conditions.

KEY POINTS :

- Stains clothes and skin – cloth stains can be removed with vinegar. Skin discoloration disappears spontaneously in 1-2 days or can be removed with oxalic acid or sodium hyposulfite.
- Risk of chemical burns when used undiluted or higher concentrations of potassium permanganate solution.

SODIUM HYPOCHLORITE SOLUTION (DAKIN'S SOLUTION) :

Diluted sodium hypochlorite (1%) solution bufferd with boric acid (available chlorine is 0.5%).

MECHANISM OF ACTION :

It is a broad-spectrum germicidal agent. Cytotoxic effects are due to oxidation of sulfhydryl groups by chloride ions. Effective against HIVs.

USES :

1. Used to sterilize flooring in wards/rooms housing patients with infected wounds.
2. Used in safe disposal of body fluids (urine, sputum, CSF) and stools of HIV infected patients.

KEY POINTS :

- It has an unpleasant fishy odor.

DINITROCHLOROBENZENE (DNCB) :

Refer to the chapter on "Topical immuno modulators" for details.

x=x=x=x=x

31
Chemical Peels

Chemical peels are controlled chemical burns that are being increasingly used for the treatment of acne, acne scars, and hyperpigmentation, dyspigmentation and facial rejuvenation. Some indications like pigmentation and inflammatory acne require superficial peeling whereas scars due to acne or other causes require deeper peels. Agents that are used for chemical peeling are as follows :

AGENTS :

Common agents used for chemical peels are :

1. Glycolic acid.
2. Trichloroacetic acid.
3. Salicylic acid.
4. Resorcinol.
5. Phenol.

INDICATIONS :

Acne :

1. Superficial acne scars.
2. Inflammatory acne.
3. Post-inflammatory hyperpigmentation.

Pigmentary disorders :

1. Melasma.
2. Postinflammatory hyperpigmentation.
3. Dyspigmentation.
4. Periorbital melanosis.

MECHANISM OF ACTION :

Peels are ("controlled chemical burns')

1. In superficial peels, they cause exfoliation due to keratolysis (phenol 44-55%) or decreased cellular adhesion.
2. In medium peels, they promote epidermal regeneration and collagen remodeling in papillary and upper reticular dermis and enhances glycosaminoglycans synthesis thereby improving superficial wrinkles.
3. In deep peels, they cause deep reticular dermal regeneration.
4. Skin lightening occurs due to the inhibition of enzyme tyrosinase leading to decreased melanogenesis.
5. Other actions :
   a. Antiinflammatory action – salicylic acid (due to inhibition of arachidonic acid metabolism).
   b. Self neutralizing action due to precipitation of proteins (phenol 88%), crystallization (salicylic acid).
   c. Local anesthetic action – phenol, salicylic acid.
   d. Comedolytic – salicylic acid (due to its lipophilicity, it can penetrate deep into follicle).

Choosing a patient for chemical peel :

1. Persons with realistic expectations.
2. Reliable with respect to follow-up and adherence to instructions.
3. Trichloroacetic acid peels can be used in all skin types though there is a risk of dyspigmentation in dark-skinned individuals. However, glycolic acid peels are suitable for skin types V-VI.
4. Peels can be avoided in cases of melasma, facial hyperpigmentation and acne in pregnant women. In

pregnancy, these conditions occur secondary to hormonal changes and are likely to subside postpartum in a majority of cases.

5. Patients should not be on medication causing phototoxicity.

GENERAL PROCEDURES OF THE PEELS :

Pre-Procedure :

1. Persons with keloidal tendency should be avoided.
2. In persons with history of herpes simplex infection, acyclovir should be started prophylactic 2 days prior to procedure and continued for 4-5 days post peel.
3. Systemic retinoids should be stopped for a minimum of 6 months prior to peel to avoid scarring and risk of hyperpigmentation due to retinoid photosensitivity.
4. Prime patients with agents like trétinoin, 6% glycolic acid or hydroquinone for 2 weeks before the procedure. Priming agent should be stopped a day prior to peeling.
5. Test patch of 1 cm^2 area in an inconspicuous location (retroauricular area) is usually chosen for 'test peel' to evaluate effects and side effects.

Peel Procedure :

1. Patient is in semi-reclining position (at an angle of 45 degree).
2. Face is cleaned with pre peel cleanser or degreasing agent like acetone.
3. Lateral canthi of both eyes, angles of mouth and nasolabial folds are covered with petroleum jelly.
4. Eyes are covered with wet gauze dipped in ice-cold water.
5. Cotton swab dipped in peel solution is applied in outward direction to different zones of the face in sequential order : forehead > cheek > chin > nose >

periorbital area. This depends upon thickness of the skin, which is thickest in forehead and thinnest in periorbital area.

6. Peel is stopped when the end point of the peel is achieved.
7. Peel is neutralized with a neutralizing solution. Normal saline or cold water is used for most of the peels. Phenol is self neutralized. Peeling solution on the forehead is neutralized in the end.
8. Apply the peeling agent beyond the desired cosmetic areas to avoid sharp demarcation lines of differential pigmentation (feathering).

Post Procedure :

1. Plain water soaks have a cooling effect, facilitate removal of crusts (in TCA peels) and allay pain.
2. Mild-moderate topical steroids are to be advocated in case of severe erythema or inflammation caused by peels.
3. Sun exposure should be strictly avoided and sunscreens need to be applied regularly even when indoors. A comprehensive sun-protection program is to be followed even thereafter oil a long-term basis.
4. Peels are generally required to be repeated every month (2 weeks for salicylic acid peels) to maintain effects.

Side Effects Associated with Chemical Peels :

1. Local irritation, burning and pain.
2. Secondary bacterial infection.
3. Reactivation of herpes infection.
4. Persistent erythema – erythema persisting for more than 5 months and 9 months in moderate and deep peels (respectively) is usually due to contact dermatitis.
5. Dyspigmentation – hyperpigmentation, hypopigmentation and depigmentation. Persons at risk are skin types IV-VI.

TABLE 31.1 : **Peeling agents and formulations**

Peeling agent	Commercial formulation	Preparations used	Methods of preparation	Shelf life	Adjuvants
Trichloroacetic acid (Blue Peel®, Accupeel)	Transparent crystals in air tight glass bottle; ready to use	Solution	TCA crystals are readily soluble in water. To obtain 30% concentration, 30 gm of TCA is dissolved in 100 ml distilled water	6 months	Glycerin
Glycolic acid Neo Strata®, Neutrogena®)	TCA solution	Solution	Ready made preparation. Distilled water/alcohol/acetone propylene glycol are used for preparation	—	Glycerin
Salicylic acid	70% stock solution in glass/plastic bottle; ready to use preparation	Solution	To obtain 20% concentration, 20 gm of SA is dissolved in 100 ml ethanol or methanol. Ten gm of SA in 10 ml of ethanol attain 10% SA peel concentration.	—	Glycerin
Resorcinol	20-30% w/v in a hydro ethanolic solution, salicylic paste (salicylic acid powder	Paste, and 53% solution	Resorcinol solution (resorcinol 24% sulfur 24%, 2.5% glycerin, 2.5% sorbitol, 1% aluminium-magnesium silicate, 0.5% carboxymethylcellulose, 45.5% deionized water) and resorcinol paste (resorcinol, olive oil, zinc oxide, wool fat, petrolatum and kaolin 5%)	6 months	—

TABLE 31.2 : **Various peeling agents and the depth of peei achieveö**

Depth of peel	Histological depth	GA	TCA	SA	Phenol	Others
Very superficial	Stratum corneum	20-35%	10-15%	10-20%	—	Resorcinol paste, Jessner's 1-3 coat
Superficial	Epidermis	50-70%	15-20%	20-30%	—	Jessner's 4-10 coats, resorcinol paste
Medium depth	Papillary dermis	70%	35-50%	30-50%	80%	Coleman Frutell peel, Monheit peel, Brody peel
Deep	Reticular dermis	—	—	—	Baker's formula	—

Females on hormonal therapy, patients who become pregnant within 6 months of the peel, patients on photosensitizing medicines and those exposed to excessive sunlight post-peel. TCA peels commonly cause hyperpigmentation dark skinned persons.

6. Milia may appear 4-6 weeks after procedure.
7. Keloids.

CONTRAINDICATIONS :

1. Presence with active infection or wound.
2. Keloidal tendency.
3. Renal, hepatic or cardiovascular disease (for phenol peels).
4. Patient with unrealistic expectations.

GLYCOLIC ACID (GA) :

Glycolic acid is an alpha hydroxy acid/fruit acid, derived from sugarcane.

USES OF GA PEEL :

Acne :

a. Superficial acnc.

b. Severe inflammatory acne.

Pigmentary disorders :

Spot peeling of hyperpigmented patches viz., melasma and postinflammatory hyperpigmentation of epidermal type, freckles and lentigines.

Facial rejuvenation :

Endpoint : Erythema or significant burning/stinging sensation.
Termination of peel : Sponging with cold water swab/sponge.

KEY POINTS :

Glycerin-improves contact of GA with skin; buffers viz., phosphoric acid, sodium hydroxide, sodium bicarbonate.

- GA has a persistent action.
- End point is erythema that is at times difficult to discern in dark patients.
- P^{ka} value is the dissociation constant of a substance and is a measure of proton donation capacity. It is the pH value at which the concentration of free acid is equal to the concentration of its salt. If, $P^{ka} > pH$, then the concentration of free acid increases leading to increased exfoliation. Ideal P^{ka} value 3.83; ideal pH value –1.5-2.5 for chemical peels, 5.0-5.5 for daily use.

TRICHLOROACETIC ACID (TCA) :

Trichloroacetic acid, a halo acetic acid, is a laboratory reagent that is irritating and corrosive.

USES OF TCA PEELS :

Acne :

- Superficial and deep acne scars.
- Severe nodulocystic acne.

Pigmentary disorders :

- Spot peeling of hyperpigmented patches viz., melasma, postinflammatory hyperpigmentation.

PEEL PROCEDURE :

End point : Frosting, a whitish discoloration of skin/lesion (due to denaturation of proteins).

Termination of peel : Sponging with cold water swab sponge.

EVOLUTION :

Within minutes—Uniform white color.

Bv 24-48 hrs—Color changes to dark brown-black.

By 5-10 days—Complete desquamation of skin.

KEY POINTS :

- Glycerin, an emulsifier, decreases TCA-induced irritation, promotes slow penetration and homogenous spread of TCA.
- TCA is also used for chemical cauterization of warts, molluscum contagiosum, seborrheic keratosis, adenoma sebaceum, trichoepithelioma, dermatosis papulosa nigra, pyogenic granuloma, xanthelasma palpebrarum.
- It is also used as a contact irritant in the treatment of alopecia areata and vitiligo.

SALICYLIC ACID (SA) :

Salicylic acid is a beta hydroxy acid derived from the willow bark wintergreen leaves and sweet birch (hydroxyl derivative of benzoic acid).

USES OF SALICYLIC ACID S :

1. Inflammatory acne.
2. Superficial acne scars.
3. Full face salicylic acid peels have been tried in patients of melasma, freckles, post-inflammatory hyperpigmentation, actinic keratoses, fine lines and wrinkles, and plane facial warts.

CONCENTRATION AND PREPARATION :

Salicylic acid 30% solution (30 gm salicylic acid powder in absolute alcohol to make 100 ml solution) is used for weekly chemical peeling sessions.

End point : Pseudo-frosting, a whitish discoloration due to crystallization of SA.

Termination of peel : Sponging with cold water swab/sponge.

KEY POINTS :

- Salicylic acid is also used for chemical cauterization of warts, molluscum contagiosum seborrheic keratosis, adenoma sebaceum, trichoepithelioma, dermatosis papulosa nigra, etc.
- Contraindications for salicylic acid peels are aspirin hypersensitivity, pregnancy and lactation.
- Salicylic acid toxicity/salicylism : Tinnitus, dizziness, headache, vomiting, hyperventilation, delirium, stupor, coma, and death. Salicylism is likely to occur when :
    1. Higher concentration of salicylic acid is used.
    2. SA is applied over a larger surface area.
    3. Abrasions or wounds increase systemic absorption of SA.

RESORCINOL :

Resorcinol peels are done with resorcinol 24% solution.

USES OF RESORCINOL PEELS :

1. ***Acne :*** Acne scars, severe nodulocystic acne.
2. ***Pigmentaty disorders :*** Spot peeling of hyperpigmented patches viz., melasma, and post-inflammatory hyperpigmentation of epidermal type.
3. ***Facial rejuvenation.***

Key Points :

- It is soluble in water, alcohol and lipid. Similar to phenol, it precipitates proteins at higher concentrations and causes keratolysis at lower concentrations.
- Side effect profile similar to phenol.
- It has antithyroid action at higher concentrations.
- Forms a thin layer on the skin which persists for 4-5 days.

PHENOL PEELS :

Phenol is an aromatic hydrocarbon derived from coal tar or manufactured from monochlorobenzene.

Indications :

1. Phenol is most commonly used for spot peels.
2. Full-face peel is used in skin types I and II, rare in Indians.

Endpoint : Frosting, a whitish discoloration due to denaturation of proteins.

Termination of peel : Sponging with methylated spirit, glycerin, vegetable or mineral oils.

Evolution :

Within minutes—uniform white color.

By 24-48 hrs—color changes to ashy gray-brown.

By 5-10 days—complete desquamation of skin.

For details, refer to the chapter "Commonly used chemical agents in dermatological practice".

COMBINATION PEEL :

In combination peeling, the combination can be either in the agent used for peeling or in the technique of peeling employed. In the former, a peeling agent that is a mixture of two or more peeling agents is used in contrast to application of two peeling agents successively during the same sitting in the latter.

COMBINATION PEELING AGENTS :

1. *Triple hydroxy acid peel* is a mixture of mono-, di- and tricarboxylic acid. This is not a very effective peel.
2. *Combination hydroxy acid peel* consists of, an alpha (glycolic acid) and a beta (salicylic acid) hydroxyl acid agent *e.g.* Jessner's solution (resorcinol 14 g, salicylic acid 14 g, 15% lactic acid 14 ml and 95% ethanol added up to make 100 ml).
3. *Other combination peel* agents are the Baker-Gordon formula (3 ml phenol 88%, 3 drops of croton oil, 8 drops of liquid hexachlorophene soap, 2 ml distilled water), Resorcinol peeling paste (resorcinol, olive oil, zinc oxide, wool fat, petrolatum and kaolin), Resorcinol peeling solution (resorcinol 24%, sulfur 24%, 2.5% glycerin, 2.5% sorbitol, 1% aluminium-magnesium silicate, 0.5% carboxymethyl cellulose, 45.5% deionized water).

COMBINATION PEELING TECHNIQUE :

1. *Monheit peel* consists of the application of Jessner's solution followed by 35% trichloroacetic acid. Of the various combinations, this is the most popular.
2. *Coleman frutell peel* consists of the application of 70% glycolic acid followed by 35% trichloroacetic acid.
3. *Brody peel* consists of the application of 35% trichloroacetic acid followed by solid carbon dioxide application. This is a very potent combination and should be used cautiously.

Principle of combination peel : One agent enhances the penetration of the other and hence obviates the need for using a higher strength of peeling agents to obtain deeper peels for better results.

Of late, chemical peels have been used in combination with laser resurfacing, manual dermabrasion and as said above, with cryo slush (*Brody peel*).

A few new peels have been added to armamentarium of cosmetic dermatologists. Some of them are briefly mentioned here.

RETINOID PEELS :

It is a superficial peeling agent.

Mechanism Of Action :

Retinoids reduce corneocyte cohesion, assists in epidermal turnover by combining with retinol receptor. It also inhibits metalloproteinases and induce collagenosis.

Uses :

- Photoaging.
- Melasma.
- Lentigens, Freckles.
- Striae.
- Axillary acanthosis, Hypermelanosis of axilla.
- Post Inflammatory Hyperpigmentation.

Key Points :

Used in the concentration of 1-5%.

They leave a temporary yellow discoloration of the skin after application.

FERRULIC ACID PEEL :

Phenolic keratocoagulant compound for superficial peeling.

> **Mechanism Of Action :**
> Acts as scavenger for free radicals thereby reducing inflammatory reaction and cellular damage.

Uses :

- Open pores.
- Uneven skin tone.
- Rhytides.
- Photoaging.

Key Points :

It is left in skin for 5-6 minutes until there is frosting.

ARGIPEEL :

20% arginine, 15% Lactic acid, regenerating agents such as aloe vera (1%) and allantoin.

Used for periorbital melanosis.

Yellow Peel :

Spot peel :

0.1% retinol, 5% salicylic acid, 13% lactic acid, !4% trichloroacetic acid, 14% resorcinol.

Uses :

Melasma, wrinkles, hyperchromic spots, skin aging, wrinkles, facial rejuvenation, stretch marks, acne scars.

Black Peel :

It is a natural organic peel containing black acetic acid. It inhibits tyrosinase activity (depigmentary) and also has antioxidant effect.

It is used as superficial peeling agent in active acne, acne with PIH and other hyperpigmentary conditions.

BLACK PEEL :

Black peel contains black acetic acid (Black vinegar), Salicylic acid, Jasmonic acid and potassium iodide. Salicylic acid and jasmonic acid have keratolytic and anti-inflammatory effects. Potassium iodide and biosulfur have antibacterial and anti-inflammatory properties. Black vinegar is rich in organic minerals and essential aminoacids.

Uses of Black Peel :

Acne and acne marks.

Superficial wrinkles.

Peel Procedure :

End point : Peel applied and observed for any erythema or edema. Transient white frost can be seen before end point. If there is no excess erythema or burning sensation or irritation, then peel left for 4-6 hours.

Termination of peel : Wash off with plain water after 4-6 hours.

Evolution :

Within 5-10 mins : Transient white frost.

By 24-48 hours : Mild exfoliation seen.

3-4 days : Exfoliation is complete.

Key Points :

- Peel can be layered over by retinol peel to enhance exfoliation.
- Due to antibacterial and anti-inflammatory actions, this can be used in acne grade III as well.

Pregnancy Category :

AHA peels are category B and hence can be used during pregnancy. Salicylic acid peels are category C and structurally related to aspirin; hence best avoided during pregnancy.

Other peeling agents	Mechanism of action	Indications	Comments
Pyruvic acid (40-70%)	Has antioxidant, sebostatic and antimicrobial properties.	Acne marks, dullness of face.	Is a keto acid, lipophilic, small molecule which penetrates deep (risk of scarring).
Citric acid (20-70%)	Is a tricarboxylic acid with antioxidant properties.	Acne marks, dullness of face.	Neutralized after 5 mins.
Mandelic acid (30-50%)	Large molecule and hence penetrates epidermis slowly Has antibacterial and exfoliative action).	Acne, acne marks.	Slow release and hence safer than Glycolic acid; Often combined with salicylic acid.
Thioglycolic acid or Mercaptoacetic acid (10%)	Thiol group chelates iron and hence reduces hemosiderotic pigmentation.	Periorbital hyperpigmentation.	Highly soluble in water and alcohol. Affinity to iron is similar to that of apoferritin. Also stimulates collagen remodeling and epidermal regeneration.
Ferulic acid 12%	Has antioxidant and tyrosinase inhibitory action.	Photoaging, photomelanosis.	Lipophilic but cutaneous penetration restricted as it is pH dependent. Hence, acts only on superficial epidermis. It's a Leave on peel. Washed off after 4-6 hours. Can be layered with retinol peel for exfoliation

BLACK PEEL

Other peeling agents	Mechanism of action	Indications	Comments
Tretinoin peel (1-10%)	Regularizes keratinization, comedolytic.	Acne, post inflammtory hyperpigmentation, fine wrinkles.	Penetrates only the stratum corneum and hence does not caused burning, stinging or irritation. Yellowish frost seen on application. Peel washed off after 4 hours.
Yellow peel	Regularizes keratization, inhibits melanogenesis	Acne, post inflammatory hyperpigmentation	Is combination of retinol, salicylic acid, phytic acid, kojic acid azelaic acid, ascorbic acid, bisabolol. Used as a sequential peel.
Lactic acid (30-92%)	Facilitate desquamation hydrates skin by increasing hyaluronic acid	Dullness of skin, dry and sensitive skin.	Large molecule AHA which penetrates slowly and has hydrating property.
Phytic acid	Subtle desquamation	Superficial hyperpigmentation	Slow release superficial peel with no visible exfoliation. Leave on peel, washed after 8 hours.
Polyhydroxy acids (lactobionic acid, gluconolatone)	Antioxidant, hydrating agent	Superficial hyperpigmentation. Sensitive dry skin	No stinging or irritation due to slow release and skin hydration property.
Tartaric and Malic acid	Subtle desquamation	Dullness of skin, dry and sensitive skin	Both are AHA and used in combination peel.

32
Wound Care Products

DRESSINGS :

Dressings can be classified based on their origin (natural/ artificial), property of occlusion (occlusive/semi occlusive), adherence to granulation tissue (adherent/non-adherent), or transparency (transparent/non-transparent). Dressings may also be wet or dry.

Dressings may be either open or closed. Open dressings readily allow for vaporization of fluids and hence dry the ulcer or erosions. Closed dressings are occlusive and protect the ulcer from external contamination.

WET DRESSINGS :

Types : When these wet dressings are wrapped with a non-permeable membrane, the process is termed as "closed wet dressing". Otherwise, it is referred to as "open wet dressing".

Agents used in wet dressing : Normal saline, various antiseptic/antibacterial agents like Condy's solution, aluminium subacetate (Burrow's solution) or acetic acid.

Method of application : Place a plastic sheet or any nonabsorbable sheet below the area to be given a wet dressing. A clean, dry thin cotton cloth (or gauze, if cloth is unavailable) is soaked with the agent to be used for wet dressing. Excess fluid is drained off by gently compressing the cloth and the cloth is now placed over the lesions or wound. The solution used can be cold/warm or tepid depending on requirement. The dressing is kept for 10-15 mins and repeated 3-6 times per day. While removing, the dressing should be moistened again with the solution to loosen the adhered dried dressing to prevent trauma to the ulcer. The solution can be used as a drip draining over the dressing to maintain continuous hydration.

USES :

Exudative ulcers, acute inflamed ulcers.

ADVANTAGES OF WET DRESSING :

1. Moistens the crust and debris and hence facilitates their removal. This is important as the crusts or debris form a culture medium for bacteria and hence promote infection.
2. Maintains a liquid phase and allows keratinocyte and fibroblast migration and hence facilitates wound healing.
3. Through evaporation of water, they induce cooling that causes vasoconstriction which is important for reducing erythema, edema and oozing.
4. They are cooling and soothing and provide symptomatic relief from discomfort, burning and itching.
5. May act as hemostatic due to its vasoconstrictive property.

DISADVANTAGES OF WET DRESSING :

1. Causes maceration.
2. Hypothermia—total body surface covered should not be more than 1/3rd of total body surface. Hence, for extensive areas, it may be used in rotational fashion.

DRY DRESSING/COMPOSITE/LAYERED DRESSING :

The layered dressing is usually 4 tiered and is made up of the following layers from the ulcer surface outwards :

contains antibiotic cream or ointment.

1. Hydrating layer.
2. Non-adherent contact layer/interface dressing.

3. Absorbent layer sterile gauze.
4. Adhesive layer adhesive plaster/Micropore 10/Jiansporey or cotton dressing bandage.

Interface dressing is a non-adherent layer of dressing, which comes in direct contact with the ulcer surface. It is usually paraffin impregnated gauze (paraffin tulle) or N-terface (thin woven dressing made of high density monofilament plastic) or Tefla® (consists of central, absorbent cellulose material sandwiched between thin, perforated polyurethane film).

Tactifiers are agents which enhance the adhesiveness of the surgical plaster or Micropore or Transpore. *Example :* Tincture benzoin.

NATURAL DRESSING :

TYPES :

Potato peel dressing, banana leaf dressing.

ADVANTAGES :

1. Occlusive and hence retain growth factors and cytokines released by the granulation tissue.
2. Semipermeable membrane and hence allows free air and vapor exchange.

DISADVANTAGES :

1. Difficult to sterilize.
2. Potato peel dressing sheets become too hard and abrasive on storage.

USES :

Used for clean erosions/superficial ulcers as in a TEN/SJS, epidermolysis bullosa, post-debridement ulcer, pyoderma gangrenosum.

Occlusive Dressings :

Here the ulcer is cordoned off from the external environment. However, these may be semi-permeable allowing gaseous exchange or non-permeable, restricting both gas and liquid transit.

Advantages :

1. Prevents microbial contamination from the exterior.
2. Prevents drying of ulcer.
3. Retains tissue fluid rich in various chemokines and growth factors that promote wound healing.
4. Decreases pain.

Disadvantages :

1. Causes maceration.
2. Promotes secondary infection of contaminated wounds.
3. Interferes with visualization of wound healing (except when transparent dressing is used).

Basic principles in choosing a dressing :

1. Use absorbent dressings (viz. alginates) for ulcers with profuse discharge of exudates.
2. If wound healing needs to be monitored with minimal intervention, then use films.
3. Absorbent dressings are contraindicated over dry/ minimally exuding ulcers.

OTHER DRESSINGS :

Anti-microbial dressings release ions or antibacterial agents slowly into the ulcer (*e.g.* cadexomer iodine dressing, slow release silver dressing).

TABLE 32.1 : **Characteristics of dressings**

Sr. No.	Characteristics of dressings		Type of dressing
1.	Origin	Natural Synthetic	Alginates, potato peels, Hydrogels, hydrocolloids, foams, films
2.	Permeability	Permeable Semi-per-permeable Impermeable	Foams, films (gas, vapor) Hydrogels Hydrocolloids, films (fluids)
3.	Adherence to granulation tissue	Adherent Non-adherent	Films, hydrocolloids Hydrogels, alginates, foams
4.	Transparency	Transparent Semi-transparent Opaque	Films Hydrogels Foams
5.	Absorbency	Absorbent Non-absorbent	Hydrogels, hydrocolloids, foams, alginates, Films
6.	Secondary dressing	Required Not required	Hydrogels, alginates, foams Films

Hydrofiber dressings are made up of cellulose and swell up to form gels on absorbing exudates.

Paraffin impregnated dressings are used to prevent adhesion of dressings to ulcers.

Hyaluronic acid dressings for gels on absorbing exudates and are said to promote granulation and wound healing.

Collagen dressings may occasionally contain alginates or hydrogels.

Activated *Charcoal impregnated dressings* are used in malodorous and/ or exudative wounds/ulcers.

Pressure dressing is a type of layered dressing in which the absorbent layer is much more bulkier. Because of the extra pressure that can be generated, it acts as an excellent hemostat and also limits the post-procedure inflammatory edema.

Composite dressings have physical properties of two or more of the occlusive dressing types.

HONEY DRESSING :

Honey is an acidic, hyperosmolar sugar solution (fructose 40%, glucose 30%, sucrose 5% and water 20%) with many enzymes, vitamins and amino acids. It improves granulation tissue, increases epithelialization and hasten wound healing. Glucose oxidase enzyme produces hydrogen peroxide. This and its osmolarity (dehydrates bacteria) contribute to its antibacterial properties. High osmolarity also draws away the accumulated lymph simulating a negative pressure wound therapy. Protease enzyme in honey acts like debridement agent. Honey used for wound care has been standardized to be equivalent to 12-16% phenol by US FDA. Manuka honey is supposed to be better than regular honey, as hydrogen peroxide produced by regular honey is neutralized by catalase enzyme in tissue but not methyglyoxal of manuka honey.

USES :

Acute and chronic ulcers or wounds.

Usage :

40% honey and 60% collagen dressing is used for oozy ulcers and 50% honey with 50% beeswax is used for maintenance therapy.

Bacterial cellulose dressing :

This is a biopolymer dressing derived from bacteria. It is more porous and robust. It can be modified to have antibacterial properties and utilized as drug delivery systems as well.

HYDROGELS :

COMPOSITION :

Made up of matrix of polymers.

TYPES :

- *Hydrogel sheets* are made up of hydrophilic polymers

which are sandwiched between thin sheets of polyethylene film.

- *Amorphous hydrogel* is composed of cornstarch-derived polymerized compound.

USES :

1. Infected ulcers.
2. Exudative wounds *e.g.* post-ablative laser resurfacing, graft donor site.

ADVANTAGES :

- Have cooling effect, decrease temperature up to 5 C for nearly 6 hours.
- Allay pain.

DISADVANTAGES :

- Though good absorbants, the rate of absorption is being absorbant but non-adherent calls for frequent change of dressing.
- Nonadherent and hence require secondary dressing to retain.
- Are poor bacterial barriers.

COMMERCIAL PREPARATION :

Flexderm®, Vigilon®.

ALGINATES :

COMPOSITION :

These are polysaccharides derived from brown seaweed. The chief constituents are mannuronic acid and guluronic acid. The enzymes in exudates easily digest mannuronic acid but not guluronic acid. Hence, if dressing contains relatively greater amounts of mannuronic acid, then the removal of dressing becomes non-traumatic as it becomes a soft gel that can be easily irrigated with normal saline.

USES :

1. Profusely exudative wounds.
2. Full thickness burns.
3. Decubitus ulcer.
4. Also used as a hemostat.

ADVANTAGES :

- Calcium released by calcium alginate dressings enhances the clotting process and hence acts as an hemostat.
- Calcium ions also improve wound healing.
- Require fewer changes of dressing.
- Non-adherent and hence non-traumatic during its removal.

DISADVANTAGES :

- Yellow-green color of the gel is often mistaken for purulent.
- Requires a secondary dressing as it is non-adherent and also to limit drying of the wound.
- Has a foul odor.

COMMERCIAL PREPARATION :

Algiderm®, Algisite®.

HYDROCOLLOID :

COMPOSITION :

Is a mixture of polymers and gels.

USES :

1. Decubitus ulcers.
2. Partial thickness wounds.
3. Erosions in epidermolysis bullosa.
4. As an occlusive dressing in psoriasis to improve efficacy of topical steroids.

ADVANTAGES :

- Has fibrinolytic property.
- Occlusive environment creates an acidic environment which sustains phagocytic cells and lytic enzymes and hence prevents bacterial growth.
- Is water resistant (the patient can have a bath with the dressing on).
- Promotes angiogenesis and wound healing.

DISADVANTAGES :

- Yellow-green color of the gel is often mistaken for purulent discharge.
- As it is completely occlusive, causes maceration of the surrounding skin.
- As it is completely occlusive, it is contraindicated in wounds with anaerobic infection.
- Leakage of accumulated excessive tissue fluids.
- Hypergranulation.

COMMERCIAL PREPARATION :

Duoderm®, Confeel®.

FOAMS :

COMPOSITION :

Is made up of polyurethane. It is a two-tiered occlusive dressing. The outer layer is composed of polyurethane, polyester or silicone and is semipermeable. The inner layer is composed of a polyurethane mesh that is permeable to gas.

USES :

1. Wound due to burns.
2. Decubitus ulcers.

3. Ulcers with deep cavities.
4. Post-laser resurfacing.

ADVANTAGE :

Silicone based foams (silastic foams) are used to pack ulcers with deep cavities like pilonidal sinus.

DISADVANTAGES :

1. As it is opaque, wound healing cannot be monitored.
2. Cannot be used in dry ulcers.

FILMS :

COMPOSITION :

Are transparent polyurethane dressings.

USES :

1. Split thickness skin grafting.
2. Superficial decubitus ulcer.
3. Post-dermabrasion.

ADVANTAGES :

1. Transparent and hence wound healing can be monitored.
2. Is water-proof and hence can protect hydrogel, alginate and foam dressings.

DISADVANTAGES :

1. It is occlusive but non-absorbant and hence needs to be changed frequently. Alternatively, it can be punctured and again resealed with a patch of film.
2. It sticks to self, causing wrinkling. This leads to leakages and bacterial penetration.

Commercial Preparation :

Tegaderm®.

UNNA BOOT :

Composition :

Paste containing zinc oxide, gelatin and glycerin applied over cotton dressing.

Action :

1. Prevents development of edema due to sustained compression.
2. Absorbs oozing fluid and dries the lesion.
3. Soothing effect.

Method of application : Applied like a plaster of Paris cast, starting from just proximal to metatarsophalangeal joints and extending proximally up to tibial tuberosity. There should be a uniform overlap of about 50% while rolling over the bandage while applying. Boot needs to be changed once in 7-10 days.

Uses :

1. Acute eczemas especially stasis dermatitis.
2. Non-elastic compression dressing in chronic venous insufficiency.

Disadvantages :

1. Irritation in hot and humid temperatures.
2. Loosening of plaster after drying of cast as well as after subsidence of edema.
3. Development of contact dermatitis.

ARTIFICIAL SKIN SUBSTITUTES :

Tissue engineered biological dressings (APLIGRAF). This is a living, bilayered dressing whose inner layer is made of human fibroblasts and bovine type I collagen and the outer layer is made of human keratinocytes. Human keratinocytes are derived from neonatal foreskin. However, they do not contain Langerhan's cells, melanocytes, lymphocytes or macrophages.

USES :

Noninfectious ulcers viz., venous ulcers, and diabetic ulcer.

N.B. : No risk of reactions to this dressing.

COMMON AGENTS USED IN WOUND CARE :

Chemical agents that are commonly used in wound care are.

1. Povidone iodine 1% solution.
2. Hydrogen peroxide 3%.
3. Chlorhexidine gluconate 4%.
4. Condy's solution (potassium permanganate 1:10,000).

Commercially available solutions of' povidone iodine and Dakin's solution have been found to be fibroblast toxic due to their higher concentrations and hence found to inhibit wound healing. Lower concentrations of povidone iodine 0.0001% and sodium hypochlorite 0.005% do not adversely affect fibroblasts and are also equally efficacious as an antibacterial agent.

HYDROGEN PEROXIDE :

Hydrogen peroxide (3% solution) is frequently used in wound care.

MECHANISM OF ACTION :

Hydrogen peroxide releases nascent oxygen by exothermic reaction. This reaction confers the following properties to hydrogen peroxide.

1. Antibacterial—due to nascent oxygen.
2. Hemostat—heat produced due to exothermic reaction seals the bleeding tiny vessels.

3. Chemical debridement—oxidation of the tissue debris and slough leads to easy removal of the same.
4. Chemical cauterization—due to heat produced as well as its hemostatic property.

Method of use : Flush the lesion with hydrogen peroxide and leave it undisturbed till the frothing ceases. If the solution is soaked in gauze, it should be kept in situ for about 5 minutes.

USES :

1. Chemical debridement of infected ulcers with slough.
2. Mouth wash – diluted (1:10) solutions in cases with oral erosions (oral pemphigus vulgaris), ulcers (aphthous ulcer herpetic stomatitis) and candidiasis.

KEY POINTS :

- The antibacterial action can be enhanced by addition of L-cysteine.
- According to one school of thought, at concentrations used for its antibacterial action, hydrogen peroxide has cytotoxic effects.

EUSOL :

Eusol is an acronym for Edinburgh University Solution and is a sodium hypochlorite solution buffered to normal pH with boric acid and contains approximately 2500 ppm of "available chlorine". The preparation is chlorinated lime 1.25, boric acid 1.25, purified water added to make 100 ml. The resultant pH is 5 (available chlorine is 0.4%). Best when used freshly prepared. But, it can be used within 2 weeks of preparation.

MECHANISM OF ACTION :

Slow release of hypochlorous acid.

USES :

1. As an antiseptic in wound cleaning and dressing.
2. Wet dressing or compresses.

SIDE EFFECTS :

1. May dissolve blood clots and cause bleeding.
2. Toxic effects on neutrophils (decreases neutrophil mobility), fibroblasts.

GENTIAN VIOLET :

This dye is available in the strength of 1% solution.

MECHANISM OF ACTION :
Used for its antifungal action.

Method of use : Gentian violet is applied with a swab stick. The swab stick should be dipped in the solution and care should be taken so that the solution does not drip while transferring the stick from the solution to the body area to be treated. The solution is applied such that the entire area turns uniformly purple. Applications are repeated at 24 hours interval.

USES :

1. Oral thrush.
2. Vaginal candidiasis.

KEY POINTS :

- *Precautions :*
  1. The solution should not be dribbling from the swab stick.
  2. Do not give an occlusive dressing after application, lest irritation occurs.

3. Stains skin, mucosa and clothes. Staining of skin and mucosa also masks the clinical findings.

- *Gentian violet* is safe in breast-feeding mothers and infants. It is also economical.

ACRIFLAVINE :

Acriflavine is a mixture of proflavine and euflavine. Glycerin flavine consists of acriflavine 0.1 g, and glycerin to make to 100 ml.

Mechanism Of Action :

Acriflavine belongs to acridine group of antiseptics that is a bactericidal due to their binding to nucleic acid. Only euflavine has antimicrobial property. It also promotes granulation tissue.

Uses :

1. As an antiseptic agent.
2. To promote granulation tissue for wound healing.
3. For the purpose of preventing infection and promoting granulation tissue, wounds are usually packed with acriflavine soaked guazes. A pack also reduces oozing and bleeding.

Key Points :

1. Acriflavine has a potential for sensitization.
2. It causes staining of clothes.

POVIDONE IODINE :

It is an iodophor (soluble complexes of iodine with organic compounds that act as carriers *i.e.*, polyvinylpyrrolidone) with slow but sustained release of free iodine.

Mechanism Of Action :

It iodinates and oxidizes various cellular components and hence acts as a broad spectrum germicides, effective against bacteria, fungi and viruses.

Uses :

1. As an antiseptic-sterilization of sharp instruments and rubber articles.
2. As a surgical scrub.
3. As an antibacterial agent in wound dressing.

Key Points :

- It is available as 5% solution for skin scrub, 5% ointment for Wound dressing, 1% solution for mouth wash and Betadine tulle (INADINAE®).
- It has an advantage of being non-toxic, non-irritant, non-staining compared to other iodine preparations.

CETRIMIDE :

1-3% solution of cetrimide is a routinely used antiseptic cleanser in dermatology.

Mechanism Of Action :

1. Quaternary ammonium (cationic) antiseptic that alter the permeability of cell membrane and hence is a bactericidal, fungicidal and viricidal. However less effective against gram negative bacteria, mycobacteria and spores.
2. Mild keratolytic.

Key Points :

- Germicidal effects are neutralized by soaps, pus (as they are anionic) and potentiated by alcohols (cationic).

CHLORHEXIDINE :

Commonly used antiseptic.

MECHANISM OF ACTION :

Is a biguanide that disrupts cell membrane and is hence a bactericidal.

Method of use :

1. As a hair wash – wet the hairs and rinse it for 5-10 min. and wash it off.
2. Mouth gargles – gargle and spit. Avoid drinking or eating for 1 hour.
3. Antiseptic gel – to be applied with fingers or a cotton swab after a thorough mouth wash and avoid drinking or eating for 1 hour.
4. As an antiseptic bath.

USES :

1. As an antiseptic hair wash in pityriasis amiantacea, tinea capitis.
2. As a mouth gargle in oral erosions/ulcers or gingivitis.
3. As an antiseptic gel in oral erosions/ulcers or gingivitis.
4. Antiseptic bath to decrease methicillin resistant *staphylococcus aureus* (MRSA) colonization.

KEY POINTS :

- Available in the strength of 20% v/v equivalent to 4% w/v.
- Persistent action of chlorhexidine is due to its retention on skin surface.
- Can cause allergic contact dermatitis.

COLLAGENASE :

COMPOSITION :

Enzyme collagenase is derived from fermentation of *Clostridium histolyticum*.

MECHANISM OF ACTION :

1. Dissolves necrotic material (chemical debridement).
2. Stimulates granulation tissue.

USES :

1. Ulcers with slough.
2. Decubitus ulcers.

Commercial formulation : SALUTYL® ointment (20 gm tube), 250 units per gram of white soft paraffin I.P.

KEY POINTS :

- Collagenase best acts at pH 6 to 8 and, hence, substances such as detergents and heavy metal ions when used simultaneously can decrease the efficacy.
- Action of collagenase can be nullified by the application of Burrow's solution (pH 3.6-4.4).

TOPICAL HEMOSTATIC AGENTS :

- Monsel's solution (20% ferric subsulfate).
- Aluminium chloride.
- Tincture benzoine.
- Hydrogen peroxide.
- Gel foam.
- Silver nitrate (Refer to Chapter 30 for details).

x=x=x=x=x

33
Baths

Baths are given for widespread dermatoses. A bathtub is used for administering baths. The bathtub should be half full with 100 liters of water to which various substances are added depending upon the dermatosis to be treated. Patients are advised to take the bath for 30 mins.

Baths are commonly used in the treatment of :

1. Eczema—soothing colloid bath.
2. Pemphigus—loosens and removes crusts, reduces bacterial colonization.
3. Ichthyosis/xerosis— oil bath.
4. Psoriasis—bath PUVA, balneotherapy.

OAT MEAL BATH :

Contents : 50% starch, 25% protein, and 9% oil (Aveeno).

MECHANISM OF ACTION :
Increase moisture uptake and retention (due to hydrophilic carbohydrates), cleanse body (due to saponins), antioxidant and anti-inflammatory (due to ferulic acid, vitamin E., avenanthramides, unsaturated triglycerides, sterols).

Preparation of bath : 1 cup of oatmeal powder thoroughly mixed with 2 cups of water and then poured into the bathtub.

Modifications : Oilated oatmeal bath contains 35% mineral oil and lanolin derivatives along with other contents.

USES :

1. Acute eczema.
2. Pityriasis rosea.
3. Atopic dermatitis.
4. Exfoliative dermatitis.

COLLOIDAL STARCH BATH :

Contents : Hydrolyzed starch.

MECHANISM OF ACTION :

Anti-inflammatory (gamma oryzanol), antiaging (phytic acid, ferulic acid, palmitic acid, gamma oryzanol.

Preparation : 2 cups of hydrolyzed starch is mixed with 4 cups of water to make a paste and then added to lukewarm water present in bathtub.

Modification : Equal amounts of sodium bicarbonate are used for soothing effect.

USE :

1. Pityriasis rosea.

OIL BATH :

Contents : Vegetable or mineral oil along with surfactant.

MECHANISM OF ACTION :

1. Water hydrates the skin.
2. Oil coats the skin and maintains moisture and prevents dryness.

Method of application : Oil is added into the bathtub along with a surfactant. This oil covers the body as a thin film that retains water and oil onto the dry skin.

USES :

1. Atopic dermatitis.
2. Psoriasis.
3. Ichthyosis.
4. Anhidrotic ectodermal dysplasia.
5. Exfoliative dermatitis.
6. Senile pruritus.

PRECAUTIONS :

1. Occlusion folliculitis if too oily.
2. Risk of slipping and sustaining fracture especially in elderly who are osteoporotic due to oiliness of skin and bathroom floor.

BATH :

Contents : Paraffin wax or match wax (melting point 42 C).

MECHANISM OF ACTION :

1. Sustained warming of the part leads to alleviation of pain.
2. Improves local blood circulation.
3. Stimulates sweating and hydrates skin.

Method of application : Wax is heated in wax bath to 49°C. Body part to be given the wax bath is immersed repeatedly in this bath so that a uniform covering of wax is formed around the part. After the outer layer of the wax solidifies, the body part with wax covering is wrapped with a polythene or grease paper. A blanket is wrapped on this to preserve the heat. After 20-30 mins, the solidified wax is removed.

Modification : If the body part cannot be immersed in the waxbath, then, the warm wax can be poured over the body part to be treated so as to achieve a uniform covering.

USES :

1. To alleviate pain in reaction hands in leprosy.
2. To improve contractures before and after surgery of hand deformities.
3. To make the skin moist and smooth.
4. Used waxing to remove unwanted hairs.

PRECAUTIONS :

1. Risk of scalds.
2. Not to use in cases with active ulceration.
3. Do not raise the temperature of the wax bath to more than 52 C.
4. Risk of causing folliculitis after waxing.

CLEANSING BATH :

Contents : Plain white soap with less than 0.0125% free alkali.

MECHANISM OF ACTION :

1. Removes dirt, scales and crusts.
2. Hydrates skin.

Method ofapplication : The patient is to take a bath in a tub with abundant lather produced by a white soap for 30 mins. Later, soap is washed off with lukewarm water initially and then with cold water. The skin is patted dry rather than rubbed to dryness; Emollients can be applied immediately.

USES :

1. Extensive acute or sub acute eczema with crusting atopic dermatitis, systemic contact dermatitis, photoallergic dermatitis.
2. Extensive erosions as in pemphigus vulgaris, Stevens Johnson Syndrome, staphylococcal scalded skin syndrome.

BATH PUVA :

Contents : 30 ml of 1% 8–methoxy psoralen solution is added to 80 lts of water to achieve a concentration of 3.75 mg/L; 5 mg/L methoxsalon concentration is substantially more effective.

MECHANISM OF ACTION :

Psoralen is adsorbed onto the skin and when exposed to UVA, leads to the therapeutic effect.

Method of application : Patient should take bath for 15 min followed by UVA exposure.

USES :

1. Psoriasis vulgaris.
2. Vitiligo vulgaris.

ADVANTAGES :

1. No systemic toxicity of psoralen.
2. No eye protection is required.
3. Greater short- or long-term safety profile.

BATH-SUIT PUVA :

This is a modification of bath PUVA in which a bath suit is soaked in the psoralen solution and is used instead of the bath tub.

ADVANTAGES :

1. Saves on the expense of the psoralen solution.
2. Does not require bath tub.

POTASSIUM PERMANGANATE BATH :

Contents : 2 tea spoon of crystals or 25 tablets of 0.3 g

strength should be added to half tub of water to achieve 1 : 10,000 dilution.

> MECHANISM OF ACTION :
>
> The oxidative property of potassium permanganate confers antibacterial properties to this bath.

Alternative antiseptic bath : 10% hexachlorophene, chlorhexidine, 2% cetrimide bath.

Method of application : Patient should take bath for a maximum 15-30 min.

USES :

Extensive exudative dermatoses.

BALNEOTHERAPY :

This is often combined with phototherapy.

Contents : Mineral rich water/mud viz., Dead sea water.

> MECHANISM OF ACTION :
>
> Calcium, potassium and phosphate in Dead sea water maintain lipid metabolism in stratum corneum and magnesium modulate calcium concentration in epidermis.

USES :

1) Atopic dermatitis
2) Psoriasis

Disadvantage :

Exact composition of Dead sea water cannot be recreated in laboratory.

BLEACH BATH :

Contents : ½ cup of 6% common household bleach in a standard 150-L bathtub full of water or 83 ml of 6% bleach added to 100L of water (thereby achieve concentration of 0.005%). Bathe for 10 mins 2-3 times per week.

> MECHANISM OF ACTION :
> Has anti-inflammatory, anti-pruritogenic properties and reduce infections by balancing skin microbiome.

USES :

1) Atopic dermatitis

Disadvantage :

Meta-analysis revealed no advantage over regular water bath.

x=x=x=x=x

34

Dermal Fillers

Fillers are products used to augment or hydrate or contour face or body parts. An ideal dermal filler should be safe, effective, noncarcinogenic, nonteratogenic, inert and durable. Dermal fillers can be classified based on :

- Origin (natural/synthetic) or
- Source (autograft/allograft/heterograft) or
- Content (collagen/fat/hyaluronic acid/others) and
- Duration of effect (temporary < 1 year/semipermanent, 1-2 years/permanent > 2 years). (Table)

PHYSICAL PARAMETERS OF HYALURONIC ACID FILLER :

1. *Crosslinking :* Interlinking of chains of hyaluronic acid to improve the strength and longevity of fillers. Common crosslinking agent is BDDE (1, 4-butanediol diglycidyl ether). Various crosslinking technologies are Hyalcross, Vycross, Cohesive polydensified matrix, non-animal stabilized hyaluronic acid (NASHA), XpresHan Technology and Resilient hyaluronic acid.
2. *Elastic modulus (G′) :* is the measure of hardness of gel. Greater the value, harder the gel and hence better for lifting. Higher G′ products are preferred for deeper deposition and facial contouring.
3. *Swelling factor :* is the ability of get to absorb water and swell. This depends on hyaluronic acid concentration and

Characteristic	Examples
Based on origin	
Natural	Zyderm®, Fibrel®, Restylane®
Synthetic	Expanded Poly Tera Fluoro ethylene (EPTFE), Silikon 1000, SL skin, Bioplastique, Pro fill
Based on sourrce	
Autograft	Fat, dermal graft
Allograft	Fascian (cadaver), AlloDerm
Xenograft	Fibroquel (bovine)
Based on composition :	
Collagen	Zydern, Zyplast, Fibroquel
Fat	Autologous fat, Frozen fat, Lipocytic dermal augmentation
Hyaluronic acid	Hylaform get, Hylan, Restylane, Belotero, Juvederm
Silicone	Silicon 1000, Biocell Ultra vitral, Bio plastique
Peptides	Fibrel
Hydroxyleythlymethacrylate and eythimethacrylate	DermaLive, DermaDeep
Autologous human fibroblasts	Laviv or Azficel-T
Calcium Hydroxyapatite	Radiesse Plus
Poly-L-Lactic acid	Sculptra
Polymethylmethacrylate	Bellafill (formerly Artefill)
Polycaprolactone	Ellanse
Based on duration of effect :	
Temporary	Zyderm, Fibrel, AlloDerm, Cymetra, Endoplast-50, Plasmagel, Restylane, Autologous fat, Frozen fat, Lipocytic dermal augmentation
Permanent	Expanded Poly Tetra Fluoro ethylene (EPTFE) Adato Sil 5000, Silikon 1000, Biocell Ultra vital
Combination of Temporary and Permanent filler	80% Bovine collagen and 20% Polymethylmethacrylate (Bellafill); 40% bacterial hyaluronic acid and 60% Hydroxyeythlymethacrylate

extent of crosslinking. Hence swelling factor varies inversely with G′.

4. *Cohesion :* is the measure of integrity of the product to resist deformation. Lower the cohesivity, easier it is for the product to spread within the tissue.

In summary, products with greater cohesion and G′ are use for facelift, deep wrinkle correction and contouring. Whereas products with least G′ and cohesion are used for skin hydration or superficial wrinkle correction.

INDICATIONS :

1. Depressed scars : acne scars, scars following surgery or trauma.
2. Wrinkles and lines (creases) due to aging.
3. Lip augmentation.
4. Dermal atrophy due to various causes e.g. morphea.
5. Facial contouring.
6. Skin hydration.

CONTRAINDICATIONS :

1. Hypersensitivity to filler
2. Pregnancy.
3. Active infection in the vicinity of filler or active acne

PROCEDURE OF FILLER TREATMENT :

PRETREATMENT :

1. Counselling regarding the expectations, achievable result, choice of product, risks and care.
2. Informed consent and documentation.
3. Anesthesia : Mostly done under topical anesthesia using EMLA. However, regional or nerve blocks are done at times for better anesthesia.

4. Asepsis is very important to prevent acute/chronic infections as well as biofilms.

TREATMENT :

1. Identify the neurovascular bundle and mark to avoid intravascular injection of fillers.
2. Filler is injected with a needle or cannula. Risk of intravascular deposition of filler is less with cannula and hence these are being used increasingly. However, fine cannulas can penetrate vessels and hence should be used cautiously.
3. Plane of injection : Filler is injected at various levels for different indications. Supraperiosteal plane of injection is usually preferred for facial contouring and intradermal injection for skin hydration or fine wrinkles.
4. Technique of injection : Bolus, small aliquots, linear threading (anterograde/retrograde), fanning, fern.
5. At the end of procedure, moulding is done to ensure uniform deposition and distribution of filler.

POST TREATMENT :

1. Do not massage the area for 2 weeks in case of hyaluronic acid fillers.
2. Avoid vigorous exercise, steam for 5 days.
3. Apply sunscreen and moisturizer regularly. Restart retinoid or other night creams after 5 days.

COMPLICATIONS :

1. ***Immediate :*** Pain, erythema, edema, bruise, xerosis, paresthesia.
2. ***Early :*** Edema, induration, bruise, nodule, pustule, Tyndall effect, avascular necrosis, blindness.
3. ***Late :*** Nodule/granuloma, Tyndall effect leads to blue color.

x=x=x=x=x

35
Botulinum Toxin

INTRODUCTION :

Botulinum toxin (BoNT) is derived from Clostridium botulinum exotoxin. There are 8 serotypes of exotoxins and among these only A and B are used for medical indications. Exotoxin A is more potent than B and is the most commonly used serotype.

STRUCTURE OF BONT :

Botulinum toxin contains botulinum neurotoxin (made of heavy and light chain bound by disulphide bond), complex proteins and excipients. Clinical effects are solely due to botulinum neurotoxin. Complex proteins have no therapeutic action and in fact contribute to antigenicity. Excipients are stabilizing agents viz., human albumin, lactose, bovine gelatin. Daxibotulinum toxin does not have any complex proteins and has a unique excipient peptide which reduces the diffusion of BoNT and increase duration of action.

MECHANISM OF ACTION :

BoNT blocks the nerve impulse transmission. The light chain of BoNT disintegrates at the cell membrane of nerve ending and is endocytosed via SV2 (BoNT-A) or synaptotagmin (BoNT-B). This light chain cleaves SNARE proteins which are crucial for release of acetylcholine into synapase. BoNT-A, C, E cleaves SNAP-25 and BoNT-B, D, F, G cleave VAMP or synaptobrevin. BoNT-C cleaves SANP-25 and syntaxin (Table 1). Motor neurons are more

TABLE 1 : **Characteristics of various botulinum toxins**

	Onabotulinum toxin A	Abobotulinum toxin A	Prabotulinum toxin A	Incobotulinum toxin A	Ianbotulinum toxin A	Daxibotulinum toxin A	Rimabotulinum toxin A
Product	Botox® (Allergan, USA)	Dysport® (Ipsen, USA)	Nabota® (Daewong, R. Korea), Jeuveau® (Evolus Alphaeon, USA)	Xeomin® (Merz, Germany)	Hengli® (P.R. China), Neuronox® (Medytox, R. Kora)	BTXA® (Intas, India), Botogenie® (BioMed, India), RTT 150 (Revance, USA)	Myobloc® (Solstice, USA), NeuroBloc® (Sloan, Europe)
Composition	BoNT-A	BoNT-A	BoNT-A	BoNT-A	BoNT-A	BoNT-A	BoNT-B
Available form	Lyophilized powder	Liquid	Lyophilized powder	Lyophilized powder	Lyophilized powder	Lyophilized powder	Lyophilized powder
Dose equivalence	1	1:2.5-5	-	1:1	-	1:1	1:50-150
Storage (unreconstituted)	2°-8°C	2°-8°C	2°-8°C	Room temperature	2°-8°C	2°-8°C	2°-8°C
Shelf life (unreconstituted)	3 years	2 years	3 years	3 years	2 years	3 years	3 years
Shelf life (reconstituted)	5 hours	4 hours	Upto 24 hours	Upto 24 hours	4 hours	4 hours	4 hours
Special feature	-	-	-	No complexing proteins	-	-	Short duration of action and higher risk of antibody formation
Specific biologic activity*	High	-	-	-	Low	-	-

* Specific biologic activity – low activity means high antigenicity.

sensitive than other neurons for all types of BoNT except BoNT-D. Amongst all serotypes BoNT-A has the longest duration of action. Duration of action is longer for autonomic neurons (6-9 months) viz., hyperhidrosis in comparison to striated muscles (3-4 months) viz, facial wrinkles. BoNT-E has fastest action (< 24 hours) and short duration (~30 days). (Table 35.1)

SPECIAL FEATURES :

Innotox® (Medytox/Allergan, R. Korea/USA) is a liquid preparation of BoNT-A and does not have biological excipients, thereby lack risk of transmission of HIV or BSE. Coretox® (Medytox, R. Korea) is BoNT-A but lacks complexing proteins and biological excipients.

NEWER FORMS :

ANT-1207 is BoNT-A and is a lotion (Anterios/Allergan, USA); MCL005 is BoNT-A and is a topical gel (Malvern Cosmeceuticals, UK), Cosme Tox® is Daxibotulinum Toxin A and is a cream (Transdermal, USA); EB-001 is BoNT-E (Bonti/Allergan, USA).

INDICATIONS :

1. Wrinkle relaxation viz., crow's feet, glabellar lines.
2. Primary palmoplantar hyperhidrosis, gustatory sweating.
3. Neuropathic pain.
4. Facial contouring viz., treating masseter hypertrophy.
5. Dystonia viz, torticollis, cervical dystonia.
6. Also, used for pore reduction and reducing seborrhea.
7. Others : Androgenetic alopecia, Hailey Hailey disease, Keloids, pompholyx.

CONTRAINDICATIONS :

1. Neuromuscular disorders viz, myasthenia gravis, Eaton Lambert syndrome.
2. Hypersensitivity to botulinum toxin A or B.
3. Concomitant use of neuromuscular blockers viz. succinyl choline.
4. Abobotulinum toxin is contraindicated in patients with cow's milk allergy.

PREGNANCY CATEGORY : C

PRE-TREATMENT :

1. Counselling of patient on their expectations, what is achievable, dosage, cost and transient nature of treatment.
2. Informed consent and clinical photography at rest and animation to document pretreatment features and also, any pre-existing anatomical variations/asymmetry.
3. ***Concomitant medications*** : Antimalarials, Aminoglycosides, cyclosporine, D-penicillamine potentiate neuromuscular blockade and hence either procedure or medication should be dropped.
4. The extent of hyperhidrosis has to be mapped with Minor's starch iodine test that involves painting the area of interest with iodine. After it dries, starch powder is sprinkled over the painted area. At sites of sweating, there is purple-blue discoloration and this is documented.

TREATMENT :

Reconstitution of BoNT :

This should be done with preservative free normal saline. Usually, Botox® is reconstituted with 2.5 ml to obtain a concentration of 4 units / 0.1 ml. The vial is gently mixed during reconstitution due to the risk of loss of potency, which may occur due to vigorous agitation. The reconstituted solution can be stored at 2-8 C for up to 4 weeks.

INJECTING BoNT :

Area to be injected is anesthetized with EMLA applied for an hour. Regional anesthesia or field blocks are done for palmoplantar hyperhidrosis. Cleanse the treatment area with spirit-iodine solution-spirit. Mark the point to be injected, Calculate the dose of BoNT required and load syringes such that not more than 3 injections are done with a syringe to reduce discomfort. Insulin or Tuberculin syringes are used for injection. Dosage of BoNT depends on indication, area and thickness of muscle.

MESOTHERAPY :

In this technique, 100 units of botulinum toxin are diluted with 5 to 10 ml of 0.9% preservative free normal saline. Botulinum toxin, 0.2 to 0.4 ml, is injected intradermally randomly into facial skin. This technique is used to treat fine wrinkles and mild sagging and has the advantage of utilizing very minimal amounts of the toxin.

POST-TREATMENT :

Apply topical antibiotic cream or a moisturizer after procedure. Animate the area injected for next 4 hours intermittently for uniform spread of BoNT in the muscle. Do not massage the area for a week. Results start as early as 2 days and optimal results seen by 2 weeks in case of wrinkle relaxation. Touch-up may be required after 2 weeks for minor corrections.

COMPLICATIONS :

1. *Immediate :* Pain, erythema, bruise. BoNT-B is associated with more pain (due to its acidic pH) and more regional and systemic anticholinergic effects. Paresthesia due to trauma to nerve.

2. *Delayed :* Diffusion or inappropriate injection leads to weakness of adjoining muscles heading to eyelid/brow ptosis, ectropion, smile distortion, cheek droop, weakness of hands (diffusion into small muscles of hands while treating hyperphidrosis), dysphagia (due to neck line injection). These are transient side effects and tend to recover spontaneously in 3-4 weeks. Infections especially mycobacterial can happen due to contamination of stored vials or improper asepsis.
3. Non-response to BoNT.

NON-RESPONSE TO BOTULINUM TOXIN :

Primary non-response : is < 25% response to first injection inspite of consecutive incremental dose of BoNT.

Secondary non-response : Failure/reduction of response with subsequent. Injections and can be due to neutralizing antibodies to core neurotoxin (binding site of heavy/light chains). Higher doses and shorter interval of treatment are associated with formation of neutralizing antibodies. Hence the minimum interval between two treatments should be more than 12 weeks. BoNT-F has been used in non-responders to BoNT-A as antibodies to latter do not block former. However, BoNT-F has short duration of action and repeated injections cause secondary non-response.

x=x=x=x=x

Appendixes

Appendix – I

Office Aids in Dermatological Practice

Various easily available materials can be utilized as extremely useful aids in dermatological practice. This chapter deals with common office aids in dermatological practice.

COMMON PIN :

The common pin has head, a body and a tip.

USES :

Head of pin :

1. To test crude touch sensation in leprosy and various neurological conditions.
2. To elicit deep dermal tenderness.
3. To demonstrate feeding vessel in spider angioma.
4. To demonstrate scales in :
   - Pityriasis versicolor (Scratch sign).
   - Discoid lupus erythematosus and pemphigus foliaceus (Carpet tack or Cat's tongue sign, tin tack sign). Psoriasis (Auspitz sign).
   - Pityriasis lichenoides chronica (Wafer like scales).
5. To stroke the skin for eliciting dermographism and Darier's sign.
6. Can be used for chemical cauterization.

Tip of pin :

1. To test pain sensation in leprosy and in other neurological conditions like Hereditary sensory autonomic neuropathy (HSAN), congenital insensitivity to pain, etc.
2. To extract mites.

Shaft of pin :

- To demonstrate in-growing hair by extracting the buried distal end from the skin in pseudofolliculitis.

GLASS SLIDE :

USES :

1. *Diascopy/Vitropression :*
   (a) To differentiate purpuric rash from erythematous rash;
   (b) To differentiate nevus depigmentosus from nevus anemicus;
   (c) To demonstrate 'apple jelly nodules' in lupus vulgaris, sarcoidosis.

   Diascopy with a glass slide can also be used for therapeutic purposes in the treatment of superficial and deep vascular malformations in the same sitting. By blanching the superficial component of malformation with a glass slide, laser light is directed to the deeper component.
2. To test the compressibility of vascular malformations.
3. To prepare various types of smears (including imprint smear, tissue smear, crush smear and slit skin smear) for Gram stain, AFB stain, Giemsa or Wright stain, potassium hydroxide (10-20% KOH) mount to demonstrate organisms.
4. Diagnosis of calcinosis cutis by demonstration of hard compact granules as irregular deep blue basophilic masses in Tzanck smear.

5. Elastosis perforans to demonstrate elastic fibers in the keratotic plug with KOH and Redi stain.
6. To transfer suction blister graft from donor area onto dermabraded recipient site.
7. To prepare hair mount.

MAGNIFYING LENS :

This can either be self-illuminating with an inherent torch or nonilluminating. Magnification of the lens may vary between 2x and 7x.

USES :

1. Study minute details about morphology of cutaneous lesions.
2. To visualize :
   - Nits and lice in pediculosis capitis and pubic louse infestation.
   - Lice in the seams of clothes in pediculosis corporis/ Vagabond's disease.
   - Burrows and mites in scabies.
   - Auspitz sign in psoriasis.
   - Nail pits in psoriasis, atopic dermatitis, alopecia areata.
   - Wickham's striae in lichen planus and hence differentiate it from lichenoid drug rash.
   - Black dots in warts and black dot tinea capitis.
   - Umbilication in molluscum contagiosum, penicilliosis, etc.
   - Carpet tack or Cat tongue sign in scales of discoid lupus erythematosus, seborrheic keratosis, Darier's disease, pemphigus foliaceus.
   - Telangiectase especially of nail folds in collagen vascular diseases.

- Furrow in the middle of ridged margins of porokeratosis.
- 'Exclamation mark' hairs at the periphery of patches of alopecia areata.

3. May be used as a diascope in the absence of a glass slide.

MEASURING TAPE :

USES :

1. Measure dimensions of various cutaneous lesions viz, ulcer, plaque and lymphadenopathy for accurate description and monitoring.
2. Measure limb hypertrophy (in Klippel Trenaunay syndrome, lymphedema), muscle atrophy (in leprosy and hereditary motor neuropathies), monitoring of limb circumference (in mycetoma).
3. Measure induration after Mantoux test or any other intradermal tests.
4. Measure chest expansion in scleroderma patients.
5. Measure hip/waist ratio in patients with lipodystrophy.
6. To measure the ratio of upper segment to lower segment (decreased) and arm span (increased) in Marfan's syndrome.

FILTER PAPER :

USES :

1. To test adherence to dapsone during leprosy treatment by testing a drop of urine on filter paper dipped in Ehrlich's reagent.
2. To test sweating by Ninhydrin test (pink color with Bromophenol blue with, blue color with sweat) in leprosy, peripheral neuropathies both acquired (mellitus, alcohol, etc.) and inherited/familial (hereditary sensory and autonomic neuropathy, porphyrias).

3. Patch testing of liquid allergens viz., formaldehyde, propylene glycol.
4. For documentation of Auspitz sign.
5. To collect and preserve hair clippings, skin scraping.
6. To sterilize tattoo pigments in autoclave by packing it in filter paper.

COTTON SWAB STICK :

Sterilization : Autoclave.

Parts : Cotton tip, wooden stick. Alternatively, ear buds can be used. Readymade cotton-tipped plastic swab sticks are also available (sterilized by gamma irradiation for the purpose of collecting specimens).

USES :

Cotton tip :

1. To prepare smear of discharges (sterile swabs for culture and antibacterial/antifungal sensitivity).
2. To apply various peeling agents viz., glycolic acid, trichloroacetic acid, phenol, salicylic acid.
3. For chemical cauterization using trichloroacetic acid, phenol.
4. Cryotherapy by dipstick method.
5. Application of podophyllin for condyloma acuminata.
6. To demonstration of subclinical condyloma acuminata by acetowhitening technique.
7. For taking cervical swab.
8. For collecting specimens for PCR studies.
9. To achieve hemostasis during hair transplantation.
10. To smear ointment over suture lines.
11. To apply topical formulations, *e.g.* psoralen lotion in vitiligo.
12. Demonstrate Nikolskiy sign over mucosal surfaces.

Stick :

1. For chemical cauterization of small lesions viz., dermatosis papulosa nigricans, digitate/filiform wart, verruca plana, molluscum contagiosum, etc.
2. Can be useful for the extraction of guinea worm.

x=x=x=x=x

Appendix – II

Common Instruments in Dermatological Procedures

COMEDONE EXPRESSOR :

Sterilization : Autoclave, hot air oven, 2% glutaraldehyde, boiling.

Parts : Central handle, two hemispherical cups at either ends with perforation in centre and blunt margins. The expressor is sinuous in shape to facilitate better handling of the instrument and aid effective extraction of contents by localizing the force/ pressure.

USES :

- To express open and closed comedones in acne.
- To express contents of nevus comedonicus, senile comedones.

Method of use :

The central perforation of the cup fits over plugged follicular ostia of open comedone and pressure is applied

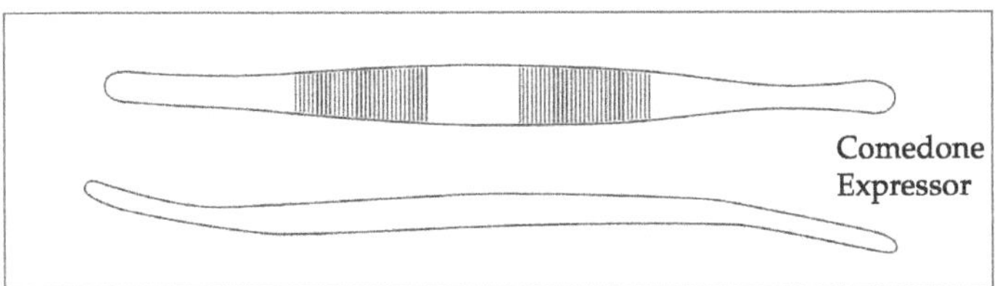

perpendicularly over the lesion. The contents of comedone collect in the cup of instrument. In case of closed comedones, an artificial opening is made using a sterile lancet or needle and then expressed as said above.

MOLLUSCUM EXTRACTOR (CURETTE) :

Sterilization : Autoclave, hot air oven, 2% glutaraldehyde, boiling.

Parts : Central handle, round'oval loop at either end.

Variants : Fox curette (round cutting edge), *Piffard curette* (oval cutting edge). Available in various sizes from I to10 mm. Commonly used curette is of 3-4 mm size.

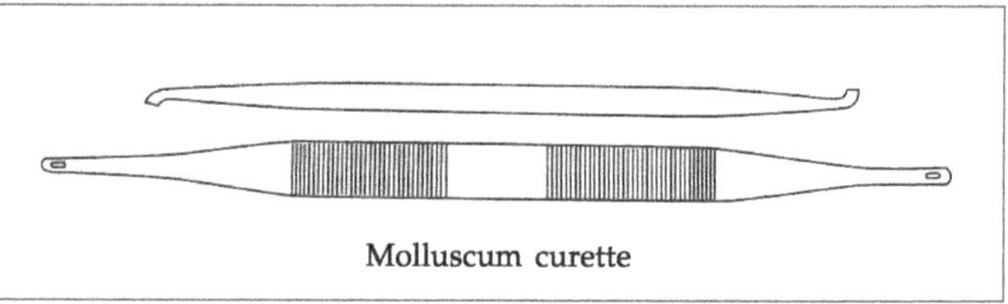

Molluscum curette

USES :

1. Extraction of molluscum contagiosum.
2. Curettage of seborrheic keratosis, stucco keratosis, verruca plana, actinic keratosis.

SCOOP :

Sterilization : Autoclave, hot air oven, 2% glutaraldehyde boiling.

Parts : Central handle; oval, spoon shaped pointed expansions at either ends.

Variants : Available in various sizes. Small to medium sized commonly used.

USES :

- To scoop out contents of cysts, abscesses, ulcers.
- To scoop out the granulation tissue in and around ingrown toe nail or any hyperplastic granulation tissue.

HYPODERMIC NEEDLE :

Sterilization : Commercially packed needles are sterilized by gamma irradiation.

Variants : Available in various sizes ranging from 18G to 30G.

USES :

1. For intramuscular/intravenous/subcutaneous (IM/IV/SC) injections.
2. For intralesional injections of drugs like corticosteroids, 5-fluorouracil, bleomycin, interferons, sodium stibogluconate etc.
3. For intramatrical injection of corticosteroids in nail psoriasis and nail lichen planus.
4. For infiltration anesthesia prior to surgical procedure.
5. To aspirate/drain bullae in vesiculobullous disorders *e.g.* bullous pemphigoid.
6. For milia extraction (Extraction of 'Rice-kernel like grain'also confirms diagnosis of milia).
7. To puncture the closed comedone and hence facilitate extraction.
8. To differentiate between papule and vesicle especially when they are smaller in size.
9. For ear and nose piercing.
10. For chemical cauterization of sebaceous cyst, steatocystoma.
11. For subcision of scar as in acne, etc.

12. For intradermal tests – Mantoux test (tuberculosis), Pathergy test (Behqet's disease, pyoderma gangrenosum, Sweet's syndrome), Kveim test (sarcoidosis), Frei test (lymphogranuloma venereum), Ito-Reenstierna test (chancroid), Montenegro test (leishmaniasis), histamine or pilocarpine test, ASST (autoimmune urticaria).
13. For needling, a therapeutic procedure for vitiligo and molluscum contagiosum.

SKIN BIOPSY PUNCHES :

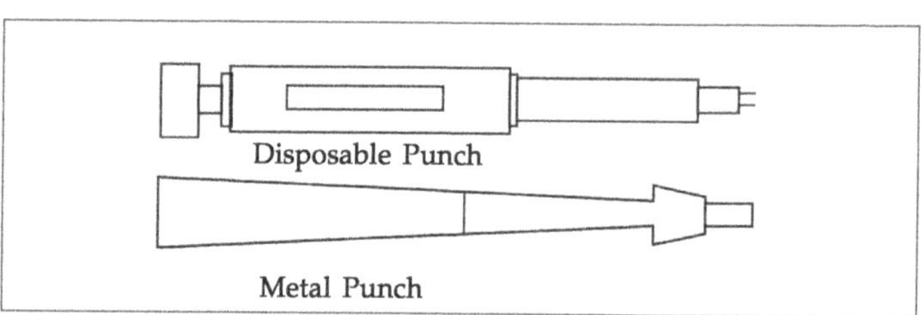

Sterilization : Metal punches – Autoclave, hot air oven, 2% glutaraldehyde, boiling; Plastic disposable punches-2% glutaraldehyde.

HAND HELD PUNCHES :

Variants : Metallic punches with tapering or cylindrical tip; Metallic handle with attachable tips (various size tips can be fitted on to the same handle). Disposable, plastic handle punches. Available in sizes 1.5 to 10.0 mm.

Parts : Metallic punches have a stylet with guard which facilitates determination of thickness of graft and also protects the sharp cutting tip from extraneous damage during storage.

N.B. : *The stylet has to be removed from the punch during biopsy and while cleaning the punch should be flushed adequately to remove all debris within its hollow.*

Power Punches :

Here, the shaft of the punch is mounted onto a hand machine with adjustable rotational speed varying from 2,000-10,000 rpm. Available in various sizes of 1.5-4.5 mm.

Uses :

1. For doing skin biopsy which has diagnostic, therapeutic (excisional biopsy of small nevus, tiny solitary molluscum pyogenic granuloma, digitate wart) and prognostic implications in dermatological practice.
2. For punch grafting in localized stable vitiligo.
3. Lipoma excision narrow hole extrusion technique.
4. For hair transplantation surgery.
5. Acne surgeries-punch excision, punch elevation, punch graft.
6. Punch excision of small tattoo and melanocytic nevus.

SCALPEL :

Parts : Consists of a surgical blade mounted on a Bard-Parker handle.

Bard-Parker Handle :

Sterilization : Autoclave, hot air oven, 2% glutaraldehyde, boiling.

Parts : Long body, grooved tapered blunt tip.

Variants : Available in various sizes. No. 3 handle accommodates surgical blades of no. 10, 11, 12 and 15. No. 4 handle accommodates surgical blades of no. 20 to 25.

Uses :

The surgical blade is mounted onto the grooved tip of handle for use in various procedures.

SURGICAL BLADE :

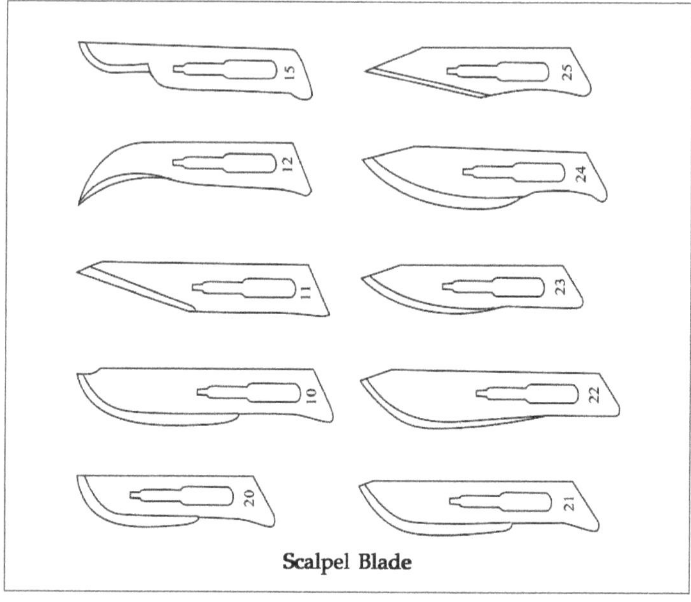

Scalpel Blade

TABLE AII.1 : **Commonly used blades and their use in dermatological Procedures**

Size of blade	Shape	Uses
11G	Triangular with narrow tip	For stab incisions
15G	Small with round belly	Slit skin smear in leprosy, leishmaniasis. For incisions over areas with thin skin viz., eyelids, face.
20-24G	Long with round belly	Incisions and excisions. Prepare Tzanck smear. Smear from molluscum contagiosum, paring of wart, corn.

Sterilization : Commercially packed blades come presterilized by gamma irradiation (cold sterilization).

Parts : Belly with one sharp edge and one blunt edge. The body has a linear slot to fit it snugly into the groove at the tip of a Bard-Parker handle.

Variants : Available in various sizes. As the number increases, the size of the blade increases.

FORCEPS :

Sterilization : Autoclave, hot air oven, 2% glutaraldehyde, boiling.

Parts : Forceps are a V-shaped metallic instrument with two blades/arms, which are fused together at one end and free at the other to clasp tissues. The free tips may be serrated, plain or toothed. Serrated and toothed forceps aid better grip.

Dissecting Forceps :

Variants :

Plain forceps – less traumatic, used to hold delicate structures like nerve or biopsy tissue.

Toothed forceps – better grip but more used to hold dermis, cyst.

Adson forceps – have wider blades with long tapered ends bearing small teeth, and are relatively less traumatic. They can be used for holding the skin except eyelids, suture removal, and punch grafts of skin.

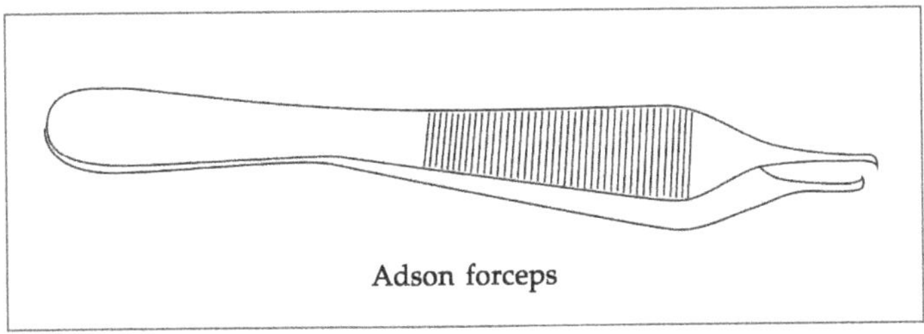

Adson forceps

Iris forceps – have a plain tip with a lock in the upper part of the instrument. They have a narrower blade with a more gradual taper than the Adson forceps, and are used in miniature punch graft, acne surgeries.

Jeweller 's forceps – have elongated plain handles which rapidly taper to a fine tip. They can be curved or straight. They are used for atraumatic handling of skin grafts, hair transplants, suture removal and clasping small bleeders during electrocoagulation.

RING FORCEPS :

Parts : This is similar to Iris forceps except that they lack both teeth and serrations and have a curved fine tip.

Uses : Hair transplantation.

EPILATION FORCEPS :

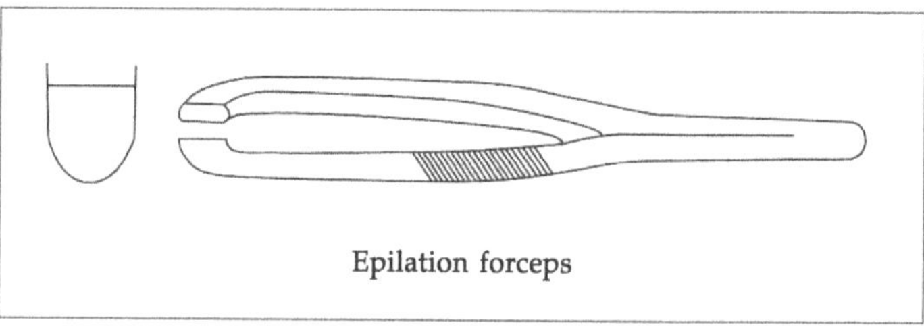

Epilation forceps

Parts : These are small forceps with serrations at the tips.

Variants : Barraquer type (rounded tip), *Bergh type* (angulated tip).

Uses : Epilation, suture removal.

DRESSING FORCEPS :

These are long, serrated forceps used for dressing.

ALLIS FORCEPS :

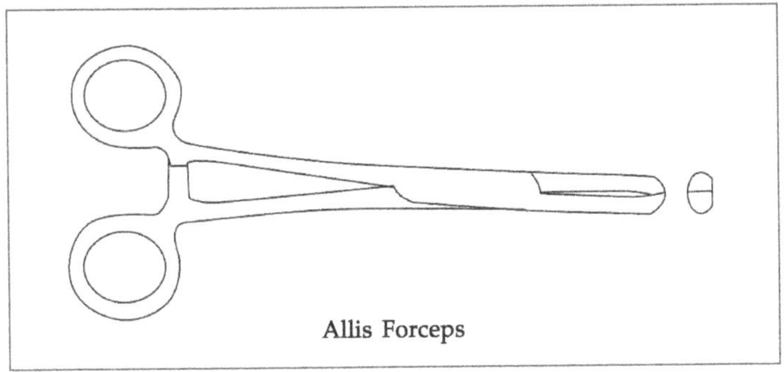

Allis Forceps

Parts : These have interdigitating tips for better grip, which is aided and secured by the lock present at the upper end of the instrument. The two prongs of the instrument are riveted at the distal end and acts as a fulcrum.

Uses : Corn enucleation, cyst excision.

CHEATLES FORCEPS :

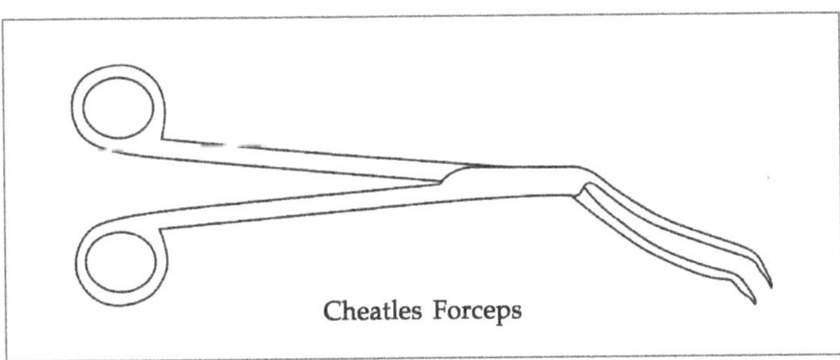

Cheatles Forceps

Parts : These are somewhat L-shaped forceps without teeth or lock. The proximal part of both arms of the forceps may have a ring to accommodate the thumb and the ring finger. Alternatively, one arm can have a ring for the thumb while the other has a V-shaped bend to accommodate fingers. The distal L-part is sinuous and always placed immersed in antiseptic solution.

Uses : Used to handle instruments, dressing material.

N.B. : *Cheatles forceps have to be kept in a bottle of Savlon.*

ARTERY/HEMOSTATIC FORCEPS :

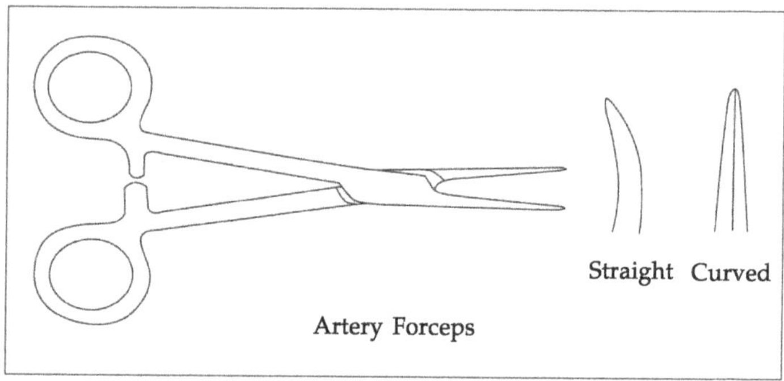

Artery Forceps

Parts : Possess blunt, tapering tips with serrations for better grip.

Variants : These are either straight or curved, the smallest are called *Mosquito forceps.*

USES :

1. Catch the bleeders.
2. Hold the free end of suture.
3. Blunt dissection of lipoma, cysts.
4. Crushing pedicle of pedunculated neoplasms *e.g.* acrochordon.
5. For removal of nail plate during partial nail avulsion.
6. For three point traction during circumcision.
7. To pluck hairs for trichogram.

SPONGE HOLDING FORCEPS :

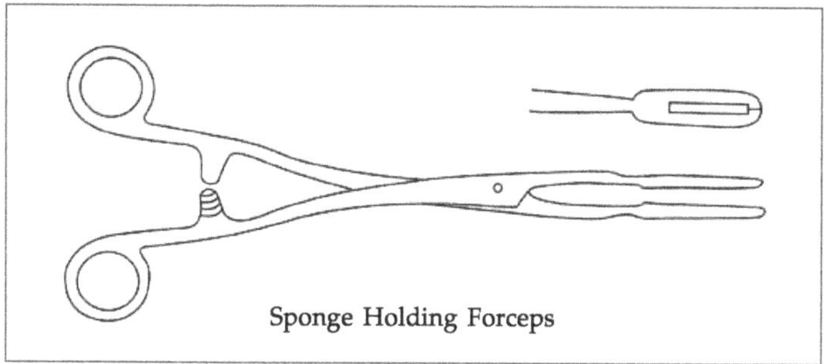

Sponge Holding Forceps

The tips of these forceps are fenestrated and serrated to aid grasping cotton swabs during preoperative antiseptic preparation of operative area.

SCISSORS :

Iris Scissors :

These have longer rivet-to-tip distance, and a short shank with a sharp tip. They can be straight or curved. One of the blades can be serrated to improve tissue grip while cutting. They are used in fine dissection; the serrated variant is helpful during procedures with thin skin.

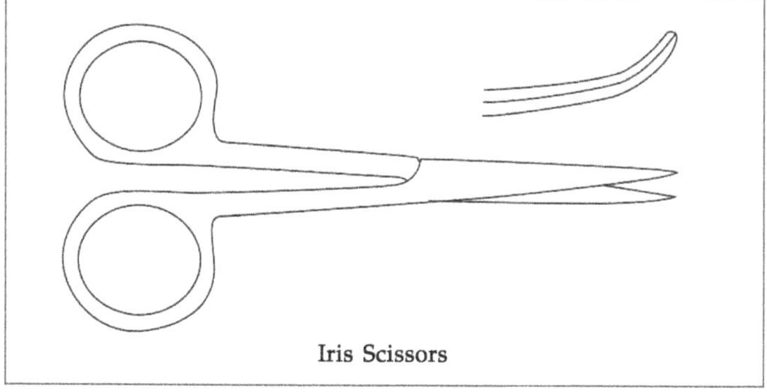

Iris Scissors

Sterilization : Autoclave, hot air oven, 2% glutaraldehyde, boiling.

Parts : These are two pronged instruments, which gyrate around a rivet which acts as a fulcrum.

Variants : They can be sharp or blunt tipped, straight or curved.

Straight Scissors/Dressing Scissors :

Used to cut dressings and suture. This has a thick, blunt blade that is introduced beneath the dressing and protects skin from injury and a sharp blade, which cuts the dressing.

Curved Scissors :

These are sharp, curved scissors used for cutting; and aid negotiation through difficult to access areas during deeper dissections.

Undermining Scissors :

These are longer with blunt and broad tips to facilitate dissection with minimal trauma to surrounding tissues. May be straight, curved or serrated (Ragnell dissecting scissors).

Castroviejo Iris Scissors :

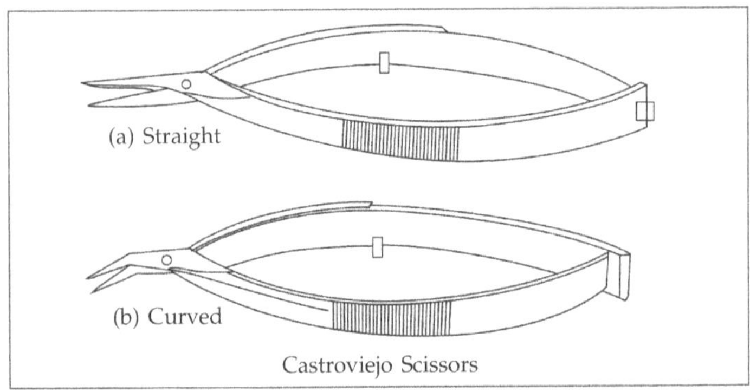

Castroviejo Scissors

These are delicate scissors with small cutting tips that can be straight or curved. Used in surgeries involving mucosa, areas with thin skin, *e.g.* eyelids, harvesting the suction blister graft.

SKIN HOOK :

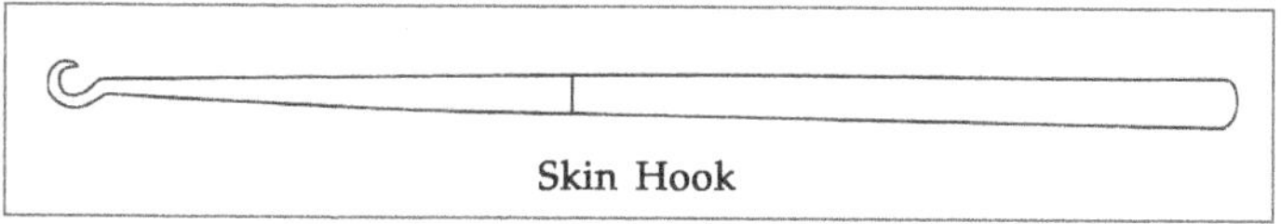

Skin Hook

Sterilization : Autoclave, hot air oven, 2% glutaraldehyde, boiling.

Parts : Handle, hook.

Variants : Fraizer skin hook (single hook), *Cottle skin hook* (bipronged hook), *Rakes* (multi-pronged skin hook).

These cause minimal trauma to delicate skin margins during suturing and handling of tissues and hence are preferred to forceps.

USES :

1. Hold skin margins during suturing especially when handling thin skin, viz., eyelids.
2. Retract skin margins during deeper dissections and undermining.
3. Hold vital structures like nerve during procedures.
4. Rakes are used for retracting large wound areas.

NEEDLE HOLDER :

Sterilization : Autoclave, hot air oven, 2% glutaraldehyde, boiling.

Parts : Its tips can be either smooth or serrated and provided with a groove. The lock present in the proximal part facilitates

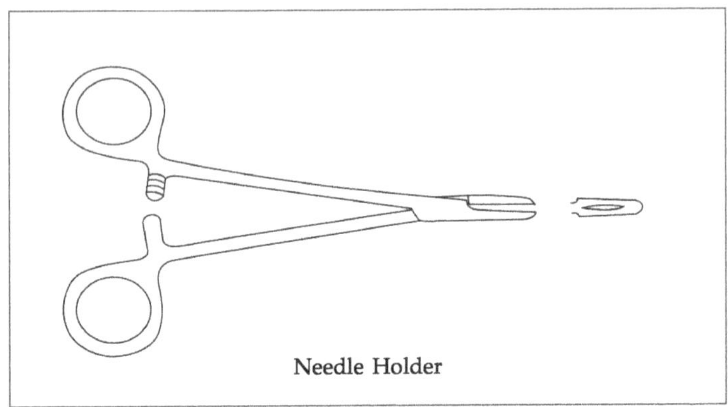

Needle Holder

better grasp of the needle. Available in various shapes and sizes.

USES :

Used for grasping the needle during suturing. Castroviejo needle holder is used during delicate surgeries like mini hair graft, acne scar revision.

SUTURING NEEDLES :

Sterilization : Autoclave, hot air oven, 2% glutaraldehyde, boiling.

Parts : Needlepoint, body and shank.

Variants : The shank can be closed (suture material is passed through it) or swaged (suture material is attached to it).

CURVED SUTURING NEEDLES :

Variants :

Based on curvature – These needles are curved and form a part of the sphere in shape that can be $1/4^{th}$, $3/8^{th}$, $5/8^{th}$ or ½ of circumference of a circle.

Based on shape – Curved needles can be cutting (triangular on cross section) or round body (spherical on cross section) type.

Conventional cutting needles have third cutting edge along the inner aspect of the curve and provides a sharp entry point for the suture that is directed towards the wound. Hence this predisposes the suture to cut through the wound margin.

Reverse cutting needles have a third cutting edge along the outer aspect of the curve and this is preferred for suturing wounds, which are under tension. Both types of cutting needles are used for suturing of skin margins.

Round body needles are similar to cutting needles but without cutting edges. These are used for suturing mucosa, taking subcutaneous sutures.

STRAIGHT NEEDLES :

These can be either round bodied or cutting type. Round type are used to suture delicate structures like mucosa and cutting type for skin.

SUTURE MATERIALS :

Sterilization : Gamma irradiation.

Variants : Available in various sizes ranging from 11-0 to 1, 11-0 being the finest and 1 being the thickest suture. Sutures thicker than 1-0 have the prefix '#'. Most dermato-surgical procedures require 3-0 to 6-0. (Table AII.2)

3-0 and 4-0 – used for scalp, back, extremities, facial wounds under tension.

5-0 – used for face, scrotum.

6-0 – used for eyelids.

Other wound closure aids :

1. Cyanoacrylate glues (N-butyl-2-cyanoacrylate, Octyl-2-cyanoacrylate).

TABLE AII.2 : **Characteristics of various suture materials**

Characteristics of of suture material	Sutures
Absorbable	Gut, polyglycolic acid (Dexon®), polyglactin 910 (Vicryl®), polydioxanone (PDS), poly-methylene carbonate, poliglecaprone (Monocryl®)
Non-absorbable	Silk, nylon (Ethilon®), polyester (Mersilene®), polypropylene (Prolene®), polybutester
Monofilament	Gut, nylon, polypropylene (Prolene®)
Multifilament	Silk, cotton, linen, nylon (Ethilon®), polyglactin 910 (Vicryl®)
Natural	Silk, cotton, catgut, linen
Synthetic	Polyglycolic acid (Dexon®), polyglactin 910 (Vicryl®), nylon (Ethilon®), polydioxanone (PDS), poly-methylene carbonate, poliglecaprone (Monocryl®)

2. Fibrin glues (obsolete in view of HIV hazard).
3. Wound closure tapes (Steri-Strip, Cover-Strip).
4. Staples.

Tactifiers are agents used to enhance adhesion of surgical tapes dressings to the skin, *e.g.* tincture benzoin.

NAIL NIPPER/NAIL SPLITTER :

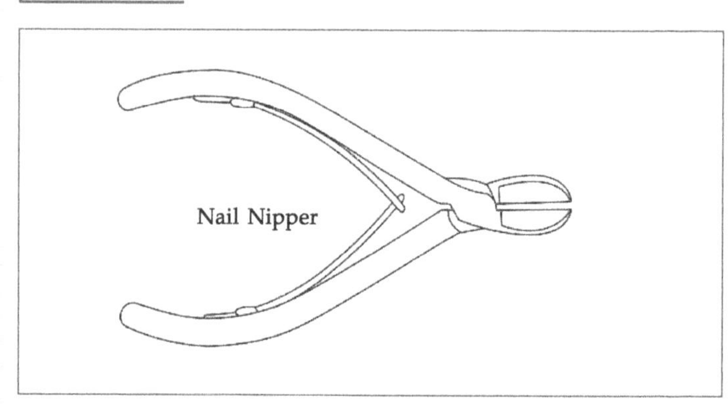

Sterilization : Autoclave, hot air oven, 2% glutaraldehyde, boiling.

Parts : Handle with stout, sharp cutting edges. In contrast, the nail splitter has one wedge-shaped blunt blade and the other sharp-cutting blade.

USES :

Cutting of nail plate during partial nail avulsion.

NAIL SPATULA :

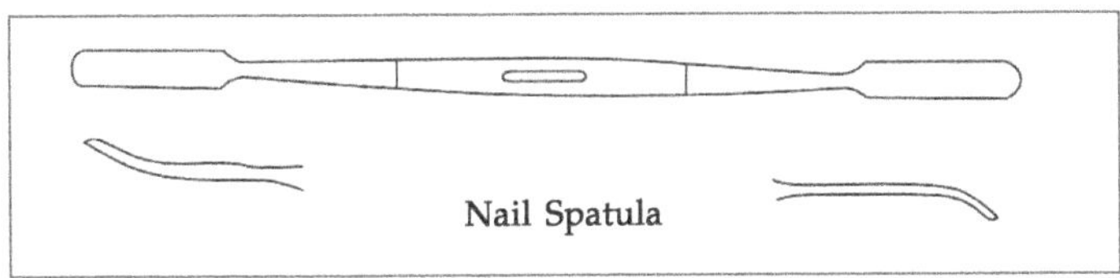

Nail Spatula

Sterilization : Autoclave, hot air oven, 2% glutaraldehyde, boiling.

Parts : Central handle, flat rectangular curved plates on either ends.

USES :

1. Separation of the nail plate from nail bed and proximal nail fold.
2. Separation of the dressing from the skin or punch grafts.

CHALAZION CLAMP :

Sterilization : Autoclave, hot air oven, 2% glutaraldehyde, boiling.

Parts : Consists of 2 arms attached at one end and free at other end; screw to approximate the clamp and retain it in that position; free ends are expanded and perforated with a large flat, thin rim. It is available in various sizes.

1/1 16 mm

1/1 20 mm

1/1 24 mm

Chalazion Clamp

USES :

1. Mucocele excision.
2. As hemostat during excision of lip pyogenic granuloma or any neoplasm.
3. To prevent excess bleeding during tongue biopsy.

DERMABRADER :

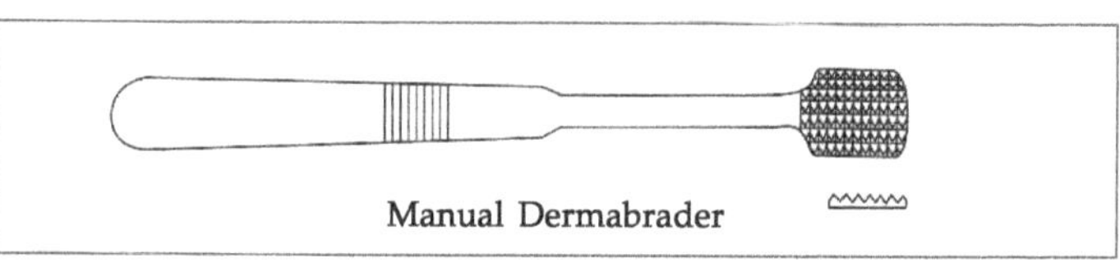

Manual Dermabrader

Sterilization : Autoclave, hot air oven, 2% glutaraldehyde, böiling.

MANECKSHA'S MANUAL DERMABRADER :

Parts : Handle with or without thumb rest, slightly curved expanded rectangular tip with sharp teeth arranged in regular rows and columns along convex surface of tip.

MOTORIZED DERMABRADERS :

Parts : These have a rotating hand piece which bears a diamond fraise or wire brushes mounted on hand engines.

Diamond fraises contain diamond chips adhered to stainless steel wheels. These are available in various sizes and shapes. ***Coarseness*** of the fraise is graded as regular, grit, coarse and extra coarse. For deeper dermabrasion coarser fraises are used.

Wire brushes have short steel wires projecting from the wheel. These achieve deeper dermabrasion than diamond fraises. They arc available in various sizes.

Hand engines are motor driven devices with 3000-30,000 rpm speed. Either of the fraises can be attached to this for dermabrasion. Bell hand engines, dental burrs are a few other devices that use hand engines.

USES :

1. *In vitiligo :*
   a. Dermabrasion of recipient areas during suction blister or split skin grafting.
   b. Dermabrasion to stimulate melanocyte proliferation and migration.
2. Dermabrasion of lichen amyloidosis, lichen simplex chronicus.
3. Spot dermabrasion for acne scars.

4. Full face dermabrasion for facial rejuvenation.
5. Debulking of rhinophymae.
6. Treatment of multiple adenoma sebaceum.
7. Tattoo removal.
8. Freshen the surface during ear lobe repair.

SKIN GRAFT HARVESTERS :

HUMBY'S KNIFE :

Sterilization : Autoclave, hot air oven, 2% glutaraldehydee.

Parts : Handle at one end and a flat, long metallic blade with adjustable screws and roller at other end. Screws facilitate adjustment of thickness of skin graft and roller flattens the skin surface before cutting the skin.

SILVER'S KNIFE :

Sterilization : Autoclave, hot air oven, 2% glutaraldehyde.

Parts : Similar to Humby's knife except smaller in size and has disposable ordinary shaving blade for harvesting skin graft.

DERMATOMES :

These are disposable split skin graft harvesting devices.

Variants : Simon Davol dermatome has a small rechargeable unit and harvest small grafts; Brown dermatome—here the thickness of the graft is adjustable (3-8 mm).

SKIN GRAFT SPREADER :

Sterilization : Autoclave, hot air oven, 2% glutaraldehyde, boiling,

Parts : It is straight metallic rod of uniform diameter with blunt ends.

Uses :

Used to spread the suction blister or split thickness skin graft over the recipient area.

Semmes-Weinstein Mono Filament (SW Mono Filament) :

These are color-coded nylon monofilaments that are used for monitoring protective sensation in leprosy and other neuropathies. Used in a standardized fashion, each filament generates predictable and graded pressure and hence filaments are classified into nearly 20 types based on this property.

History : Designed by Josephine Semmes and Sidney Weinstein.

Composition of filament : Polyhexamethylene dodecandiamide (nylon 612).

Technique :

The filament is held at right angles to the skin surface and pressed gently until it forms a "C" shaped curve. At this moment, the patient is asked about the perception of the sensation. There is regional variation in the perception of minimal force. The fact that curving occurs on application of the same amount of force, makes this test objective. The testing is done at specific mapped points. Graded monofilaments are supposed to be the most objective test for the monitoring of sensory testing, with a loss of sensation at any of the five points tested being a 'positive' result.

Although detailed testing with all filaments at all standard testing points on the palms and soles is the preferred method of monitoring of silent neuritis in leprosy, the inability to perceive the purple filament is taken as an indicator of loss of protective sensations. Similarly, the loss of the ability to perceive a thicker filament will be taken as a mark of progression of silent neuritis.

TABLE AII.3 : **Various types of nylon monofilaments and their characteristic**

Sr. No.	Colour of filament	Force applied (in grams)	Extent of sensation perception
1.	Green	0.05	Normal
2.	Blue	0.2	Decreased light touch
3.	Purple	2.0	Decreased protective sensation
4.	Red	4.0	Loss of protective sensation
5.	Orange	7.5	Residual deep pressure

Number of sites to be tested :

Hands *:* 7 (3 sites for ulnar nerve, 3 sites for median and 1 site for radial nerve).

Foot *:* 8 (7 sites for common peroneal nerve, 1 site for posterior tibial nerve).

USES :

1. Screening for sensory neuropathy.
2. Measuring sensory neuropathy in leprosy, diabetic neuropathy and other peripheral neuropathies.
3. Monitoring for development of silent neuropathy in leprosy Testing should be every fortnight for initial 4 months and later monthly.

INSTRUMENTS IN STI PROCEDURES :

SIM'S ANTERIOR VAGINAL WALL RETRACTOR :

This elongated thin instrument with expanded ends that bear an oval fenestration aids vaginal examination by retracting the anterior vaginal wall. It is used in conjunction with Sim's speculum during gynecological examination and procedures.

Sterilization : Autoclave, hot air oven, 2% glutaraldehyde, boiling.

Parts : Central elongated metal arm with expanded, oval,

fenestrated ends that make an angle with the body of instrument. Expanded ends have serrations for better grip.

USES :

1. Used along with Sim's speculum during various gynecological examinations and procedures.
2. Facilitates visualization of cervix and fornix.

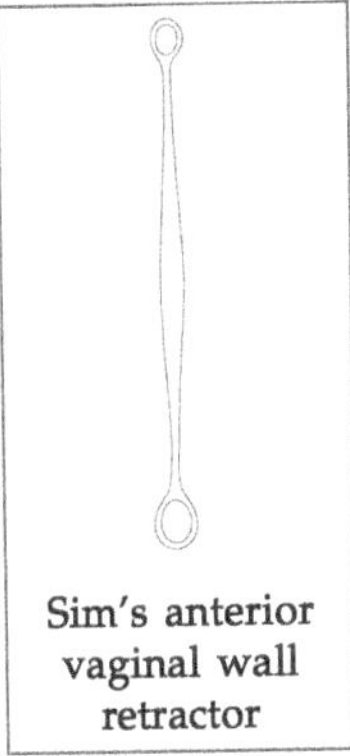

Sim's anterior vaginal wall retractor

SIM's SPECULUM :

This smoothly curved plate with central depression facilitates visualization of cervix and posterior fornix and aids collection of vaginal discharge from the posterior fornix.

Sterilization : Autoclave, hot air oven, 2% glutaraldehyde, boiling.

Parts : It has two horizontal plates of differing sizes and a vertical handle in-between. There is a trough along the entire length of instrument.

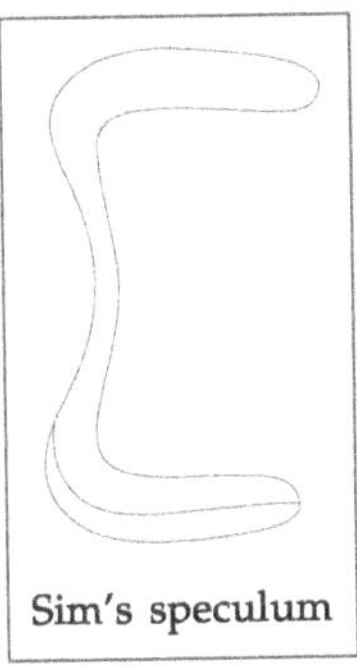

Sim's speculum

Variants : Available in various sizes (26 and 31 mm, 31 and 36 mm, 36 and 42 mm) and types (single ended or double ended).

Method of use : The instrument is dipped in warm water prior to use. One of the blades is introduced into the vagina while holding the blade vertically and then, this is rotated at right angles so that the posterior vaginal wall is depressed with it. The anterior wall is then retracted using the Sim's anterior vaginal wall retractor. In conditions with profuse vaginal discharges, viz., trichomoniasis, the secretions readily collect in the depressed central part of the plate.

USES :

1. Facilitates visualization of anterior and lateral vaginal walls, vaginal fornix, cervix, cervical orifice.
2. Distinguish cervical discharge from vaginal discharge.
3. Visualization of punctate hemorrhage in cervix 'Strawberry cervix' in trichomoniasis.
4. Collection of vaginal discharge for :
   - Demonstration of 'wobbling motility' of *Trichomonas vaginalis* by wet mount/hanging drop preparation.
   - Demonstration of budding yeast in candidiasis by 1000 KOH preparation or Gram smear.
   - Demonstration of vaginal epithelial cells with blurred margins due to coating by numerous *Gardnerella vaginalis* ('Clue cells') in vaginal discharge.
5. For Pap smear preparation.
6. For treatment of cervical or vaginal condyloma acuminata by podophyllin/cryotherapy.
7. During 'Aceto test' (acetowhitening) for visualization of incipient condyloma acuminata (3-5% acetic acid causes white discoloration of condyloma acuminata).

DISADVANTAGES :

1. The patient needs to be brought to the margin of the examining table.
2. The clinician's hands are not free to carry out a problem-free procedure.

CUSCO'S SELF RETAINING VAGINAL SPECULUM :

This is an instrument that resembles the beak of a bird. It opens when fastened and close when the screw is loose. By fixing the screw, the speculum can be made self-retaining and hence facilitates the attending clinician to do procedures, viz., chemical cauterization of condyloma acuminata with minimal assistance.

Sterilization : Autoclave, hot air oven, 2% glutaraldehyde, boiling.

Parts : Consists of two blades with handles at right angles which are riveted together. The handles can be approximated with a screw lock to hold the blades apart. Blades are concave inside and have round distal free margin.

Variants : Available in 3 sizes (small, intermediate, and large). Intermediate is the most commonly used. Small sized may be used for nulliparous females and larger sized for multiparous females with prolapse of uterus and vagina.

Method of use : With the 2 blades closed and oriented vertically, speculum is introduced into the vagina and once the instrument is inserted completely within the vagina, the speculum is rotated anticlockwise by 90 degrees, and the handle is pressed to the desired extent that opens up the 2 blades. This position is then fixed by tightening the screw fitted on the handle.

ADVANTAGES :

1. It is a self retaining speculum and hence the clinician's hands are free to carry out procedures like chemical cauterization, Pap smear, biopsy.
2. No need for the patient to move till the edge of the table.

DISADVANTAGES :

Anterior and posterior vaginal walls cannot be visualized.

USES :

Similar to Sim's speculum with the exception that anterior and posterior wall lesions cannot be visualized well or accessed for procedures.

x=x=x=x=x

Appendix – III

Apparatuses in Dermatological Practice

WOOD's LAMP :

Wood's Lamp is a handy instrument of great diagnostic value in dermatological practice. Fluorescence produced due to absorption of short UVA aids in diagnosis of cutaneous and systemic diseases. Various infections or conditions produce a characteristic color of fluorescence. In addition to the ultraviolet lamp, most Wood's lamp models have a white light source and a magnifying glass, making it a self-illuminating magnifying lens.

History : Robert W Wood, a physicist, devised the lamp in 1903. It was initially used for epidemiologic screening of school children for the detection of tinea capitis.

Parts : High pressure mercury arc lamp with Wood's filter (made up of 9% nickel oxide and barium silicate).

Power supply : Alternating current.

Power output : < 1 mW/cm^2.

Wavelength of ultraviolet light : 365 nm (320-400 nm).

IMPORTANT FACTS DURING WOOD'S LAMP EXAMINATION :

1. Use the instrument in a dark room. If a dark room is not available, a hood can be used.
2. Pre-warm the instrument for 1 minute before use.

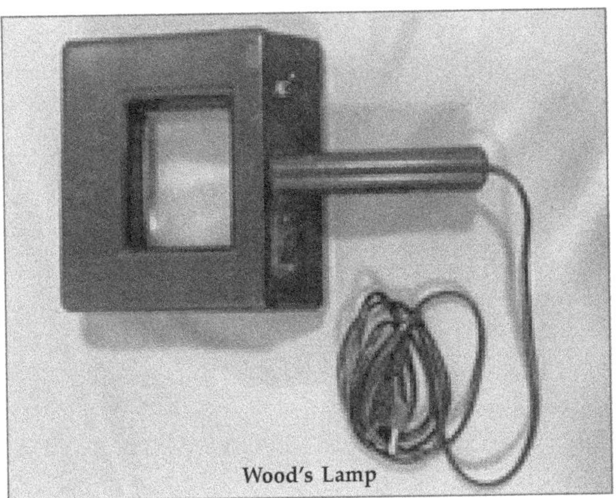
Wood's Lamp

3. Hold the lamp 4-5 inches away from the skin.
4. Having bath/cleaning the lesion before examination gives false negative result in erythrasma due to washing off of water-soluble coproporphyrin III.
5. False positive fluorescence could be due to reflection from white apron (light blue), due to presence of scales, salicylic ointment (green), or petrolatum (bluish/purplish).

USES :

Diagnostic :

1. ***Diagnosis of fungal infections :***
   - ***Pityriasis versicolor*** – Golden yellow fluorescence due to presence of porphyrin.
   - ***Tinea capitis*** – Due to presence of pteridine.
2. ***Diagnosis of bacterial infections :***
   - ***Pseudomonas infection*** – Greenish fluorescence (pyoverdin).

- *Erythrasma* – Coral red (coproporphyrin III).

3. To differentiate vitiligo (chalky white fluorescence) from other hypopigmented lesions.
4. To differentiate nevus depigmentosus from nevus anemicus.
4. To categorize melasma – epidermal type shows accentuation (more useful in fair skinned individuals).
5. Urine in porphyrias (except erythropoietic protoporphyria) reveals pink fluorescence.
6. Pink fluorescence of tears, saliva, blister fluid, teeth and bones in porphyrias.
7. Acne lesions reveal orange-red fluorescence due to coproporphyrin produced by *Propionibacterium acnes.*
8. Uniform application of glycolic acid peel can be detected by using salicylic acid in the peel (salicylic acid gives green fluorescence).

TABLE AIII.1 : **Fluorescence obtained on Wood's lamp examination in various conditions**

Sr. No.	Condition	Color of fluorescence
1.	**Fungal infections :**	
	Pityriasis versicolor	Golden yellow
	Tinea capitis : *M. canis, M. audouinii, M. distortum, M. ferruginum, M. felineum*	Blue-green
	M. gypseum	Dull-yellow
	T. schoenleinii	Dull-blue
2.	**Bacterial infections :**	
	Pseudomonas infection	Greenish (pyoverdin, fluorescein)
	Erythrasma	Coral red (coproporphyrin III)
3.	Vitiligo	Bright blue white (collagen)
4.	Porphyrins	Pink (porphyrin)
5.	Tetracycline	Yellow

9. Detection of burrows in scabies by applying tetracycline paste (green fluorescence) or fluorescein dye (yellow orange fluorescence).
10. To detect adequacy of barrier cream application in contact allergic dermatitis.

Therapeutic :

1. Treatment of vitiligo (if UV light is not available, longer exposure times are required which is not usually recommended).

Non-dermatological uses :

1. Eradication of *Staphylococcus aureus and Mycobacterium* contaminants in culture media.
2. For the detection of cracks in prosthesis or metal parts.
3. Detection of semen in cases of sexual abuse.
4. Calculation of circulation time by injection of fluorescein.
5. Detection of fake currency and forgeries.
6. Verification of signatures.

DERMOSCOPE :

(*Synonyms* : Skin surface microscope, Dermatoscope, Epiluminescence microscope or Episcope).

A dermoscope is a non-invasive diagnostic tool for in vivo examination of skin and subsurface structures of the skin that are not normally visible to the unaided eye. Some dermatoscopic patterns are observed consistently with certain diseases and these then could be used for their diagnosis.

The dermoscope is functionally similar to a magnifying lens but with the added features of an inbuilt illuminating system, a higher magnification which can be adjusted, the ability to assess structures as deep as in the reticular dermis, and the ability to record images.

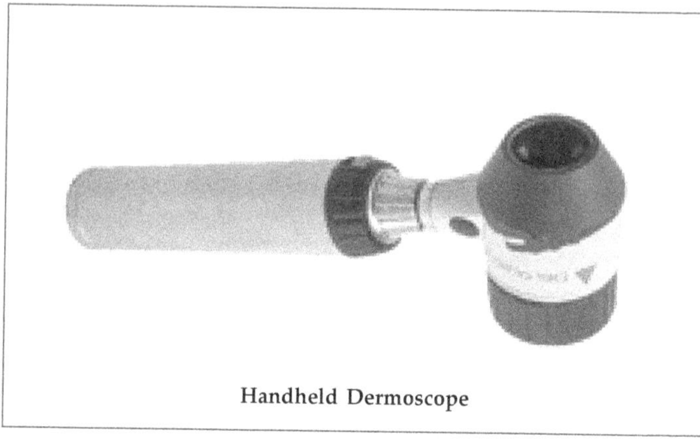

Handheld Dermoscope

COMPONENTS OF DERMATOSCOPE :

Achromatic lens : Varying magnification.

Inbuilt illuminating system : Halogen lamp, light emitting diode (LED).

Power supply : Lithium/AA battery, rechargeable handles.

Additional facilities in some dermoscopes are an inbuilt photography system, either an attachable conventional or digital camera or an inbuilt camera, and supporting software, for the capture, storage, retrieval and even interpretation of images.

TYPES OF DERMOSCOPY INSTRUMENTS :

a. *Instruments without image capturing facility, e.g.* DELTA 10©, Mini 2000 Dermatoscope©.

b. *Instruments with image capturing facility, e.g.* Derma scope©, Derm lite Foto©, Derma photo©, Delta 20©, and Video episcope©.

c. *Instruments with image capturing facility and analytical capability, e.g.* DermoGenius Mole Map©, Fotofinder dermoscope©, Mole max 11©.

TECHNIQUE OF DERMOSCOPY :

TWO techniques : Non-contact or the contact technique.

In the *contact technique,* the glass plate of the instrument comes in contact with the surface of the linkage fluid applied lesion. In contrast, in the *non-contact technique,* there is no contact of the lens with the skin; the cross-polarized lens absorbs all the scattered light and hence allows only light in a single plane to pass through it. While the non-contact technique ensures that there are no nosocomial infections, this advantage is overshadowed by the disadvantages of decreased illumination and poor resolution.

CONTACT PLATES :

1. Made of multi-coated silicone glass.
2. Are graduated/non-graduated plates.
3. May be regular/small plates (to facilitate use in difficult to access regions like the web spaces, flexures and for nail fold capillaroscopy).
4. Sterilized by using 2% glutaraldehyde, methylated spirit, boiling or autoclaving.

USES :

1. Used mainly in diagnosis of pigmented lesions (nevi and melanoma) especially for early diagnosis of melanoma in the white-skinned individuals.
2. It may also be used in diagnosis of psoriasis, lichen planus, dermatofibroma, Darier's disease, cicatricial alopecia, seborrheic keratosis and urticarial vasculitis.
3. Calculate the follicular density in the donor area before follicular unit hair transplantation.

ELECTROCAUTERY/ELECTROSURGERY :

HISTORY :

William Bovie is considered to be the 'Father of modern

electrosurgical unit'. *Cautery* means hot iron *(Gk. Kauterian)* The variety of procedures that can be carried out makes it all essential apparatus in any dermatological care center. The improvement in technology with introduction of radiofrequency equipment is now pushing this instrument to the backyard. However, it is still one of the most commonly used equipment in dermatological offices.

PRINCIPLE OF ELECTROCAUTERY :

The machine modifies the alternating current (240 V, 6A) to achieve high voltage (550V), high frequency and low amperage current to generate oscillating radio waves referred to as *'Sine waves'* using the oscillating circuit (Oudin coil). These sine waves could be damped (un-rectified), non-damped (pure/rectified) or blended (mixture of damped and pure). Tissue destruction occurs due to the påssage of oscillating radio waves through the tissue.

Spark gap type is the most easily accessible and the most widely used type of instrument by dermatologists throughout India. Even though the electrocoagulation achieved by this is inadequate, it is sufficient for most office-based dermatological procedures. (Table AIII.2)

TABLE AIII.2 : **Types of oscillatory circuits**

Type of oscillatory circuit	Basic component of circuit	Type of oscillatory wave	Type of electrosurgery
Spark gap circuit	Spark gap	Damped sine Wave	Electrofulguration Electrodesiccation Electrocoagulation
Vacuum tube circuit	Thermionic vacuum tube	Pure sine wave	Electrosection
Solid state Circuit	Transistor circuits	All types of waves or blended waves*	Electrocoagulation Electrosection

* Blended waves are the combination of damped and pure sine waves that offer both coagulation and cutting facility.

MECHANISM OF TISSUE DESTRUCTION :

Tissue destruction is the collective effect of,

Ohmic heat – is the heat produced due to tissue resistance to the flow of current

Convective heat – is due to dissipation of thermal and electrical heat from the spark.

Mechanical energy – electromagnetic waves produced at the tip of electrode cause disruption of cells.

Energy thus generated causes denaturation of proteins, cell wall damage, enzyme deactivation, dehydration of cells, steaming of intracellular water leading to bursting of cells.

PARTS OF ELECTROCAUTERY INSTRUMENT :

Power regulator : By turning round this knob, power output can be adjusted between 1-10 for procedures (electrofulguration < electrodesiccation < electrocoagulation).

Sockets : These accommodate the non-treating ends of terminals and are following types :

- Monopolar socket are of two types. Low type is used for fulguration and high for desiccation and coagulation.
- Bipolar socket is used for electrocoagulation and electrosection. This is usually accompanied by a socket for ground electrode.
- Epilation socket is used for epilation.

Terminal : This refers to the treating electrode :

- Monoterminal are the most common type with single electrode.
- Biterminal literally means two electrodes (forceps like), but is commonly used when a grounding/earthing plate is used in addition to the treating electrode. Ground plate is usually required when greater amperage is used as in electrocoagulation or electro dissection.

Pole : It is a term used for electrode of a direct current driven instrument where there is unidirectional flow of current. Hence, this term should not be used for commonly used electrocautery machine.

Electrode probe : These are the detachable terminal parts of the terminals. They are of various shapes and sizes to suit different function viz., pointed, sharp bent tip (fulguration, desiccation); straight, tapering, sharp tip (desiccation and dissection); sharp, expanded, plate-like (electrosection), round (coagulation); fine, thin wire-like (epilation). Also available are, Teflon coated probes (epilation, telangiectasia), forceps electrode (coagulation).

Ground/dispersive plate : This is a metal plate which is placed in contact with the patient during procedures involving greater amperage. This plate acts as an exit for the excess current flowing through the body and hence prevents undesired electrical trauma. It also recycles the current and improves the efficacy of the instrument.

Footpad : The circuit is completed on pressing the footpad once the main switch is on.

Cleaning and sterilization of electrode probe :

Cleaning of tissue debris adherent to the probe is done with a scalpel blade/sand paper/files or steam cleaning using wet gauze. Electrode probes do not require sterilization, as the heat generated is self-sterilizing. However, some dermatologists prefer using a disposable electrodes.

Types Of Electrosurgery :

Electrofulguration (Lt. Fulgur Lightning) :

This is a no touch procedure, in which the probe is held away from the skin (1-3 mm) and the long thick spark jumps from the tip onto the skin causing destruction of superficial tissue.

Dispersion of spark can be restricted by using fine probes (epilation probe).

Advantages : There is no scarring during healing, as the damage is restricted to the epidermis.

Power specifications : Power output 1-2, high voltage and frequency; duration 2-3 sec.

Uses : Verruca plana, stucco keratosis, dermatosis papulosa nigra, milia, tiny molluscum to dry).

Electrodesiccation (Lt. Dessicare = To Dry) :

The probe touches the skin and the short fine sparks cause tissue charring extending up to papillary dermis. It coagulates tiny capillaries in papillary dermis. Larger lesions 'bubble' due to separation at dermoepidermal junction by the steaming of interstitial fluids.

Advantages : Scarring is minimal.

Power specifications : Power output 5-7, high voltage and frequency; duration 2-4 sec.

Uses : Seborrheic keratoses, warts, pyogenic granuloma, acrochordons, molluscum contagiosum, xanthelasma palpebrarum, spider angioma, superficial BCC.

Electrocoagulation (Lt. Coagulare To Clot) :

This may be no touch or touch procedure mediated by short thick sparks which coagulate medium sized blood vessels (1-2 mm). A biterminal forceps can also be used for this. A high current flows through both the tips of forceps that act as poles alternatively.

Precautions : There is obvious scarring due to damage to reticular dermis. Due to higher amperage/current employed, ground plate should be used.

Power specifications : Power output 7-10, low voltage and frequency.

Uses : Telangiectasia, trichoepithelioma, BCC, nail matrix destruction during partial nail avulsion, coagulation of bleeders during various procedures like excisions.

Electrosection :

Here, high amperage and low voltage is used to generate pure sinewaves that cut rather than desiccate/coagulate the tissue. Ideal speed of electrosection should be 5-10 mm/sec. If excess spark occurs during sectioning, then it implies that either the speed is slow or current is too high.

Types : Pure cutting type and cut and coagulate type.

Precautions : Coagulation of vessels prolongs wound healing. Rarely used in India by dermatologists.

Uses : Keloids, acne keloidalis, rhinophyma.

CONTRAINDICATIONS FOR ELECTROSURGERY :

1. Patients with pacemaker implantation (risk of precipitating arrhythmias).
2. Patients with keloidal tendency.
3. H/o seizures.

PRECAUTIONS :

1. Do not use/keep inflammables (alcohol, ether) near the cautery site.
2. Avoid using spirit for local disinfection and if used, wait till it evaporates completely.
3. Never forcibly extract the eschar.
4. Use fumes evacuator or at least face mask to prevent transmission of diseases due to *HPV, HBV, and HIV* Evacuators should be placed within 2 cm of surgical site.

5. Ensure proper body contact of dispersive plates when used.
6. Avoid infiltrative local anesthesia when treating telangiectasia (may blanch the vessels leading to partial treatment).

ELECTROLYSIS :

Electrolysis (or chemolysis) is a commonly used method of electroepilation that involves ionization in the presence of water and sodiun) chloride under the influence of direct (galvanic) Current. This ultimately leads to recombination of ions and synthesis of sodium hydroxide (NaOH) that is caustic to hair bulb resulting in permanent destruction.

The treating electrode is attached to the negative pole (cathode) and is inserted into the hair follicle while dispersing electrode is attached to the positive pole (anode) that is held against the patient's bare skin to complete the circuit.

Steps Involved In Electrolysis :

Ionization :

$H_2O \longrightarrow H^+ + OH^-$

(Water)

$NaCl \longrightarrow Cl + Na$

(Sodium chloride)

Recombination of ions :

(At negative electrode)

$Na^+ + OH \longrightarrow NaOH$

(Sodium hydroxide or lye which is caustic to hair bulb)

$H^+ + H^+ \longrightarrow H_2$ (hydrogen gas)

(At positive electrode)

$H^+ + Cl^- \longrightarrow HCL$ (Hydrochloric acid)

$Cl^- + Cl^- \longrightarrow C1_2$ (Chlorine gas)

RADIOFREQUENCY :

Radiofrequency is a form of electrosurgery like electrocautery. However, its electrical unit converts the wall outlet alternating current to very high frequencies, producing a high voltage and low amperage current. As the unwanted frequencies are not produced' there is lesser tissue destruction and better control of the procedure. The frequency of radiofrequency waves is 500-4000 kHz. The use of radiofrequency also depends on the predominant waveform that is employed. Damped sine waves are used for procedures, which deal with superficial lesions. Pure sine waves, due to their minimal lateral spread, are used for taking incisions. Varying combination of these two types of waves are used for electrocoagulation.

USES :

Uses are similar to those of electrocautery, however radiofrequency has a choice of selecting treating mode.

ADVANTAGES :

Less lateral spread of energy and hence decreased destruction of normal surrounding tissue. This results in :

1. Cosmetically scars are more acceptable.
2. Lesser chance of secondary bacterial infection.
3. Bleeding can be controlled more easily. (Table AIII.3)

DISADVANTAGES OVER ELECTROCAUTERY :

1. Expensive.
2. Probes are very fragile and add to consumable cost.

CRYOTHERAPY :

Cryotherapy is a unique therapeutic modality that has an inherent anesthetic property. Decreasing the temperature decreases nerve conduction too and hence makes this

TABLE AIII.3 : **Modes of radiofrequency**

Type of mode	Clinical indication
Cut mode	• Removal of skin tags/pedunculated tumors, nevi, cysts. • Shave removal of xanthelasma palpebrarum, verruca plana
Cut and coagulate mode	• Curettage of hypertrophic granulation tissue. • Removal of seborrheic keratoses, keloids, warts etc. • Removal of cutaneous malignancies viz., Bowen's disease, superficial BCC, small squamous cell carcinoma, Paget's disease. • Debulking of rhinophyma, large pyogenic granuloma.
Coagulation mode	• Pyogenic granuloma, hemangioma, telangiectases.

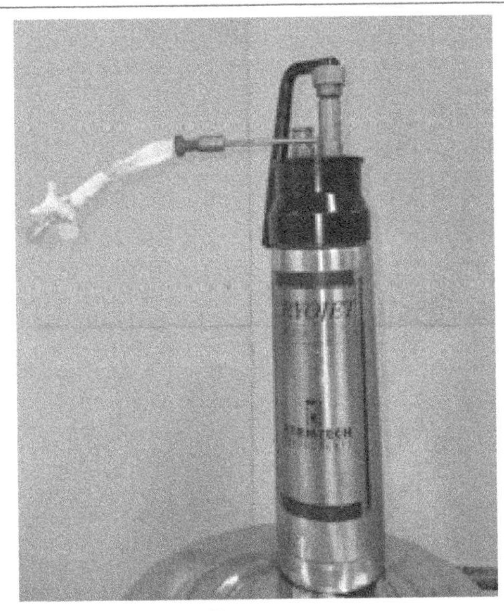

Cryospray

procedure painless. This property can be used as primary objective as in case of injecting intralesional steroids into firm keloids and allaying pain in sprain or may be a secondary benefit obtained while treating hypertrophic scars and keloids with cryotherapy.

History : James Arnott is considered the 'Father of modern cryosurgery'.

MECHANISM OF ACTION :

1. Freezing of tissue :
   - ***Intracellular ice formation*** – damages cell organelles.
   - ***Extracellular ice formation*** – damages cell membrane.
2. Osmolarity increases in extracellular compartment causing disruption of cell membrane.
3. Local ischemia occurs due to vascular spasm and small vessel microthrombi formation.
4. Thermal shock.
5. Denaturation of lipoprotein complex.
6. Immunologic (applicable to warts) :
   - ***Local*** – destruction of affected cells and stimulation of immune system and generation of long term memory cells.
   - *Systemic* – destruction of distant affected cells by the circulating stimulated lymphocytes.

TERMINOLOGY :

Cryogens : These are agents used for cryotherapy.

Target area : Lesion to be treated.

Cryoprobe : Unit coming in contact/delivering the cryogen to the target area.

Ice ball : The ball of frozen cryogen that precipitates on the lesion treated.

Freeze time : It is the duration of freezing measured after the formation of ice ball.

Thaw time : It is the time required for restoration of normal skin temperature in the lesional area after the cessation of freezing. It is approximately twice the freeze time.

Depth of freeze : Maximal vertical dimension of ice ball formation/freeze.

Lateral spread of freeze : Extent of extension of peripheral margin of freeze.

Freeze – Thaw cycle : Total duration of freezing followed by thawing.

Halo – Thaw time : Time required for the restoration of normal skin temperature in the marginal area adjacent to the lesion after the cessation of freezing.

FACTORS AFFECTING EFFICACY OF CRYOTHERAPY :

1. *Rate of fall in temperature :*
   - Rapid, lesser duration efficacious than slower, longer freeze.
   - Slow freeze promotes extra cellular ice formation.
   - Fast freeze promotes intracellular ice formation and produces better tissue destruction.
2. Rate of re-warming.
3. Rapid freeze, slow thawing is more efficacious than slow freeze, rapid thawing.
4. Duration of freezing exposure.
5. Lowest temperature attained in the target area.
6. Application of pressure increases rate and depth of freeze.
7. *Number of freeze* – thaw cycles; greater the number, the tissue destruction.

8. Inter-cycle thaw duration : Shorter the duration. better the tissue destruction.
9. *Solute concentration* – ice formation leads to increase in extracellular solute concentration and increased osmotic gradient across the cell wall causing destruction of the cell organelles. When the ice melts, water enters the cell causing the cell to swell up causing further damage.

TABLE AIII.4 : **Characteristics of cryogens**

Cryogen		Effective temperature	Mode of application
Ethyl chloride		+13.1°C	Spray
Salt ice		-20°C	Gauze
CO_2 slush		-20°C	Gauze
Fluorocarbons	Frigiderm (dichlorotetrafluorofluoroethane)	+3.6°C	Applicator, Probe,
	Freon 22	-30°C	Spray
	Freon 12	41°C	Spray
CO_2 snow		-79°C	Gauze, Spray (gaseous CO_2)
Liquid nitrous oxide		-89°C	Probe
Helium		-185°C	
Liquid nitrogen		-20°C (swab)	Applicator,
		-196°C (spray)	Applicator spray, intralesional

TABLE AIII.5 : **Thermal sensitivity of various tissues**

Cells/tissue	Thermal sensitivity
Melanocytes*	–4 to –8°C
Keratinocytes	–20 to –30°C
Dermal connective tissue, fibroblasts	–30 to –40°C

* This high sensitivity to negative temperatures is the cause of increased incidence of depigmentation associated with cryotherapy.

USES :

1. ***Cryocauterization :***
   - *Benign lesions :*
     i. ***Infective*** – warts, molluscum.
     ii. ***Non-infective*** – keloid, hypertrophic scar, pyogenic granuloma, skin tags, seborrheic keratosis, mucous and myxoid cyst angioma.
   - *Premalignant lesions* – Leukoplakia, Bowen's disease, actinic keratosis, Erythroplasia of Queyrat.
   - *Malignant lesions* – BCC (except morpheiform), SCC, LMM, palliative therapy for inoperable carcinomas.
2. ***Superficial acne scars*** – cryo roller (liquid nitrogen).
3. ***Inflammatory acne*** – cryo slush (solid carbon dioxide), cryo roller (liquid nitrogen).
4. To soften keloid and decrease pain during intralesional steroid injection.
5. Non-surgical facial rejuvenation.
6. For cooling the skin surface during laser therapy for hair reduction and telangiectases and hence protect the epidermis from heat damage.
7. Increases laser fluence and irradiance.
8. Frozen sectioning of skin biopsy for rapid diagnosis of staphylococcus scalded skin syndrome.
9. Cryopreservation of fragile vesicle during biopsy (ethyl chloride).
10. As a topical anesthetic (ethyl chloride).
11. Freezing of cutaneous myiasis (chronic migratory type) and extraction of the larva.
12. Moh's microsurgery.

CONTRAINDICATIONS :

1. Cold aggravated/precipitated conditions, viz., cold intolerance Raynaud's phenomenon, cryoglobulinemia, cold urticaria.
2. Undiagnosed lesion.
3. Multiple myeloma, agammaglobulinemia, CTD.
4. Atherosclerosis.
5. Concurrent immunosuppressives.

COMPLICATIONS :

Acute : Pain, headache, edema, blister formation, syncope, fever.

Chronic : Hypo/depigmentation, hyperpigmentation, milia, hypertrophic scar/keloid arthralgia, nerve damage, paraesthesia, atrophy, cicatricial alopecia, ectropion, notching of eyelid, necrosis of cartilage.

Others : Infection, hypertrophic granulation.

PRE-PROCEDURE PREPARATION :

- Hydration improves the efficacy of cryotherapy by enhancing cryoball formation. Hence, moisten the lesion with saline/hydrating gels.
- Local anesthesia required in the following circumstances : Lesions are overlying a peripheral nerve, large, bulky lesions and apprehensive patients.

METHODS OF CRYOSURGERY :

CRYO SLUSH :

Cryogen : Solid CO_2 (–20°C)

Solid CO_2 is mixed with,

1. ***Acetone***—When added to dry ice, it lowers its

temperature. It also prevents CO_2 from sticking to the skin and thus protects from superficial burns and allows free movement of the gauze ball over skin.

2. Sulfur—comedolytic.

Indications : Acne scars, wrinkles, acne grade III-IV.

Endpoint : Crackling white frost formation.

DIPSTICK METHOD :

Cryogen : Liquid nitrogen.

Method of application : Cotton tipped applicator is dipped in the cryogen and is then applied firmly to lesion till a narrow halo of white ice forms around the bud.

DISADVANTAGES :

1. Dribbling from the stick can lead to superficial burns.
2. Cannot achieve < 20°C beyond 2-3 mm depth.
3. Viral contamination may occur.
4. Slow freeze speed.

CRYOSPRAY METHOD :

Open Method :

Method of application : Fill the cryo jet unit with liquid nitrogen till 2 inches from the brim. Wait for 34 mins to pressure to build up. Select the appropriate cryoprobe.

Mark the periphery of the lesion and spray at the centre of lesion from a distance of 1 cm. Confirm the complete melting of ice ball before starting 2nd freeze thaw cycle.

Spray technique :

1. ***Spot*** – here spraying is done over the centre of lesions < 2

cm, 40°C to - 60°C attained till 5-6 mm. If lesions are > 2 cm, then the total area is subdivided into overlapping circles of 2 cm diameter and treated separately.

2. ***Paintbrush*** this technique is employed for large irregular lesions. Spraying is done as in painting moving vertically with simultaneous forward progression.
3. ***Spiral*** – employed for larger lesion where spraying is started in the center of the lesion and gradually moving out to periphery in a spiral fashion.
4. ***Rotatory*** – in large lesion, spraying is done along concentric circular pathways with gradually increasing diameter moving from inside to outside.

Advantage : This is a 'No-touch' technique and hence ideal for treating *HIV/HBV/HCV* affected patients.

Closed method :

Method of application : Here cones and cylinders (plastic, metallic) are used to restrict the lateral spread of the spray and hence should be used when working adjacent to eyes.

Advantages :

1. Prevents lateral spread.
2. Concentrates the freeze.
3. Achieves rapid fall in temperature.

CRYOPROBE :

Method of application : The tip of the probe is cooled by circulating liquid nitrogen and the probe is placed over the lesion to be treated.

Choosing the probe : Probe size = lesion size.

Precaution : Probe should be removed after sufficient thawing.

Advantage : Pressure can be applied and hence greater depth of freeze can be achieved.

Disadvantage : Slower rate of freeze.

CRYOROLLER :

Method of application : Here metallic roller (stainless steel/ brass) is dipped in liquid nitrogen and is rapidly rolled over the treatment area.

Indications : Acne scars, hypertrophic scars, keloids.

FORCEPS TECHNIQUE :

Method of application : Forceps is dipped in cryogen and then the pedicle of the pedunculated is compressed with its tip.

Uses : Used for pedunculated lesions.

Advantage : Acts both mechanically by crushing the lesion as well as by cold cautery due to cryotherapy.

INTRALESIONAL CRYOTHERAPY :

Method of application : Long metallic Luer lock spinal needles passed through and through the deeper part of lesion. Cryogen (liquid nitrogen) is passed through this needle.

Uses : This technique employed for thick lesions, as other modalities are ineffective below 2 cm depth like keloids.

Advantage : It spares the surface epidermis and hence lesser chance of depigmentation.

Disadvantage : Necrosis of overlying tissue.

ACCESSORIES OF CRYOTHERAPY UNIT :

1. *Cryoprobes :*
   - Open end—spiral tips, truncated neoprene cones, cylinders.

- Closed end—flat (keloids), pointed (verruca plana, milia), rounded (cysts, pyogenic granuloma).

2. *Protective Devices :*
   - Eyes – Jaeger's eye retractor, eye goggles.
   - EAC – cotton plugs.
   - Anterior nares – tongue depressor.
3. *Temperature Monitoring Devices :*
   - Thermocouple needles.
   - Electrical impedance measurement device.
4. *Chamois Bag :*
   - To collect CO_2 gas from a CO_2 cylinder for cryo slush preparation. Alternatively CO_2 may be obtained as dry ice from an ice-cream shop.

Sterilization of accessories—dry heat, autoclave, or chemical (2% glutaraldehyde).

MACROSCOPIC CHANGES AFTER CRYOTHERAPY :

During and immediately post-op : White ice field.

Few Minutes of Thawing :

1. Purplish-violet color develops at periphery, moves centrally.
2. Deeper tissues become pale.

About 12-48 hours : A hemorrhagic blister on an erythematous base develops in the center of the treated zone.

The blister forms an eschar over a period of 1 week.

The eschar separation occurs spontaneously but the time taken for it differs according to the depth and site of treatment as well as the type of lesion. As a rough guideline, it separates for :

1. Benign and premalignant lesions—10-14 days.
2. Malignant lesions—34 weeks.
3. Lesions on back and leg may take up to 3 months.

LASERS :

Lasers have become the therapeutic modality of choice in the present age for many conditions, dermatological and non-dermatological. Its use has been mainly harnessed in the cosmetic and surgical dermatology. This relatively painless procedure is also easy to execute and hence used mostly as an office procedure.

Laser is an acronym for *"Light Amplification by Stimulated Emission of Radiation."* Lasers act by specifically targeting different chromophores in the skin. Since the disease pathology and consequently the target chromophore may differ in various conditions it is imperative to have a different laser for treating each condition.

Lasers are characterized by a coherent, collimated monochromatic light beam of high intensity.

Collimated lights are those whose cross sectonal diameter is constant throughout.

Coherence means all light particles/photons are in the same plane, traveling in the same direction and are in the same phase.

Monochromatic implies light of single wavelength. Tissue penetration is directly dependent upon wave length.

Basic Components of Lasers :

1. *Gain medium or lasing medium : e.g.* carbon dioxide, argon etc.
2. *Optical resonators :* Comprises a 100% reflecting mirror and a partially reflecting mirror.
3. *Power source :* This can be either of the following :
   - ***Electrical*** – radiofrequency (argon laser, carbon dioxide laser), pulsed flash lamp pumping (ruby laser, dye laser, Nd:YAG, Ho:YAG, Er:YAG).
   - ***Chemical*** – hydrogen fluoride laser.
   - ***Other laser powered*** – diode laser pumped Nd :YAG laser, argon laser pumped dye and titanium sapphire laser.

Mechanism Of Action Of Lasers :

Selective photothermolysis : different wavelengths of lasers are varyingly absorbed by various chromophore producing localized and selective tissue destruction.

Photothermal effect : heat produced by the laser produces destruction of tissue.

Thermo-mechanical effect : attainment of very high temperatures rapidly causes disruption of cells due to pressure, cavitation and differential expansion.

Photoacoustic effect : high energy pulses cause fragmentation and shattering of pigments.

Terminology in Laser Therapy :

Energy : It is proportional to total number of photons incident on the target (joules).

Power : Energy delivered per unit time (joules/sec or watt).

Irradiance : Power per unit area (watt/cm^2).

Fluence : Actual amount of energy irradiated on unit area (joules/cm^2).

Pulse duration : Duration of incident laser beam (in milli, micro or nanoseconds).

Pulse frequency : Number of repetitions of laser beams per unit time (Hertz).

Thermal relaxation time : It is the time required for dissipation of 50% heat gained by the tissue (in milli or microseconds) during irradiation.

Spot size : Thickness of laser beam (in millimeters).

Modes of output : Output of laser energy can be :

Continuous wave: Continuous delivery of laser in seconds to milliseconds.

Pulsed wave: Intermittent delivery of laser in very short time of milliseconds

Ultrapulse wave: pulse width is in microseconds

Pseudocontinuous wave: very short pulses of laser delivered at very high repetition rates

Superpulsed CO_2 Laser: very short duration pulsed delivery such that the peak power is higher than continuous wave but has same average power over time

In Q switch laser, pulse duration is in nanoseconds; in Picoseconds laser, pulse duration is in 10^{-12} seconds and in mode-locked technology, it is in femtoseconds (10^{-15})

Chromophore : Selectively laser energy absorbing target molecule *e.g.* melanin, water, hemoglobin, pigments.

Fractionated laser: Larger laser beam is divided into multiple smaller laser beams leading to microthermal zones of ablation with skip areas of normal skin for faster regeneration and healing. Distance between the adjoining beams is called Pitch. Greater the pitch, lesser is the laser treated area.

Techniques of Laser Hair Reduction: Stamping technique involves delivery of energy in single shot. ***In-Motion*** technique is deliver of low doses of energy at high repetition rates which slowly heat the skin to desired level. This reduces pain of procedure.

Techniques of QsNd:YAG laser: Q-PTP (Quick Pulse-To-Pulse): In Q switch Nd:YAG laser, if one pulse is subdivided into 2 pulses at a very short interval of 80microseconds and these two weak energy pulses create a higher peak power energy. This method is used for melasma, lichen planus pigmentosus.

Laser peel / Carbon peel: Carbon dye applied on skin absorbs QsNd:YAG laser and prevents its deeper penetration. The energy transmitted superficially rejuvenates skin.

Techniques of Tattoo Removal: R20 Technique: 4 sessions of laser are done in succession at 20 mins interval (if whitening is not present or resolved). ***R0 Technique:*** Perfluorodecalin is applied immediately after laser to prevent whitening. Second and subsequent sessions are done in immediate succession without any interval.

TABLE AIII.6 : **Classification of lasers based on the lasing medium**

Solid laser	Ruby laser (sapphire host contains chromium impurity), YAG group of lasers (Yttrium-Aluminium-Garnet host contains erbium/neodymium/holmium impurities)
Liquid laser	Dye laser
Gaseous laser	Argon laser, Krypton laser, Excimer laser, Carbon dioxide laser
Vapor laser	Copper vapor laser, gold vapor laser
Non-taser laser	IPL (Intense pulsed light) laser

TABLE AIII.7 : **Indications for laser therapy**

Indication	Laser
Laser hair reduction	**Single wavelength technology** Long pulsed Nd:YAG laser (1064 nm) – for skin types III-VI Diode laser (810 nm) Alexandrite laser (755 nm) Ruby laser (694nm) – for skin types I-III IPL **Triple wavelength Technology** 755/810/1064nm; 810/940/1064nm
Hyperpigmentation	**Epidermal** Q switched, double frequency Nd : YAG laser (532 nm) PDL(510 nm) **Dermal type** Q switched Nd:YAG laser (1064 nm) **Mixed type** Q switched Ruby laser (694 nm) Alexandrite laser (755 nm) IPL(515-2100 nm)
Vascular Lesions	**Port wine stain** PDL Alexandrite laser (755 nm) Nd:YAG laser (1064 nm) **Small caliber telangiectasia** PDL **Large caliber telangiectasia** Argon pumped tunable dye laser (577 and 585 nm) Krypton laser (568 nm)

TABLE AIII.7 : *(Continued)*

Indication	Laser
	Nd:YAG laser (1064nm) Copper vapor laser (578 nm) PDL-Nd:YAG dual wavelength **Bulky malformation** Alexandrite laser (755 nm) Nd:YAG laser (1064 nm)
Scars	**Ablative:** Carbon dioxide laser (10,600 nm) (both superficial and deep) Erb:YAG laser (2940 nm) (only superficial) **Fractional Ablative** Carbon dioxide laser (10,600 nm)Erb:YAG laser (2940 nm) 2790 Erb:YSGG (Erb:Yttrium Scandium Gallium Garnet) **Non-Ablative** Diode laser (980, 1450 nm) Long pulsed Nd:YAG laser (1320, 1450 and 1540 nm) PDL (585 nm) Q switched Nd : YAG laser (1064 and 532 nm) Erb:Glass (1540, 1550nm) fractional, non-ablative KTP (532nm) IPL (550, 590 and 755 nm) **Fractional Non-Ablative** Fractional 1550nm Erb-doped laser

TABLE AIII.7 : *(Continued)*

Indication	Laser
	Fractional 1540nm Erb:Glass **Picosecond Lasers** Alexandrite (755nm) Nd:YAG laser (532, 730, 785, 1064nm)
Tattoo	**Red/orange/yellow** PDL Frequency doubled Nd:YAG laser (532 nm) **Green** Q switched alexandrite laser (755 nm) **Black/ blue-black** Q switched (5-100ns): Ruby laser (694 nm), Nd:YAG laser (1064 nm) Subnanosecond (350 – 900ps): 694, 755, 1064, 1064/532nm **Any color** Carbon dioxide laser (10,600 nm)
Acne	PDL (585, 595, 1319 nm) Diode laser (1450 nm) Erb:Glass laser (1540 nm) Nd:YAG laser (1320 nm)
Psoriasis	Xénon chloride excimer laser (308 nm) PDL (585 nm)
Vitiligo	Xénon chloride excimer laser (308 nm) Fractional Carbon dioxide laser (10600 nm)
Laser lipolysis	Nd:YAG laser (1064 nm) Diode laser (924, 975, 1060 nm)
Benign neoplasms, Verruca	Carbon dioxide laser (10,600 nm)
Hemostasis	Carbon dioxide laser (10,600 nm)

TABLE AIII.8 : **Commonly used lasers in dermatological practice and their uses**

Nd:YAG laser Q-switch (1064 nm)	**Q Switch** Tattoo removal, hyperpigmentation, **Double frequency** Tattoo removal, psoriasis, hyperpigmentation (epidermal) **Long pulse (1064 nm)** Hair reduction, mature Port wine stain, bulky vascular malformation **Long pulse (1320, 1450, 1540 nm)** Non-ablative laser resurfacing
Erb:YAG laser	Ablative laser resurfacing, hair reduction
PDL	Vascular lesions, keloids, warts, nonablative laser resurfacing, acne, tattoo removal
Carbon dioxide laser	Keloids, hypertrophic scars, ablative laser resurfacing, warts, vitiligo, pyogenic granuloma, surgical incisions, control of hemorrhage in patients with pacemaker
IPL	Non-ablative laser resurfacing, hair reduction, hyperpigmentation, acne
Erb:Glass laser	Acne, scars
Diode laser	Hair reduction, acne, laser lipolysis
Alexandrite laser	Hair reduction, scars
Picosecond laser	Tattoo removal, acne scars, post inflammatory hyperpigmentation, facial rejuvenation
Triple wavelength laser	Hair reduction

Side Effects Of Lasers :

Immediate :

- Pain, burning sensation, edema.

Early :

1. Oozing, crusting.
2. Secondary infection.
3. Reactivation of herpes simplex infection. (Table AIII.8e)

Late :

- Dyspigmentation (hypopigmentation, hyperpigmentation or depigmentation).
- Change in skin texture.
- Demarcation lines (common in facial rejuvenation).
- Keloids and hypertrophic scars.
- Scarring.
- Hypertrichosis.
- Milia.
- Persistent erythema.
- Dilated follicular ostia.

COOLING SYSTEMS :

As the laser passes through the skin, most of the energy is absorbed by epidermis and this damages the sensitive melanocytes. This problem is more common when the target is in deep dermis viz., laser hair reduction. By reducing the surface epidermal temperature or by using a cooling agent, this damage can be prevented.

Various agents used are as follows :

1. Ice pack.
2. Cryo slush.
3. Layer of cooling gel.
4. Cooled glass chamber.
5. Cooled sapphire tip.
6. Pulsed cryogen spray.
7. Cold air.

Most lasers have an inbuilt cooling system.

DEVAOURIZER :

Plume evacuator can be inbuilt or external.

PRECAUTIONS :

1. Do not keep or store combustible agents in and around the laser equipment.
2. If spirit has been used to degrease, then, wait until the alcohol vaporizes completely.
3. Use physical protective measures like eye goggles, face mask, gown and head gear/cap.
4. Plume evacuator is necessary especially when working on large lesions or warts.
5. Do not use instruments/equipment with reflective surface.

NON-LASER LIGHT SYSTEMS :

INTENSE PULSE LIGHT (IPL) :

Light source : Xenon flash lamps.

Characteristic of light : This is a non-monochromatic light with a mixture of wavelengths ranging from 500 to 1200 nm.

Advantage : With the use of appropriate filters, undesired wavelengths can be cut off. Hence, wide range of procedures requiring varying wavelengths can be treated with single equipment.

BLUE LIGHT :

MECHANISM OF ACTION :

Propionibacterium acnes synthesize porphyrins especially corproporphyrins. On photoexcitation with blue light, there is destruction of cell membrane leading to death of bacteria. Synthesis of porphyrins is enhanced by 5-

aminolevulinic acid. Bacteria have a peak at 400 nm (Soret band).

USES :

1. Inflammatory as well as non-inflammatory acne.
2. Photodynamic therapy.

RED LIGHT :

Light source : Light-emitting diode.

Characteristics of light : It has a wavelength of 660 nm.

MECHANISM OF ACTION :

Similar to blue light except for better penetration by red light.

USES :

1. Photodynamic therapy.
2. Inflammatory as well as non-inflammatory acne.

NON-INVASIVE FACE AND BODY CONTOURING TECHNOLOGIES

Non-invasive face and body contouring is achieved through various technologies namely monopolar radiofrequency (refer section on Radiofrequency Treatment), cryolipolysis, high-intensity focused ultrasound, high intensity focused electromagnetic therapy, low level laser therapy and extracorporeal shock wave therapy.

NON-ABLATIVE RADIOFREQUENCY

Radiofrequency waves are electromagnetic waves with frequency varying from 3kHz to 1GHz (above 1GHz is referred as microwave).

Principle: Skin and deeper tissues offer resistance to flow of radiofrequency and this creates heat which stimulate collagen. Ideal heat to be created in dermis is 55–68^{0}C.

Amount of heat generated depends on,

Amount of current used: intensity and duration of current

Resistance offered by target tissue: Fat offers maximum resistance and hence maximum heat generated

Characteristics of electrode: monopolar/bipolar radiofrequency energy, type of needle (insulated/non-insulated)

Effects of RF

Immediate: Collagen denaturation and fibril contraction – gives rise to immediate skin tightening

Delayed: Inflammatory response stimulated leading to neocollagenogenesis – gives rise to delayed skin tightening

Long term: Tightening of fibrous septae – leads to anti-sagging effect. Also, lower temperatures created for longer duration has lipolytic effect. This leads to changes in contour

Types of Radiofrequency (RF)

Radiofrequency energy is delivered through treating electrodes or through needles which penetrate into skin.

Monopolar RF: there is single treating electrode. Radiofrequency energy passes through the body and hence there is an earthing plate in contact with body to complete the circuit. Hence, the energy passes deep and used for deep tightening and body contouring.

Bipolar RF: there are two electrodes in treating tip. Radiofrequency energy passes between the electrodes through the skin. Energy is distributed more superficially and hence used for treating scars.

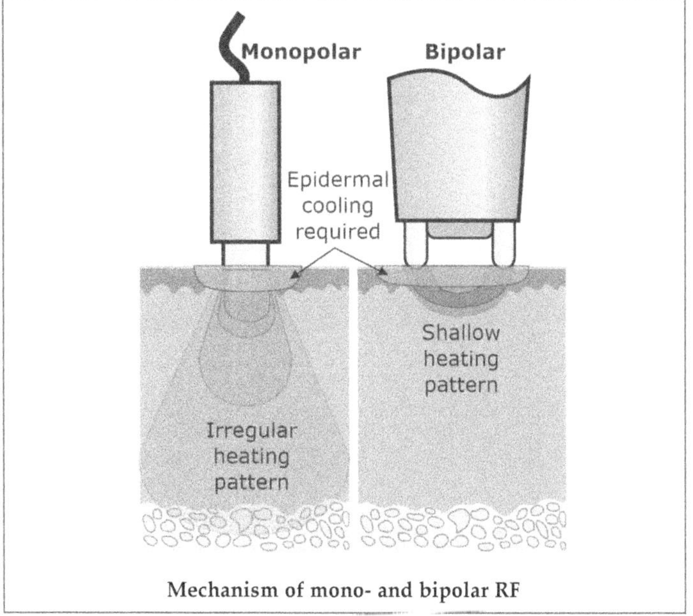

Mechanism of mono- and bipolar RF

Variants of Bipolar RF

Fractionated microneedle RF: Treating hand piece has a set of needles (1x10, 5x5, 7x7). Needles (200 – 300ìm) penetrate the skin (upto 3.5mm) and then the energy is delivered. As the total energy gets split through these needles, it is referred as Fractionated RF.

Needles can be insulated (needle is coated all over except the tip so that energy passes through only the tip) or non-insulated (needle is non-coated and hence energy passes through the entire length of needle). Due to the needles, radiofrequency energy penetrates deeper and hence used to treat scars as well as for deep tissue tightening and contouring.

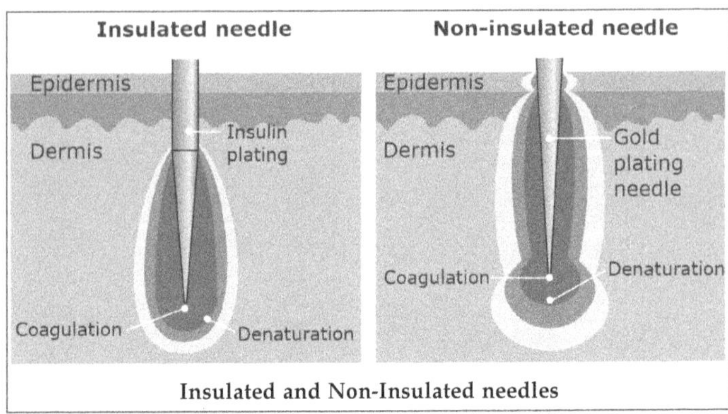

Insulated and Non-Insulated needles

Deeper needle penetration and higher intensity of RF leads to deeper delivery of energy and hence apt for deep tissue tightening or contouring. Longer duration of RF and lower intensity of RF leads to more collateral heating and hence apt for treating scars.

Sublative RF: RF energy is delivered multi-electrode pins

Indications

1. Acne scars (bipolar RF, microneedle RF, sublative RF)
2. Striae (microneedle RF, sublative RF)
3. Facial and body contouring (monopolar RF, microneedle RF)
4. Facial rejuvenation (microneedle RF, sublative RF)
5. Topical drug delivery (microneedle RF, sublative RF)

Side effects

1. Immediate: pain, erythema, edema
2. Early: scabbing (microneedle RF, sublative RF), ulcers
3. Late: post inflammatory hyperpigmentation

CRYOLIPOLYSIS

Fat cells are more sensitive to temperature changes than water rich cells. Vaccuum cup sucks target area to constrict blood vessels (increases cooling effect) and then tissue cooled to -11°C

Principle

1. Cryolipolysis: Cooling leads to crystallization of fat and disruption of fat cell membrane leading to fat loss
2. Cryothermogenesis: Cooling induced thermogenesis leading to fat reduction
3. Cryolipolysis was also found to stimulate neocollageno-genesis leading improvement of skin as well

Indications: Body contouring, Cellulite

Contraindications: cryoglobulinemia, cold urticaria, cold agglutinin disease, paroxysmal cold hemoglobinuria, Raynaud's disease

Side effects: Early - Erythema, myalgia, transient muscle spasm, transient arthralgia, tendinitis; Late - Paradoxical adipose hyperplasia

HIGH INTENSITY FOCUSED ULTRASOUND (HIFU)

Ultrasounds are sound waves beyond the human hearing frequency and range from 20KHz to several gigahertz. HIFU is delivery of focused high intensity ultrasound energy (3MHz – 10MHz) to deep dermis, subcutaneous fat, fascia and superficial musculoaponeurotic system (SMAS) through transducers. Target area is visualized upto 8mm depth by ultrasound and energy is delivered to various depths viz., 1.5mm (superficial dermis), 3mm (deep dermis) and 4.5mm (SMAS). Epidermis and muscles are unaffected by HIFU.

Principle

Tissue coagulation: Focused ultrasound beams travel deep and heat the deep tissues upto 65^0C causing tissue coagulation. This leads to collagen contraction, neocollagenogenesis and tightening of deeper tissues including SMAS. This leads to tightening of deeper tissues.

Cavitation: Pressure of sound waves break down fat to glycerol and free fatty acids. This leads to body fat reduction.

Indications: Facial and body contouring, Cellulite

Side effects: Pain, erythema, edema, tenderness, ecchymosis, lumps

HIGH INTENSITY FOCUSED ELECTROMAGNETIC THERAPY

Unlike all other noninvasive body contouring techniques, this technology not only addresses fat but also strengthens and tones the muscle to contour body.

Principle: There is supra maximal stimulation of muscle due to high stimulation of muscle (20,000 times/30 mins leading to muscle hypertrophy and hyperplasia. Simultaneous lipolytic action leads to fat loss.

When body fat is more, the stimulation from magnetic coil cannot effectively reach the motor neurons and hence the muscle contractions become suboptimal. Persons with less than once inch pinchable fat is the ideal candidate for this novel therapy.

LOW LEVEL LASER THERAPY

Low level laser therapy (LLLT) for body contouring is done with 635nm lasers. Upto 52gm of fat is lost in a single laser therapy.

Principle: LLLT dilates the tiny temporary openings in the cell membrane of adipocytes leading to outflux of lipids into interstitum and thereby its clearance through lymphatics. It also stimulates the respiratory chain in cell by its photoexcitation effect by stimulating cytochrome C in mitochondria.

EXTRACORPOREAL SHOCK WAVE THERAPY

Defocused, low energy shock waves are employed for body contouring incontrast to focused high intensity shock waves used in other fields of medicine.

Principle

1. Disruption of fat cells and hence lipolysis
2. Weaken the thick fibrotic subcutaneous septae leading to smoothening of cellulite
3. Improve lymphedema by stimulating neolymphangio-genesis
4. Stimulates adipose stem cells

THERMO-MECHANICAL FRACTIONAL ABLATION

This is a novel technology for treating scars/ striae and mode of transdermal drug delivery.

Principle

Pure thermal energy is delivered through a metallic tip consisting of an array of pyramids with a mechanical impact. The heat and impact leads to:

1. Dehydration of tissue: creating a diffusion gradient (aids transdermal drug delivery)
2. Impact creates transient micropores: acts as transient channels for diffusion (aids transdermal drug delivery)

3. Ablation and tissue vapourization of tissue similar to fractional ablative lasers viz., carbon dioxide laser (collagen remodelling)

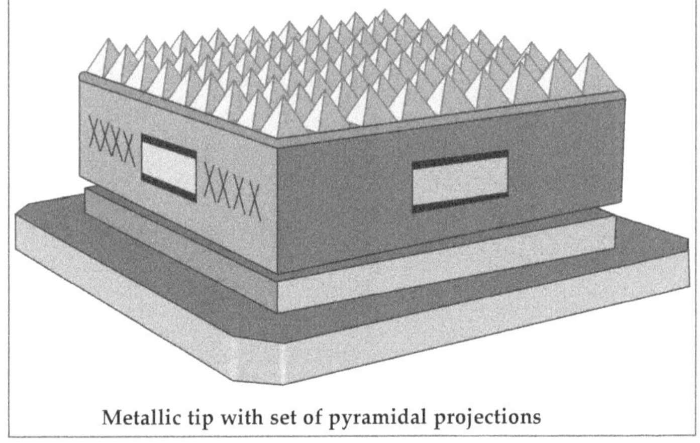

Metallic tip with set of pyramidal projections

Characteristics of Treating Tip

1. Metallic tip (1x1 cm) has 81 (9x9) titanium coated pyramidal projections (Figure 1)
2. Pyramid are 1.25mm and 100ìm at the tip
3. Tip is heated to about 400^{0}C

Characteristics of treatment

This technology works in non-ablative (5ms - 8ms) or ablative (9ms - 16ms) mode depending upon the pulse duration. On face, average thickness of epidermis is 0.04mm and dermis is 1.3mm. Protrusion of tip into skin can be varied between 0.1mm – 1mm. So, the energy can reach upto deep reticular dermis. Tip is autosterilized by heating of tip to 350^{0}C for 3mins. Tissue debris can be cleaned with isopropyl alcohol.

Indications

1. Acne scars
2. Striae
3. Topical drug delivery (aids to treat melasma, haemagioma)

Side effects

Immediate: pain, burning sensation, erythema, edema

Early: scabbing, post inflammatory hyperpigmentation

Late: post inflammatory hyperpigmentation

APPARATUSES FOR INDUCTION OF SUCTION BLISTER :

Blisters can be induced 'With the help of suction equipment with some modifications or through a set up of syringes.

SUCTION MACHINE :

Apparatus required : Suction equipment, glass cup with non-traumatic rim.

The suction end is attached to a specially designed glass cup with non-traumatic rim via a vacuum gauge. Suction pressure of 250-500 mm of Hg is used.

DISADVANTAGES :

1. Requires expensive and bulky equipment.
2. Requires designing special cups.
3. Glass cup needs to be sterilized before use.

SYRINGE TECHNIQUE :

Apparatus required : Disposable syringes of 20, 50 or 100 ml three way cannula (Disofix®).

Fixing the apparatus and generating a blister : Three-way cannula is connected to the tip of each syringe whose piston is removed Two or three 10/20 ml syringes with cannula are to be placed on the donor area. Two or three such syringes can be interconnected. Three way of the distal-most syringe is locked to exterior and a 50 or 100 ml syringe is attached to the three-way cannula present at the other end of the setup. This makes the equipment airtight when the open syringes are placed on the skin surface.

The donor area is cleaned and sterilized with an antiseptic scrub. Hairs should be shaved. The whole setup is placed on the donor area with the open posterior wide part of the syringe coining in contact with the skin. Firm pressure is applied on the setup and the 50 or 100 ml attached to the end of the 3-way cannula is retracted to create negative pressure within the setup. Once the piston of the syringe is retracted to the maximum possible, the 3-way to which the syringe is connected to the syringe is closed. This creates a negative pressure that holds the setup in place without the need for any fixtures.

The negative pressure creates a blister in 1-2 hours due to disruption at dermo-epidermal junction. If the pressure is adequate, then a single blister filling up the lumen of the syringe is formed.

Sites for generation of blister : Anterolateral thigh, flexural fore-arm, abdomen.

ADVANTAGES OF SYRINGE TECHNIQUE :

1. Inexpensive.
2. Less painful.
3. No need for sterilization (use of disposable syringes).
4. Ease of preparation of assembly.

ADVANTAGES OF SKIN GRAFTING BY SUCTION BLISTER TECHNIQUE :

1. Faster (but not immediate) pigmentation.
2. Suitable for areas with thin skin viz., eyelids, lips, glans penis.
3. Good cosmetic result. No risk of pebbling (unlike punch grafting), dyspigmentation (unlike with tattooing) or change in skin texture (unlike split thickness skin graft).
4. Minimally invasive.

IONTOPHORESIS :

Iontophoresis is a procedure of driving ionic agents of therapeutic relevance into skin by employing direct current.

Principle : Acidic agents (cations) are repelled by cathode; similarly alkaline agents (anions) by anode. Hence the agent is driven effectively in to the skin. These charged ions penetrate the skin either through the natural shunts for example hair follicles and ducts (or) through the pores which are formed in the skin due to molecular reorientation of proteins and lipids and Iontophoresis also works thought the occurrence of chemical gradient at the tip of electrodes (polar effect).

Cathode generates tiny bubbles when placed in weak salt solution and turns moist litmus paper red. Anode generates large bubbles and turns litmus paper blue.

INDICATIONS :

1. Palmoplantar hyperhydrosis.
2. Delivery of medication viz., tretinoin for scars, glycolic acid for facial rejuvenation, retinoids for melasma, warts (sodium salicylate), no-healing ulcer (zinc oxide), scars (iodide), herpes labialis (idoxuridine).
3. Patch test.
4. Pilocarpine test.

Procedure : Area is cleaned with spirit, if acidic agent is applied than cathode becomes the treating electrode, anode becomes indifferent electrode. Vice versa occurs for alkaline agents. Current is gradually increased from 0 to 3.8 mA with continuous circular stroking movements of electrode. Full face is done in 25-20 minutes. Clinical end point is mild erythema. Current is gradually decreased to zero and then is reversed for few minutes.

PRECAUTIONS :

1. At the end of procedure, current reversal is done to reverse the polarity of electrodes to neutralize the chemical reaction and prevent sticking of electrode to the skin.
2. Grease any abrasion, wound or cut present to avoid electrical injury because of enhanced conductivity of such areas.
3. Stop the procedure immediately and reverse the current on complaints of severe pain/burning.

CONTRAINDICATION :

1. Anaesthetic skin.
2. Cuts/wounds/ulcers.
3. Dermatitis.

COMPLICATIONS :

1. Immediate-erythema, urticaria.
2. Delayed-burns (chemical), follicle irritation, irritant and allergic dermatitis.

PATCH TESTING :

Patch testing is the only safe, objective, painless and easy to perform investigative tool to confirm allergic contact dermatitis. It also helps in the diagnosis of photoallergic dermatitis. Its use also extends into research for investigating

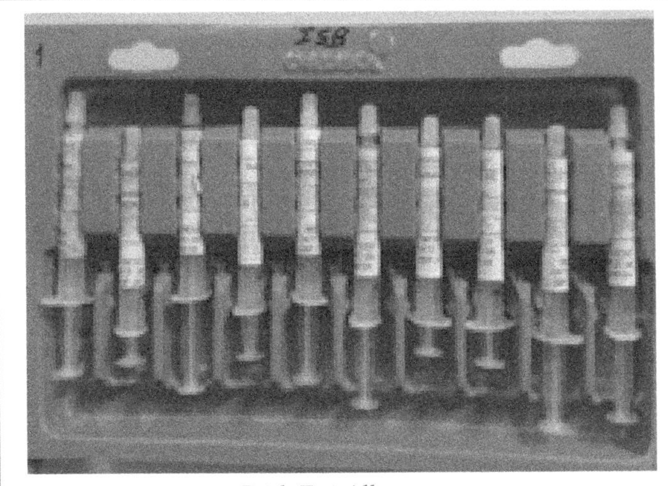

Patch Test Allergens

the irritancy potential of various topical agents. With the availability of TRUE test kit, the execution of patch testing has become more user-friendly. Also, the pain of pricks associated with intradermal tests is absent in this technique.

History : Jadassohn, who introduced patch test in 1895, is considered to be the 'Father of patch testing'.

PRINCIPLE OF PATCH TESTING :

Patch test is used for the demonstration of delayed contact hypersensitivity (Type IV hypersensitivity) in cases of suspected allergic contact dermatitis. Allergens are applied in a patch to the upper back/outer arm/outer thighs in that order of preference. The patch is removed after 48 hours and then read for any reaction.

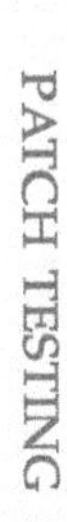

KITS FOR PATCH TESTING :

Indian standard series : Devised by Contact Dermatitis Forum of India (CODFI), these kits contain allergens including plantgens required in the Indian settings. Additional cosmetic and footwear series allergens are also available. Aluminium 'Finn chambers Inounted on micropore tape are available with the kit.

TRUE test kit : TRUE test is an acronym for *Thin-layer Rapid Epicutaneous test* and was devised by Fischer and Maibach. Its main advantage is that the allergens are available *ready to use* form. It has a standard set of 20 allergens coated onto polyester patches in a hydrophilic vehicle. However some of the allergens like *Parthenium* are missing in this series.

Chenzotechnique diagnostics patch test kit has hypoallergenic polyethylene plastic chambers that are mounted on tape. More than 25 different series are available with this kit including the International Standard Series and the European Standard Series.

METHODS OF PATCH TESTING :

1. *A1 test :* made of aluminium foil covered with polythene. Allergens are adsorbed onto a centrally placed filter paperdisc of 10 mm diameter.
2. *Finn chambers :* made of aluminium wells of 8 mm diameter and 0.5 mm depth. Plastic coated Finn chambers are preferred for testing sensitivity to metals viz., nickel, cobalt, mercury as these interact with aluminium.
3. *Plastic chambers :* are of 10-15 mm diameter accommodating 15-100 µl of allergen.
4. In *TRUE* test, allergens are available ready to use form coated onto polyester patches in a hydrophilic vehicle.
5. In the absence of these standardized kits, patch test can still be done using simple gauze piece and sticking

plaster. However, the chance of false negative or false positive reactions is higher.

PROCEDURE OF PATCH TESTING :

Site of patch testing : paramedian juxta-scapular area or outer arms or anterolateral thigh.

Patch test strips are applied over back and have to be retained in place for 48 hours without wetting them. The patch is removed after 48 hours (or sometimes at 72 hours) and the first reading is taken half an hour after removal (Table AIII.9). Two late readings are usually taken to check for allergens, which react late viz., Kathon CG, neomycin, cobalt salts, formaldehyde resins, para tertiary butyl phenol, tixocortol –21 pivalate and nickel. The first late reading is taken after another 48-72 hrs and the second late reading after 4-7 days of applying the test patch.

False positive reactions are due to :

Excited back syndrome/angry back syndrome/status eczematicus—false positive reactions to multiple allergens.

TABLE AIII.9 : **Reading patch test (International Contact Dermatitis Research Group, ICDRG guidelines)**

Clinical signs	Reading of of test	Interpretation of test
Faint erythema only	± or ?	Doubtful reaction (Janes reaction)
Erythema, edema, discrete papules	+	Weak/Non-vesicular
Erythema, edema, papules and vesicles	++	Strong/Vesicular
Intense erythema, edema and coalescing vesicles	+++	Extreme/Bullous

Key : (+), positive reaction; (–) negative reaction.

VEHICLES USED FOR PATCH TESTING :

Petrolatum (used for most of the allergens), acetone, ethyl

ether, ethanol, methyl ketone, hydrophilic lanolin, and plastibase are observed.

1. Retesting after the subsidence of reaction reveals true hypersensitivity to allergens.
2. Misreading of irritant reactions as positive reactions.
3. Too much amount or concentration of allergen.
4. Testing of whole product instead of specific/purified allergen.
5. Scratching of the site.
6. Malingering.
7. Rarely sensitivity to the vehicle in a patch (control patch shows reaction).

False Negative Reactions are due to :

1. Inappropriate selection of allergens.
2. Too little amount or concentration of allergen in a test strip.
3. Loosening of patch.
4. Impaired release of allergen due to use of inappropriate vehicle for allergen.
5. Lack of natural contributing factors like moisture etc. required for the elicitation of allergic reaction.
6. Systemic corticosteroids in a dose greater than 20 mg/day or any other immunosuppressants.
7. Refractory state after severe allergic reaction.
8. Testing of wrong allergen.

Complications Of Patch Testing :

1. Exacerbation of existing contact allergic dermatitis.
2. Persistent positive reaction – persistence of positive reaction for more than 1 month.
3. Active sensitization to a host of allergens to which host

was not sensitive before the patch test. Positive patch test after 10-14 days indicates active sensitization.

4. Contact urticaria that may spread beyond the site of application and rarely even anaphylaxis.
5. Plaster reaction—is due to irritant contact dermatitis because of the adhesive in plaster *e.g.* Colophony.
6. Focal flare—active eczematous reaction at the site of completely subsided positive reaction following activation of patient's eczema.
7. Dyspigmentation and rarely scarring or keloid formation.

PHOTOPATCH TEST :

Here, patch tests are applied in duplicate for 24-48 hrs. At the end of 48 hrs, patches are removed and the test is read. One of the sets is exposed to 5-15 joules/m^2 of UVA and further observed for 48 hrs. Positive reaction in photo-exposed set implies a photoallergic reaction while positive reactions in both the sets indicate allergic contact dermatitis.

OTHER TESTS FOR CONTACT ALLERGIC DERMATITIS :

1. *Open test :* Used for screening purpose. Allergen is applied on skin and left to dry and read as for a standard patch test. (Table AIII.10)
2. *Repeat Open Application Test (ROAT) :* Allergen is applied repeatedly (daily once or twice) over ante-cubital fossa for fixed duration (5-7 days) or until elicitation of positive reaction. This test is employed to determine the relevance of doubtful positive reactions.
3. *Usage test :* Suspected product is used in its usual manner for several days and the sites of application observed. Employed in cases of negative patch test but with strong history suggestive of contact allergic dermatitis.
4. *Prophetic patch test/repeat insult patch lest :* Test agent is applied repeatedly (10-14 applications) under occlusion

TABLE AIII.10 : **Differentiating irritant and allergic reactions**

Features	Irritant reaction	Allergic reaction
Incidence	Occurs in most individuals tested	Occurs in few sensitized individuals only
Onset of reaction on contact with test agent	Immediate (minutes to hours)	Delayed (2-7 days)
Symptoms	Burning greater than itching	Itching greater than burning
Signs	Brown erythema, minimal edema, tiny follicular papules and pustules	Bright erythema, variable edema, vesicles. Pustule occurs only in ACD to metals
Exposure	Occurs with first exposure	Reactions occur only after a prior sensitizing exposure
Desensitization	Cannot be done. However, with repeated exposure, skin hardening occurs, which can decrease the severity of reaction	Possible but unpredictable outcome
Biopsy	Mixed infiltrate with neutrophilic spongiosis and necrotic keratinocytes in epidermis	Infiltrate of lymphocytes and occasional eosinophils with spongiosis
Further testing	Open application test, patch test	Patch test

(patch test). After a 1-week of test free period, individual is challenged with the test agent again by application of test agent and readings for erythema, edema and vesiculation is taken at 24, 48 and 72 hours after of removal of patch. If the test is positive at anytime during repeat application but does not show reaction after challenge, then it implies that the test agent is a mild irritant. On the contrary, if the reaction develops after challenge, then it implies that the agent tested is an allergen. Hence this test gives prediction of possible allergenicity of the test agent before it is used/ marketed widely.

5. *In vitro tests :* Leukocyte migration inhibition test,

lymphocyte transformation test.

Spot tests are used to detect the presence of allergens in suspected contactants :

- Dimethyl glyoxime test for nickel.
- Lutidine test for formaldehyde.

PRICK TEST :

Prick testing for the demonstration of type I hypersensitivity reactions is done using pre-dissolved antigens for the diagnosis of respiratory allergies and chronic urticaria mediated by immediate or Type I hypersensitivity reactions. The kit consists of different antigens including positive (Histamine) and negative (normal saline) controls. Available kits for prick testing differ in number of antigens.

THE KIT OF PRICK TESTING :

1. Allergens in the solution form in small bottles.
2. Blood lancets – to introduce the allergen in the superficial

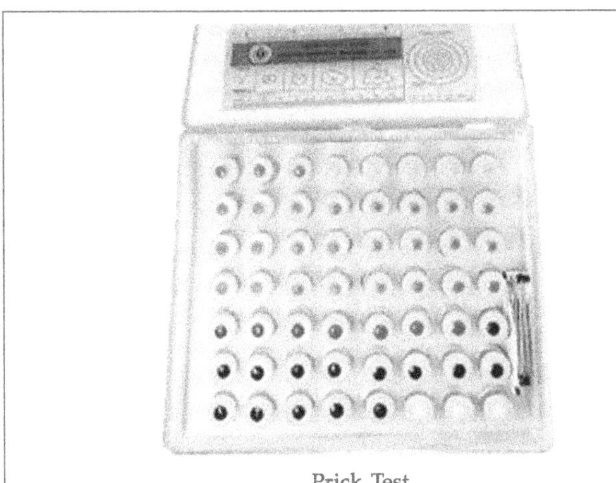

Prick Test

skin.

3. Stencil for the measurement of erythema/wheal.

PROCEDURE :

1. Detailed history of exposure to allergens-inhalation or ingestion of allergens is obtained in a given patient.
2. Prick test is usually done over the flexural aspect of forearm; it can also be done over the back, which is a preferred site for younger children.
3. Allergens in the solution form are applied over the skin, drop by drop, each separated by about 1 inch. Positive and negative controls are also placed.
4. The skin is now pricked superficially (not to cause bleeding) through the solution of antigen using the lancet. It is relatively painless procedure provided that the prick is given superficial. Lancet has to be wiped off using a dry sterile gauze after every prick.

INTERPRETATION :

Reading of prick test is done after 20 minutes with the help of stencil that is used to measure erythema/wheal for each allergen and control.

Reading	Results	Interpretation
+	No wheal, Have 3 mm more than negative control	Mild sensitivity
+ +	2-3 mm wheal	Moderate sensitivity
+ + +	3-5 mm wheal	Severe sensitivity
+ + + +	> 5 mm wheal	Very severe sensitivity

RELEVANCE :

Positive prick testing has been correlated with allergen exposure in the given patient to demonstrate its relevance for the causation of allergy.

TABLE AIII.11 : **Types of allergens**

Type of allergens	Examples
Mite	*D. pteronyssinus, D. Farinae* etc.
Fungi	*Aspergillus* sp. *Penicillium* sp, *Rhizopus, Fusarium* sp., *Candida* etc.
Pollen	*Xanthium strumarium, Parthenium hysterophorus, Sorgum vulgare, Eucalyptus spp, Ricinus communis* etc.
Dust	Wheat, cotton, house dust, paper dust, hay dust, saw dust, grain dust etc.
Epithelia	Dog epithelia, sheep's wool, pigeon feather, human dander
Insect	Ant, mosquito, cockroach, honey bee, cricket, grass hopper, house fly etc.
Food items :	
Food	Rice, Wheat, Bajra, Jowar, Bengal gram, Maize, Masoor dal, Urad dal, Kabuli gram, Soybean, Rajma, Vinegar etc.
Vegetables	Spinach, Cabbage, Cauliflower, tomato, Onion, Brinjal, Carrot, Lady's finger, Beet, Pea, Bean, Mushrooms etc.
Non-vegetarian food	Whole eggs, Egg white, Egg yolk, Chicken, Mutton, Sardine (fish), Salmon, Prawn, Lobster, Crab etc.
Miscellaneous	Latex
Control solution	Saline (Negative control) and Histamine (Positive control)

KEY POINTS :

- Anti-histamines, oral or injectable steroids, mast cell stabilizers (ketotifen and disodium cromoglycate) are stopped prior to testing as they effectively block the wheal and flare reaction. The time duration of stopping of these drugs varies according to their half-life.
- An emergency kit containing hydrocortisone acetate, adrenaline, chlorpheniramine maleate and bronchodilator should be kept ready in case of anaphylaxis following prick testing.

x=x=x=x=x

Index

A
Abacavir 80-81
Accompanied Multidrug Therapy (A-MDT) 117, 131
Acetic acid 417
Acitretin 184
Acne lotion 295
Acriflavine 451
Actinomycetoma *Drugs* 16–18, 22
Actinomycosis *Drugs* 8
Acyclovir 64-66
Adalimumab 213
Adapalene 356
Albendazole 104
Alefacept 210
Alginate 443
Alitretinoin 186
Allopurinol 114
Alpha lipoic acid 409
Alpha lipoic acid 409
Altazanavir 89
Amebiasis cutis *Drugs* 103
Ames test 349
Amikacin 18
Amino acid fillagrin based anti-oxidants (AFA) 400
Aminoglycosides 15
Amitryptiline 268
Amorolfine 310-313
Amoxicillin 11
Amphotericin liposomal 56
Amphotericin-B 55
Amphotericin-B *Topical* 113
Ampicillin 11, 12
Amprenavir 88
Amprinavir 88
Anaphylaxis 11
Ancylostomiasis *Drugs* 103
Anthralin 296, 353, 394, 395
Antiacne *Topical* 308
Antiandrogens 267
Antibacterial *Topical* 298
Antibiotics 37
Antibiotics 37
Antifungal agents *Systemic* 58
Antifungal agents *Topical* 311
Antifungals 309-315
Antifungals 42, 43
Antihistamines 255-261
Antiinflammatory agents 273-276
Antileprosy drugs 29, 117-132
Antioxidants 400
Antioxidants topical 405
Antiparasitic 102-116
Antiparasitic agents 102, 103
Antiparasitic *Topical* 325-334
Antiperspirants 272
Antipsychotic agents 152, 269
Antiretroviral 73-101
Antiretroviral drugs 73-101
Antituberculosis 127
Antituberculous agents (ATT) 29, 36, 114, 133-147
Antituberculous therapy (ATT) failure 146
Antiviral
Antiviral agents *Systemic* 64
Antiviral *Topical* 316
APLIGRAF 447
Apparatuses in dermatological practice 506-549
Appendix II 481-505

Appendix III 506-549
Apremilast 216
Arbutin 409
Argireline 405
Arsenic 205
ART failure 99
ART failure 99
ART First line 95
ART for prevention 94
ART Guidelines
ART in hepatitis 98
ART in tuberculosis 97
ART PPTCT 96
ART regimens 95
ART resistance 92
ART Resistance 92
ART Second line 99, 100
Aspergillosis *Drugs* 49, 55
Astemizole 257, 261
Atazanavir 89
Atypical mycobacterial infections *Drugs* 146
Avobenzone 362
Azathioprine 169, 170
Azatadine 256
Azelaic acid 369, 3710
Azithromycin 28

B

Bacitracin 299
Baricitinib 222
Basic fibroblast growth factor 393
Baths 457
  Cleansing bath 458
  Colloidal starch bath 456
  Oat meal bath 455
  Oil bath 456
  Potassium permangnate bath 459
  Wax bath 457
BCG vaccination 227
BCG vaccine 354
Benzoyl peroxide 298, 299, 301, 307
Benzyl benzoate 331
Beta fibroblast growth factor 393, 394
Betacarotene 192
Betamethasone dipropionate 338
Betamethasone propionate 338
Betamethasone *Systemic* 157
Betamethasone valerate 338
Bexarotene 185
Bidaquiline 130, 140
Bifonazole 311, 313,
Bifonazole 311, 313, 314
Biologicals 208, 210, 211
Biopsy punch 484
Biotin 244
Biphasic vehicles 294
Black peel 434-436
Blastomycosis Drugs
Bleomycin 321
Blue light therapy
Botulinum toxin 466–471
Brimonidine 391
Buproprion 269
Burrow's solution 296, 418
Buspirone 268

C

Calamine lotion 295
Calcipotriol 352, 388
Calcium dobesilate 285
Candidiasis Drugs 47, 48, 49, 51, 53–55

Cantharidin 319, 323
Capreomycin 134, 142
Carbapenems 37
Castellani's paint 296
Cat scratch disease 3
Cephalosporins 12
Cetirizine 255, 257
Cetrimide 452
Chalazion clamp 497
Chancroid Drugs 5, 14, 17, 19, 21, 25, 26, 29, 36,
Chaulmogra oil 129
Chemical agents in dermatological practice 412–420
Chemical Peels 421-436
Chemical peels 421–436
Chicken pox Drugs 66
Chlorhexidine 448
Chloroquine 187, 192
Chlorpheniramine 256
Chromoblastomycosis Drugs
Ciclopirox olamine 309–10, 312–13
Cidofovir 64, 69–70, 316–18
Cidofovir 69
Cimetidine 227, 261–262
Cinnamates 362
Ciprofloxacin 36, 134, 142
Citalopram 269
Clarithromycin 30, 117, 134, 146,
Clarithromycin *Topical* 299, 301, 308
Clemastine 256
Clindamycin 26, 30–31, 299, 307–308
Clindamycin *Topical*
Clobetasol propionate 338
Clofazimine 122–123
Clomipramine 269
Clotrimazole 311, 313
Coal tar lotion 296
Coccidioidosis Drugs
Colchicine
Collagenase 454
Comedone expressor
Condy's lotion 418
Contact sensitizers 320, 344, 347
Copper 249, 252, 403–4, 531–32
Copper peptides 403
Corticosteroids 148
Cosmeceuticals 399-411
Cosmeceuticals 399–411, 468
Cosmeceuticals for acne 410
Cosmeceuticals for antiaging 411
Cosmeceuticals for hyperpigmentation 410
Cotrimoxazole 3–5, 77, 94, 146
Creams 294, 340, 408
Crotamiton 325, 331
Cryotherapy 479, 518
Cryptococcosis Drugs
Cusco's vaginal speculum
Cyclophosphamide 167
Cycloserin 140
Cyclosporine 60, 162, 171–73
Cyproheptadine 256, 258
Cyproterone 270
Cysticercosis cutis Drugs 103
Cytomegalovirus infections Drugs 69, 71

D

Dakin's solution 419

Dapsone 118, 273–277
Dapsone syndrome 277
Daptomycin 38
Deflazacort 149, 151, 153, 155
Delaviridine 73
Demelanizing agents 308, 374
Denileukin Diftitox 210
Dermabrader 498–500
Dermal fillers 462–465
Dermatome 500
Dermatophytosis Drugs 44, 49, 54
Dermoscope 509, 510
Desloratidine 261
Desonide 338
Desoxyfructoserotonin
Dexamethasone cyclophosphamide pulse therapy (DCP) 158
Didanosine 78
Diethylcarbamazine (DEC) 108
Dinitrochlorbenzene (DNCB) 227, 228
Diphenhydramine 256, 398
Diphenyl cyclopropenone (DPCP) 349, 350
Disulfiram-like reaction 13
Dithranol pomade 297
Diuciphon 130
Dolutagravir 91
Donovanosis Drugs 5, 14, 17, 21, 26, 28, 36,
DOTS 147
Doxepine 268
Doxycycline 21, 22
Dupilumab 221

E

Ebastine 257
Eberconazole 309
Echinocandins 59, 60
Echinococcosis Drugs 103
Econazole 311, 313,
Eflornithine 391
Eflornithine 391–92
Efulizumab 210
Efuvirenz 311, 313
Electrocautery 511–517
Electrolysis 517
Emmolients 378, 379
Emtricitabine 81
Emtricitabine 81
Emulsifying agent 293
Emulsion 293
Enfluvirtide 89, 90
Enfuvirtide 89
Engineered peptides 400
Enterobiasis Drugs 103
Epidermal exfoliants 400, 401
Epidermal growth factors 402
Erythromycin 26, 27
Erythromycin *Topical* 299, 301, 308
Essential fatty acids 253, 254
Etanercept 214–215
Ethambutol 134, 138–40, 144
Ethionamide 117, 125, 134, 140, 141, 144
Etretinate 180, 184–85
Eumycetoma Drugs
EUSOL 449
Excimer laser 203, 531
Extracorporeal photochemotherapy 203, 204

F

Famciclovir

Famcyclovir 64, 67–68
Famotidine 261
Fexofenadine 257, 261
Filariasis Drugs 103
Films 441
Filter paper 478
Finasteride 271
Fluconazole 47, 311
Fluconozole *Topical*
Flucytosine 43
Fluocinolide 338
Fluocinolone acetonide 338
Fluoroquinolones 3, 34–36, 130, 299, 304
Fluorouracil 321–322
Fluoxetine 268–69
Flutamide 270
Fluticasone propionate 338
Foams 441
Folic acid 165, 234, 246–47
Folinic acid 165
Forceps 487, 489–491, 527
Fosamprenavir 89
Foscarnet 64, 68, 316
Foscarnet 68
Fosfomycin 39
Framycetin sulfate
Furopenem 37
Fusidic acid 130, 299, 306–307
Fusion inhibitors 74, 89

G

Gamma-benzene hydrochloride 325
Ganciclovir 64
Ganciclovir 64
Gel 311, 454
Gentamicin 18, 299
Gentian violet 450–451
Glass slide 450–551
Glutaraldehyde 450–51
Glycerin 376, 380–81, 425, 427–28, 451
Glycolic acid 368, 371–72, 421, 425–26
Glycopyrrolate 272–73
Gonorrhea Drugs 8, 26, 28, 36
Green tea 408, 410
Green tea 410
Griseofulvin 43, 45
Guinea worm infestation *Drugs* 106, 480

H

Halcinonide 338
Halobetasol 338
Hamycin 311
Hemostatic agents 454
Herpes genitalis *Drugs* 64
Herpes labialis *Drugs* 65
Herpes meningoencephalitis 65
Herpes simplex infections *Drugs* 64, 70
Herpes Zoster *Drugs* 64, 65, 67
Highly active antiretroviral therapy (HAART) 93, 94
Histoplasmosis *Drugs* 46, 49, 52, 55
Hoigne syndrome 7
Hook worm infestation *Drugs* 102, 103, 105
Humectants 376
Humby's knife 500
Hydrocarpus oil 129
Hydrocolloid 444, 445
Hydrocortisone 149, 151, 157, 218, 338, 340, 342
Hydrocortisone acetate 338

Hydrocortisone acetate depot injection 549,
Hydrocortisone butyrate 338
Hydrocortisone valerate 338
Hydrogel 442
Hydroquinone 368–369
Hydroxychloroquine 187–89, 191–92
Hydroxyurea 74, 92
Hydroxyzine 256

I

Imiquimod 318
Immune reconstitution inflammatory syndrome 100
Immunobiologicals 208–232
Immunomodulators *Topical* 344–354
Immunostimulants 344
Immunostimulators 351, 352
Immunosuppressive *Drugs* 148
Indinavir 87
Infliximab 211
Ingram's dithranol paste 297
Instruments in dermatological practice 481–506
Instruments in STI Procedures 502–504
Intense pulse light 535
Interferons 223–228
Interferons *Topical* 319, 353
Intralesional BCG 354
Intralesional steroids 353
Intramuscular dapsone 120
Intravenous immunoglobulins 229–232
Iontophoresis 538–539
IRIS 100
Iron 251–252
Isoflavin genistin 410
Isoflavone 409
Isoniazid 133–136
Isotretinoin 182–184
Itraconazole 47–51
Ivermectin 108, 109
Ivermectin 108–110

J

Jarisch-Herxheimer reaction 6

K

Kanamycin 142
Keratolytic agents 319, 320, 380, 381
Ketoconazole 51–53, 113
Ketoconazole *Topical* 313
Ketolides 30
Ketotifen 263, 264
Khellin 195, 196, 200
Kinerase 402
kinerase 402
Kojic acid 368, 372, 373

L

Lactic acid 383
Lamivudine 76
Larva currens *Drugs* 103, 105
Larva migrans cutaneous *Drugs* 103, 105
Larva migrans visceral *Drugs* 105
Lasers 202, 203, 528–534
Lasser's paste 296
Leflunomide 176, 177
Leishmaniasis *Drugs* 103, 110, 113–115
Levamisole 227

Levamisole 264
Levocetirizine 257
Levofloxacin 142
Licorice 406
Lincomycin *Topical* 299, 308
Linezolid 32
Liniment 294, 296
Liposomal Amphotericin 56
Liposomal amphotericin, leishmaniasis 112
Loaiasis *Drugs* 108
Lopinavir 74, 96
Loratidine 261
Low molecular weight dextran 282, 283
Luliconazole 309, 311
Luliconazole 309, 311
Lymphogranuloma venereum *Drugs* 5, 26

M

Macrolides 301
Magnesium ascorbyl phosphate 368
Magnifying lens 477
Meglumine antimoniate 111
Malathion 332
MESNA 169
Meso botulinum toxin therapy 470
Methemoglobulinemia 4, 118, 121
5-methoxypsoralen 195, 196
8-methoxypsoralen 195, 196
Methotrexate 162
Methyl prednisolone 149
Methyl prednisolone aceponate 338
Metronidazole 305
Metronidazole *Topical* 305
Miconazole 311, 313
Miltefocine 115, 116
Miner greases 376, 378
Minocycline 22–24
Minoxidil 390
Miscellaneous topical agents 323
Mizolastine 257
MMR vaccine 228
Moisturizers 376–380
Molluscum extractor 482
Mometasone furaote 338
Monobenzyl ether of hydroquinone (MBH) 373, 374
Monoclonal antibodies 209–211
Monophasic vehicle 293
MRSA *Drugs* 5, 31
Mucormycosis *Drugs* 49, 55
Multibacillary leprosy *Drugs* 122, 127
Mupirocin 302
Myco W vaccine 228
Mycophenolate mofetil 175, 176

N

Nadifloxacin 304
Naftifine 42, 43
Nail spatula 497
Nail splitter 496
Natamycin 42, 309
Natural moisturizing factor (NMF) 289, 380
Needle holder 493
Needles 494, 495
Nelfinavir 87
Nelfinavir 87, 88
Neomycin *Topical* 298–300

Neurocysticercosis *Drugs* 105
Nevirapine 82
Newer antileprosy *Drugs* 129
Nocardial mycetoma *Drugs* 5
Nongonococcal urethritis *Drugs* 26, 36
Non-nucleoside reverse transcriptase inhibitors (NNRTI) 73, 81
Non-steroidal immunosuppressive agents 162-177
Norfloxacin 34, 36
Nucleoside reverse transcriptase inhibitors (NRTI) 73, 74
Nystatin 43, 311, 313, 314
Nystatin *Topical* 309, 310, 311, 313, 314

O

Office aids in dermatological practice 475–480
Ofloxacin 117, 118, 122, 129, 130, 134, 142
Ointment 385
Omalizumab 220
Onychocerciasis *Drugs* 109
Onychomycosis *Drugs* 46, 51, 417,
Oral minipulse therapy (OMP) 155
Oral retinoids 178–186
Oxenoxacin 304
Oxiconazole 309, 311, 313
Oxybenzone 362
Ozenoxacin 304

P

P. carinii *Drugs* 4, 5, 94
Paint 292, 294, 296
Para amino benzoic acid (PABA) 118,
Para-amino salicylic acid PAS 320
Paracoccidioidomycosis *Drugs* 48, 56
Paromomycin sulfate 334
Patch testing 540–544
Paucibacillary leprosy *Drugs* 118, 127
Pediculosis *Drugs* 103,
Pelvic inflammatory disease *Drugs* 14
Penciclovir 317
Penicillin desensitization 12
Penicillins 6–12
Pentamidine 111
Pentapeptides 404
Permethrin 325
Phenol 415, 416
Photodynamic therapy (PDT) 204
Pimecrolimus 346
Pimozide 268
Pin 475, 476
Pityrosporum infections *Drugs* 53, 54
Placental extract 392
Podophyllin 322
Polymixin B
Posaconazole 62, 63
Post exposure prophylaxis *Drugs* 132
Post herpetic neuralgia *Drugs* 65
Post kala azar dermal leishmaniasis (PKDL) *Drugs* 113–115
Potassium hydroxide 412, 413
Povidone iodine 451, 452

Praziquantel 103, 105
Precipitated sulfur 385
Prednisolone 7, 100, 128, 149, 151, 153, 155
Prednisone 149
Prick testing 546–549
Procaine psychosis 7
Promethazine 255, 256, 259
Propantheline bromide 272, 273
Propylene glycol 293, 376, 379, 381, 384, 388, 479
Protease inhibitors (PI) 84
Protease pouch 87
Prothionamide 125
Psoralens 194–200
Psychotropic agents 266
PUVA 194–200
PUVA Bath PUVA 459
PUVA Bath Suit PUVA 459
Pyrazinamide 137
Pyridoxine 234, 242, 243
Pyrrolidone 376, 380

Q

Quinacrine 187, 191
Quinine 187

R

Radiofrequency 518
Ranitidine 61, 262
Red light 206, 207, 536
Red man syndrome 32, 124, 136
Re-PUVA 182
Resorcinol 429, 430
Retapmulin 303
Retinoids *Systemic* 202
Retinoids *Topical* 355–359, 384
Retinol 401
Rhinoscleroma *Drugs* 35,
Rifabutin 84, 98, 130, 134, 137, 144, 146, 182
Rifampicin 114, 123, 136
Risperidone 269
Ritonavir 86
Rituximab 218, 219
ROM therapy 129
Rosacea 307
Rosacea *Drugs* 21
Round worm infestation *Drugs* 102, 105
Roxithromycin 27, 28
Ruxolitinib 222

S

Salicylates 362
Salicylic acid 320, 381
Salicylism 320, 382, 429
Saquinavir 85
Scabies *Drugs* 103
Scalpel 485
Schistosomiasis *Drugs* 103
Scissors 491, 492
Scoop 482, 483
Secukinumab 213
Selenium 253
Selenium sulfide 253, 312, 313
Sertraline 268, 269
Shake lotion 291, 292, 294
Silver nitrate 413–315
Silver sulfadiazine 298, 299, 302
Silver's knife 500
Sim's anterior vaginal wall retractor 502
Sim's vaginal speculum 503
Siplizumab 210
Sirolimus 347
Sisomycin 298–300
Skin and soft tissue infections

Drugs 8, 14, 28, 36
Skin graft spreader 500
Skin hook 493
Sodium hyposulfite 415, 419
Solution 292, 296
Soy 409
Sparfloxacin 34–37, 130, 198
Spectinomycin 19
Spironolactone 270, 272
Sporotrichosis *Drugs* 46, 55
Squaric acid dibutyl ester (SADBE) 351
Stanozolol 284
Stavudine 77
Steroid equivalence 151, 157
Steroids *Topical* 337-343
Stibogluconate 110
Streptomycin 139
Strongyloidiasis *Drugs* 103,
Suction blister grafting 493, 536–538
Sulfadoxine pyrimethamine 247
Sulfamethoxypyridazine 117
Sulfur 295, 315, 329, 385, 525,
Sun protection factor (SPF) 361, 362
Sunscreens 360–367
Suturing materials 495, 496
Suturing needle 494
SW monofilament 496, 501, 502
Swab stick 479, 480
Syphilis *Drugs* 8, 14, 21, 26

T

Tacrolimus 174
Tacrolimus 174, 345, 346
Tape 478
Tape worm infestation *Drugs* 102, 105
Targetted UVB phototherapy 200–202
Tazarotene 357
Tedizolid 33, 34
Teicoplanin 32
Teicoplanin 32
Telithromycin 30
Telithromycin 30
Tenofovir 80
Tenofovir 80
Terbinafine 53, 54
Testosterone *Topical* 397
Tetracycline 19, 20
Tetramethyl thiuram monosulfide 325
Thalidomide 280–282
Thiabendazole 105, 333
Thiacetazone 125
Thiambutosine 126
Tigecycline 24
Tincture 292
Tinea corporis *Drugs* 43, 54, 382
Tinea manuum *Drugs* 43
Tinea pedis *Drugs* 43, 54, 382
Tinea unguium *Drugs* 44
Titanium dioxide 362
Tofacitinib 222, 223
Tolnaftate 313
Topical therapy 289-297
Topical zinc 353
Torsades de pointes 260,
Toxoplasmosis *Drugs* 3, 4, 5, 103
Tretinoin 356
Triamcinolone acetonide 157, 338
Triamcinolone 149, 151, 156, 157, 338, 342,
Trichenellosis *Drugs* 102, 103, 105

Trichloroacetic acid 319, 421, 422, 427, 428
Trichomoniasis *Drugs* 103
Trichuriasis *Drugs* 102, 104, 105
Trimethoxypsoralen 196
Triphasic vehicles 295

U

Undecycleinic acid 309, 312, 313
Uniform multidrug therapy (U-MDT) 131
Unna boot 447
Urea 383
UVA protection factor 363
UVB phototherapy 200–202

V

Valacyclovir 66–68
Vancomycin 31, 32
Vehicle 290–297, 543
Venlafloxine 269
Vit C topical 406
Vit K topical 238, 239
Vitamin A (Retinol) 233–235
Vitamin B12 (Cyanocobalamin) 234, 247
Vitamin B2 (Riboflavin) 234, 239
Vitamin B3 (Niacin) 240, 241
Vitamin B3 *Topical*
Vitamin B5 (Pantothenic acid) 387, 242
Vitamin B6 (Pyridoxine) 242, 243
Vitamin B9 (Folic acid) 246, 247
Vitamin C (Ascorbic acid) 244
Vitamin C *Topical* 245
Vitamin D (Cholecalciferol) 235, 236
Vitamin E (Tocopherol) 236–238
Vitamin E *Topical* 234, 245
Vitamin H (Biotin) 234, 244
Vitamin K (Menedione) 238
Voriconazole 60, 61

W

Wart lotion 297
Whitfield's ointment 296, 309
Wood's lamp 506–508
Wound care products 437–454

Z

Zalcibitane 79
Zidovudine 75
Zinc 249
Zinc oxide 362
Zinc sulfate 227, 250
Zinc *Topical* 353

www.ingramcontent.com/pod-product-compliance
Ingram Content Group UK Ltd.
Pitfield, Milton Keynes, MK11 3LW, UK
UKHW062253290726
14090UKWH00017B/665